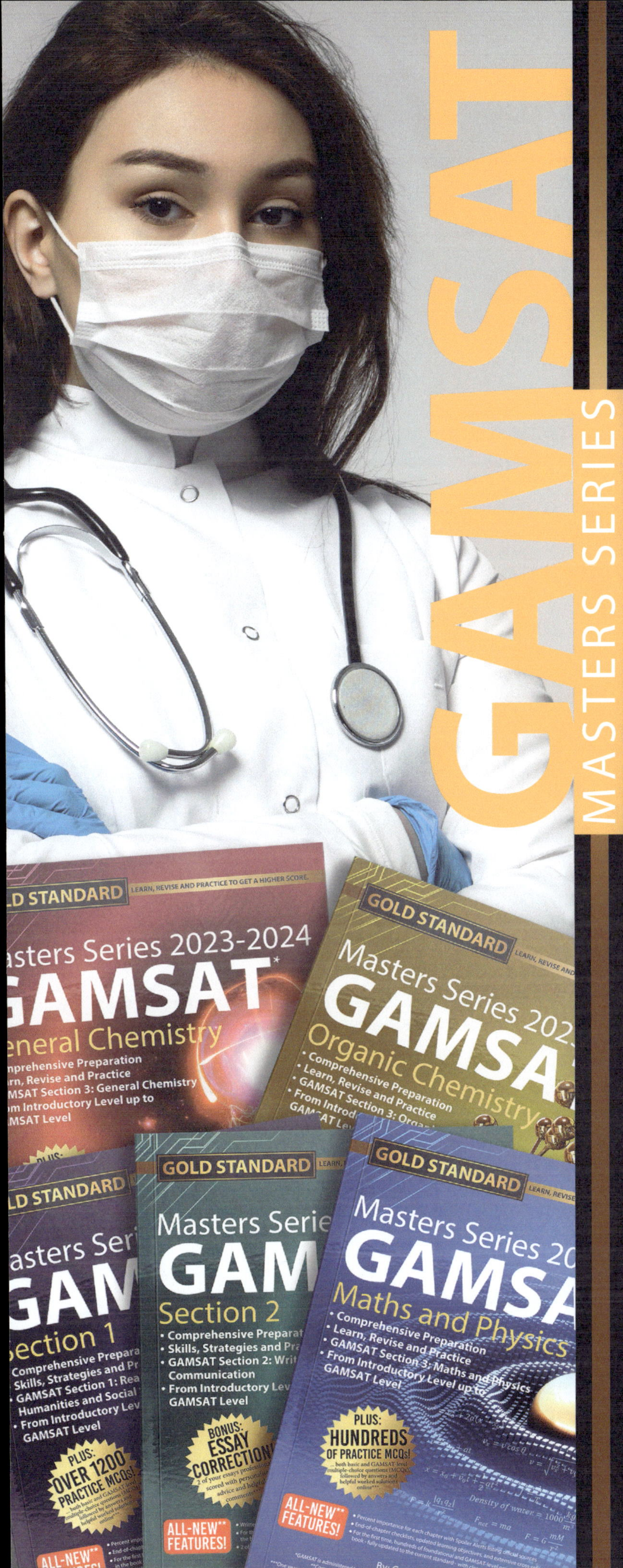

GOLD STANDARD

01 Editor and Author

Brett Ferdinand BSc MD-CM

02 Contributors

Lisa Ferdinand BA MA
Sean Pierre BSc MD
Kristin Finkenzeller BSc MD
Ibrahima Diouf BSc MSc PhD
Charles Haccoun BSc MD-CM
Timothy Ruger BA MA
Jeanne Tan Te

03 Illustrators

Harvie W. Gallatiera BS CompE
Gilbert Rafanan BSc

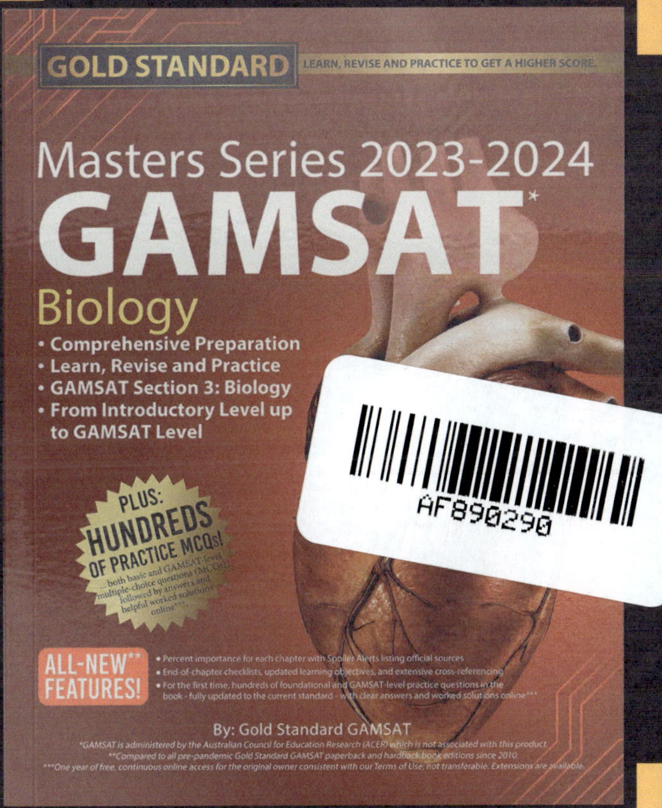

Free Online Access*

Answers and detailed worked solutions for hundreds of end-of-chapter practice questions, as well as the full-length practice test GS-Free which has the new digital GAMSAT format and cross-references to this Masters Series book.

*One year of continuous access for the original owner of this textbook upon online registration at www.gamsat-prep.com/gamsat-biology
If you purchased this textbook or the eBook directly from www.gamsat-prep.com, then your online access is automated.

Please note: Benefits last for one year from the date of online registration, for the original book owner only, and are not transferable; unauthorized access and use outside the Terms of Use posted on GAMSAT-prep.com may result in account deletion; if you are not the original owner, or if you are seeking an extension, you can purchase your virtual access card separately at GAMSAT-prep.com.

Online access: reduces digital piracy; allows the addition of relevant multimedia including videos; permits the updating of strategies and content to reflect the evolving GAMSAT; permits more detailed worked solutions; reduces the retail price; and ultimately, saves trees!

Visit The Gold Standard's Education Center at www.gold-standard.com.

ISBN 978-1-927338-72-8

Address all inquiries, comments, or suggestions to the publisher. For Terms of Use go to: www.GAMSAT-prep.com

Gold Standard GAMSAT Product Contact Information

Distribution in Australia, NZ, Asia

Woodslane Pty Ltd 10 Apollo Street
Warriewood NSW 2102 Australia
ABN: 76 003 677 549
learn@gamsat-prep.com

Distribution in Europe

Central Books 99 Wallis
Road LONDON,
E9 5LN, United Kingdom
orders@centralbooks.com

Distribution in North America

RuveneCo Publishing
334 Cornelia Street #559
Plattsburgh, New York 12901, USA
buy@gamsatbooks.com

GAMSAT (Graduate Medical School Admissions Test)

Computer-based exam held at test centres internationally for graduate-entry medicine

Section I

Reasoning in Humanities and Social Sciences

multiple-choice section with stimulus materials requiring comprehension and analysis of non-science content

poetry • proverbs cartoons • novels or play excerpts • travel and/or medical journal entries • social science graphs

Section II

Written Communication (Writing Tasks A & B)

2 essays responding to 2 different themes using sound reasoning and competent English-writing skills (essays must be typed)

Writing Task A: sociocultural theme (e.g., free speech, justice, social media)
Writing Task B: personal-social themes (e.g., humour, love, happiness)

Section III

Reasoning in Biological and Physical Sciences

multiple-choice section with questions mostly based on science passages that require problem-solving and graph analysis

first-year undergraduate level Biology (40%), General Chemistry (20%) & Organic Chemistry (20%) • A-level/Leaving Certificate/ Year 12 level Physics (20%)

Top GAMSAT Score: 100
Average GAMSAT Score: 57

Summary of the new Digital-format GAMSAT Exam Day

	KEY POINTS	EVENT	DURATION
Arrival and Sitting of Exam	Bring only the acceptable ID documents and permitted items to the test centre as specified in ACER's GAMSAT Information Booklet	Security, identification, health protocols	45-60 minutes
Section 1: Reasoning in Humanities and Social Sciences	Key skills are reading speed and comprehension of information within socio-cultural contexts	62 MCQs* (the test centre will provide you with 2 sheets of A4 scratch paper to be used for both Section 1 and 2; *option*: whiteboard)	100 minutes
Section 2: Written Communication	Produce ideas in writing with clarity and soundness; essays are typed with no copy/paste function	2 essays typed on a computer (for all sections including the essays: no longer is there a formal, dedicated reading time)	65 minutes
Lunch	Consider packing your own lunch to avoid queues with nervous chatter	–	60 minutes
Section 3: Reasoning in Biological and Physical Sciences	Analyse and solve problems: 40% Biology, 40% Chemistry (equally split between General and Organic); 20% Physics	75 MCQs* (the test centre will provide you with 2 new sheets of A4 scratch paper to be used only for Section 3; *option*: whiteboard)	150 minutes
Total Test Time	–	–	5 hours, 15 minutes
Total Appointment Time	Success requires stamina; stamina improves with practice.	–	7-9 hours**

*MCQs: multiple-choice questions, 4 options per question with only 1 best answer. Note that the 'old' GAMSAT had a dedicated 'reading time' of 10 minutes for each of Section 1 and 3, and 5 minutes for Section 2. During that reading time, students were not permitted to write or mark their exam paper in any way. The new digital GAMSAT has added time for each of the 3 exam sections as a legacy to 'reading time'; however, in practice, you can use your exam time in any way that you see fit.

**It might be a good idea to allocate a whole day to sit the GAMSAT test to allow for any contingencies and/or technical issues that you might encounter. Safety measures and health protocols should be carefully anticipated when making travel arrangements and accommodations to and from the testing centre.

<u>Common formula for acceptance</u>:

GPA + GAMSAT score + Interview = Medical School Admissions

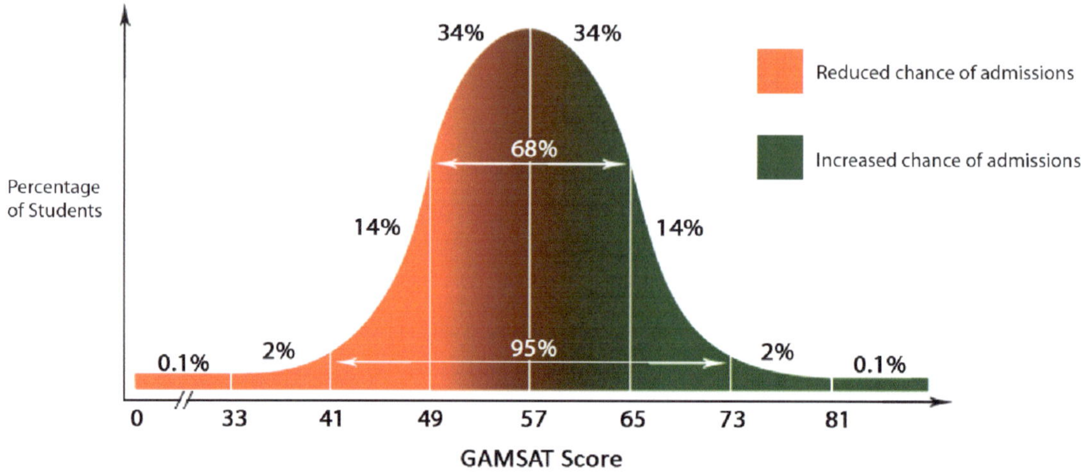

Typical Overall GAMSAT Score Distribution (Approx)

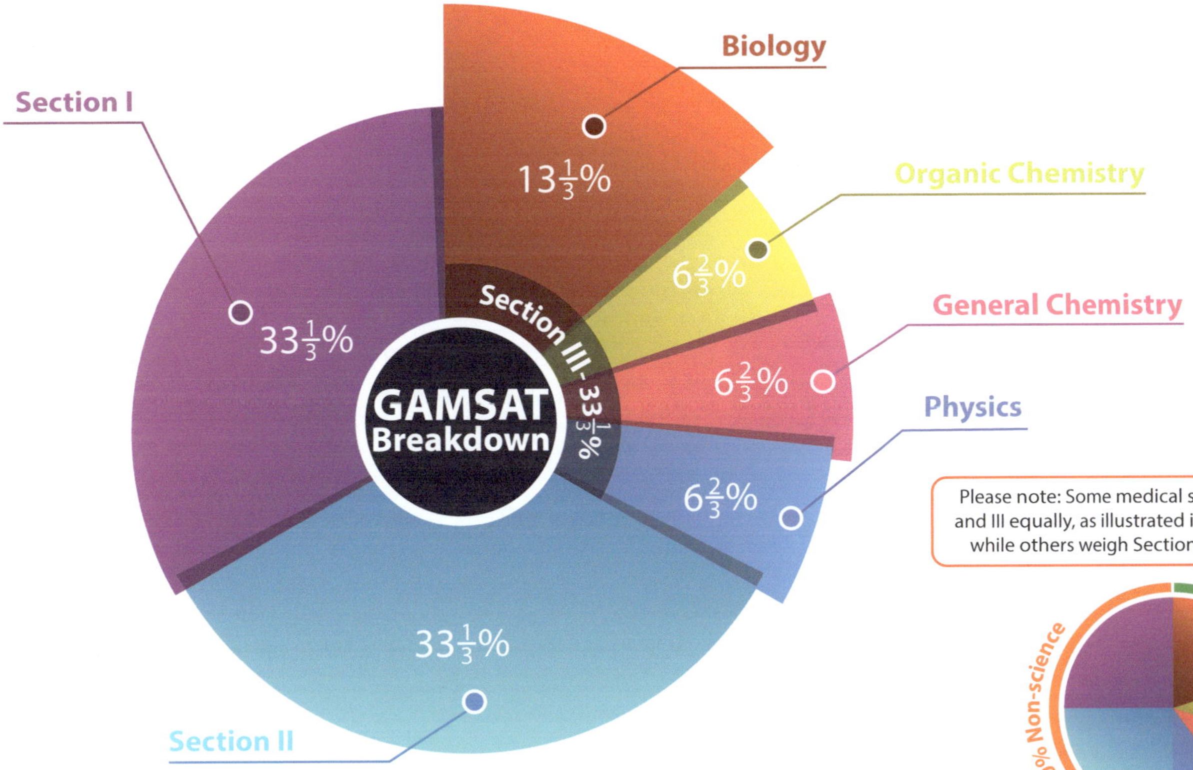

Please note: Some medical schools weigh Section I, II and III equally, as illustrated in the pie chart to the left, while others weigh Section III twice as seen below.

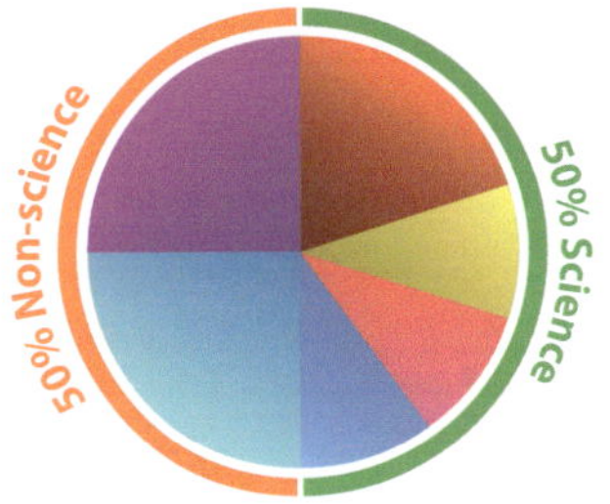

GAMSAT is challenging, get organised.

gamsat-prep.com/free-GAMSAT-study-schedule

1. How to study

- Learn, revise and practice using the GAMSAT Masters Series book(s) and/or videos.
- Complete all exercises and multiple-choice practice questions in this book.
- Consolidate: create and study from your personal summaries (= Gold Notes) daily. Create study cards or audio files from your Gold Notes to increase your study efficiency.

2. Once you have completed your studies

- Sit a full-length GAMSAT practice test.
- Analyse mistakes and all worked solutions.
- Consolidate: Revise all your Gold Notes and create more.

3. Sit multiple mock exams

- ACER GAMSAT practice exams with free Gold Standard worked solutions on YouTube
- Free full-length Gold Standard (GS) mock exam GS-Free with helpful, detailed worked solutions
- HEAPS: 15 full-length exams, 5 in the book and 10 online with the new, digital GAMSAT format

4. How much time do you need to study?

- On average, 3-6 hours per day for 3-6 months; depending on life experiences, 2 weeks may be enough and 8 months could be insufficient.
- Try to study full on for 1-2 weeks and then adjust your expectations for your personal, ideal study time.

5. Recommended GAMSAT Communities

- All countries (mainly Australia): pagingdr.net
- Mainly the UK: thestudentroom.co.uk (Medicine Community Discussion)
- Mainly Ireland: boards.ie (GAMSAT and GEM forum)

Is there something in the Masters Series that you did not understand? Don't get frustrated, get online:

gamsat-prep.com/forum

Table of Contents

Note that: H = High-level Importance; M = Medium-level Importance; L = Low-level Importance.

Note that: H = High-level Importance; M = Medium-level Importance; L = Low-level Importance.

Note that: H = High-level Importance; M = Medium-level Importance; L = Low-level Importance.

Note that: H = High-level Importance; M = Medium-level Importance; L = Low-level Importance.

INTRODUCTION

GAMSAT Section 3, Reasoning in Biological and Physical Sciences, is the longest of the 3 subtests on exam day. 'Biological Sciences' refers to Organic Chemistry and Biology. 'Physical Sciences' refers to Physics and General Chemistry.

Essentially, 40% of Section 3 is Biology. Officially, the level of assumed knowledge is first-year university. With time, it may become clear to you that despite the preceding statement, the assumed knowledge for Biology is mostly consistent with A-Level/Leaving Certificate/Year 12 courses. However, the topics explored in the stimulus material during the exam can be quite advanced with the aim being to test your ability to learn on the spot and apply your reasoning skills to novel scenarios.

What is so *new* about the new GAMSAT Biology Masters Series?

As compared to pre-pandemic softcover and hardcover Gold Standard GAMSAT books, over 50% of this book contains brand new content and that does not include all of the text improvements. The great majority of the new content is related to practice questions. Each chapter begins with an updated list of what to commit to memory, what you should understand (*your learning objectives*) and the Percent Importance of that chapter based on the number of times content in that chapter would have been helpful to solve specific problems among ACER's officially released 440 Section 3 multiple-choice questions (MCQs).

Each chapter ends with: **1)** Spoiler Alerts listing official MCQs to continue your chapter-specific practice and to confirm, through examples, the data that we have presented to you in this Introduction and in each chapter; **2)** Chapter Checklists to further guide your note-taking and confirm that you have met your learning objectives for that chapter.

MCQs are now, for the first time, in the book with answers, helpful worked solutions and free discussion boards for all worked solutions online (*free access for the original owner for 1 year; dozens of hours of relevant teaching videos also free; extensions available*); also new: Dimensional-analysis, graph-analysis, flow-chart and research chapter-ending practice questions. Regarding the latter, also for the first time for GAMSAT Biology, the practice questions are divided into 2 sections: **(1)** foundational (*basic understanding*) MCQs to ensure that you are grounded in the fundamentals; and **(2)** GAMSAT-level MCQs which have been tailored to reflect the most current exam trends.

Note that about 5 exams from our new 15 full-length exam book *HEAPS* are the source of many of the chapter-ending MCQs, and they are identified as such.

What is Biology?

Biology is the study of life and living organisms. This includes the physical structure, chemical processes, molecular interactions, physiological mechanisms, development and evolution of organisms. Biology basics include the recognition of the cell as the fundamental unit of life, genes as the basic unit of heredity, and evolution as the mechanism driving the creation and extinction of species. Living organisms are systems that survive by transforming energy and decreasing their local randomness (*entropy*) to maintain a vital circumstance known as *homeostasis* (i.e. the ability to maintain a relatively stable internal state).

What is GAMSAT Biology?

GAMSAT Biology is primarily concerned with graphs, tables and diagrams (the latter includes flow charts). Undoubtedly, GAMSAT Biology success requires a foundation in GAMSAT Maths (this is especially true for students with a non-science background, NSB). Should you have any concerns regarding your basic algebra skills, either you should brush-up on your skills in maths through other resources, or revise the knowledge you once had in secondary school with the GAMSAT Maths and Physics Masters Series book. There are 2 chapters in that book that will have the greatest effect on your GAMSAT score - GM Chapter 2: Scientific Measurement and Dimensional Analysis, and GM Chapter 3: Algebra and Graph Analysis.

Even if you do not have the GAMSAT Masters Series Maths and Physics book, we have created a brand new section of gamsat-prep.com which you can access for free with your GS Online Access: GAMSAT Biology Chapter 0. We have placed over 50 MCQs - mostly in video format - with step-by-step worked solutions exploring graph analysis and flow charts.

"over half (even a bit more) of my exam questions had a graph to refer to"
"biol - tonnes of complex graph interpretations, especially multiple graphs which somehow correlate to each other"
"Punnet squares!"
"Mainly graphical interpretation where (for bio) knowledge would help but wasn't 100% vital"
"Had a lot of physiology related questions, most of them contained graphs or diagrams"
From a very small number of students:
"Surprisingly not a lot of graphs/tables"
"I think less biology than I expected, I didn't really get any graph questions"
"I got 0 Punnet squares in my test"

Student "Debriefs": Comments from recent GAMSAT sittings left in online forums about GAMSAT Biology shortly after the real exam. Note that for exam security and other reasons, not all exams are identical even when students sit the real GAMSAT on the same day in the same city. {FYI NSB candidates: We will address Punnett squares in Chapter 14, Genetics.}

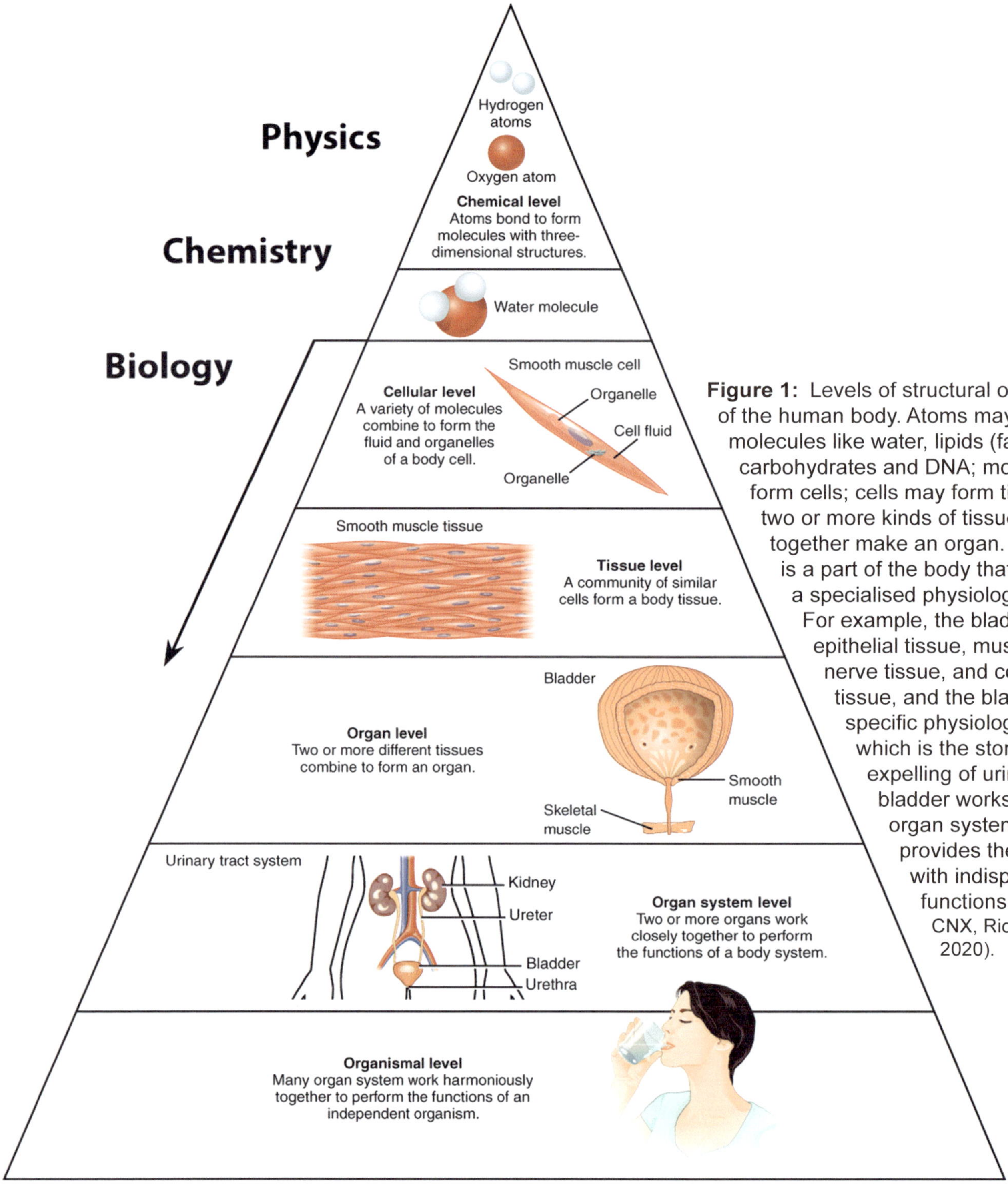

Figure 1: Levels of structural organisation of the human body. Atoms may form molecules like water, lipids (fats), protein, carbohydrates and DNA; molecules may form cells; cells may form tissues; and two or more kinds of tissues working together make an organ. An *organ* is a part of the body that performs a specialised physiologic function. For example, the bladder contains epithelial tissue, muscle tissue, nerve tissue, and connective tissue, and the bladder has the specific physiologic function which is the storing and expelling of urine. The bladder works within an organ system which provides the organism with indispensable functions (OpenStax CNX, Rice University; 2020).

We are not trying to suggest that all assumed knowledge for GAMSAT Biology is irrelevant. A very basic understanding of cell biology, the circulatory system, and genetics have been proven to be quite helpful topics. However, the majority of questions in the science with the greatest impact on your Section 3 score requires little to no biology-specific assumed knowledge.

As many of you may know, Gold Standard GAMSAT was the first company to create step-by-step worked solutions to all of the over 400 multiple-choice Section 3 official ACER GAMSAT practice questions, and then we put them on YouTube for free access through the Gold Standard GAMSAT Channel. In addition, we carefully re-examined all of ACER's practice materials multiple times and compared the data generated with students' experiences as publicly reported in online forums. If we have erred, it is on the side of conservative estimates.

The percentages below reflect the number of instances specific information in a specific chapter would have been helpful to solve a question among ACER's official materials. Here is the summary of the level of importance for the 16 GAMSAT Biology chapters in this book:

Chapter	1	2	3	4	5	6	7	8	9	10	11	12	13	14	15	16
Percent Importance	15%	8%	6%	7%	1%	1%	19%	6%	6%	2%	6%	8%	0%	5%	10%	0%
Relative Importance	H	M	M	M	L	L	H	M	M	L	M	M	L	M	H	L

Note that: H = High-level Importance; M = Medium-level Importance; L = Low-level Importance.

The data is real but, of course, the labels representing 'relative importance' are subjective. Note that approximately 75% of ACER's chapter-related Biology questions are based on less than half of the 16 chapters. Specifically, the following 7 chapters are above average: 1, 2, 3, 4, 7, 12 and 15.

Note: If you are also using other Masters Series books you might notice that the subjective labelling is not the same for all chapters because it depends on the number of chapters in that GAMSAT subject. The more chapters, the lower the threshold for the subjective label. For GAMSAT Biology, at least 10% is high; at least 3% but below 10% is medium; and below 3% is labelled as low importance.

It is also important to note, that of the hundreds of official ACER MCQs, not one single question required assumed knowledge that was not clearly presented in a GAMSAT Masters Series book.

An existential question: Why have a chapter in a book with a 0% "Importance" rating? The chapters in question are traditional, introductory-level university subjects in Biology consistent with ACER's official line (Chapter 16 has the title Evolution; in a modern curriculum, how could one not discuss evolution?). Although any facts contained in low-importance chapters would be extremely unlikely to be necessary to answer a question correctly during the real exam, there is value in reading Biology content within the context of traditional subjects, there might be some value in having a little degree of familiarity, but very importantly: the practice questions at the end of those chapters are definitely at the calibre of the real GAMSAT. In other words, the least that you should consider for "0-1% chapters," would be to complete the GAMSAT-level practice questions found at the end of those chapters.

Breaking the Wheel: Problem-based Learning

In this Introduction, we will apply problem-based learning (PBL) to explore 2 very common GAMSAT Biology question types: **(1)** graph analysis, and **(2)** reasoning through diagrams, a subset of which includes flow charts. If you happen to have a strong science background, then the following exercises would be more helpful if you restrict yourself to a maximum of 2 minutes per question which is the new digital-GAMSAT timing. Otherwise, take your time and try your best before exploring the worked solutions. We understand that some of you may have little or no background for the following questions. But keep in mind: The real exam is designed to expose you to new content on the day of the exam to see if you can reason through to a solution. In keeping with 'learning is better by doing', let's begin.

> **Student:** *Teach me everything I need to know then test me on exactly that material.*
> **GAMSAT:** (giggles)
> **PBL:** *Hold my beer…*

UNIT 1, Questions 1-3

Marine biologists have determined that there is a relatively high concentration of predator fish like tuna, and large fish such as swordfish and marlins that are characterised by long sword-like bills (i.e. *billfish*), commonly found in biodiversity hotspots. In other words, the abundance (or species density) of tuna and billfish are good indicators of overall marine biodiversity.

Although environmental change is often responsible for fluctuations in the sizes of fish communities from year-to-year, global declines in the abundance of fish over longer timescales are believed to be primarily driven by overfishing. Consider the data in Figure 1.

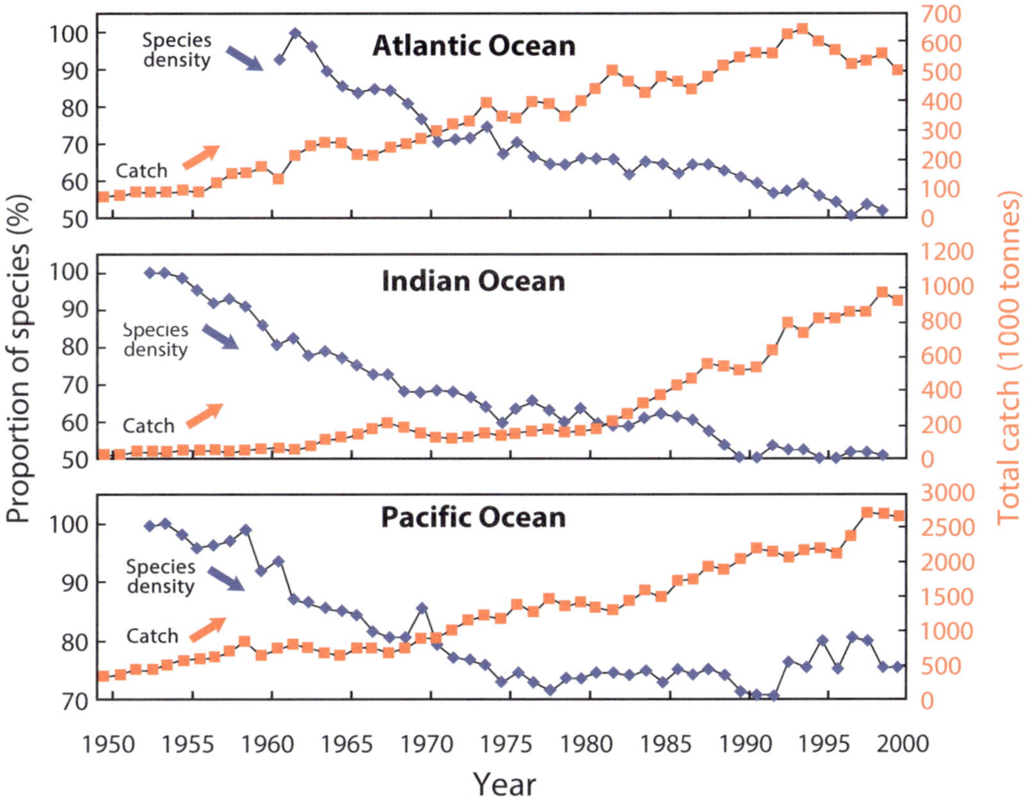

Figure 1: Changes in species density (the number of species caught on a standard fishing line with 1000 hooks) and total catch of tuna and billfish by ocean. (Ref.: Science Education Resource Center at Carleton College carleton.edu)

Note that: 1 tonne (also known as a 'metric ton') = 1000 kilograms

1. According to Figure 1, which of the following is most consistent with the increase in the total catch of tuna and billfish in the Indian Ocean between 1980 and 1987?

   A 3.0×10^2 kg
   B 3.0×10^5 kg
   C 3.0×10^6 kg
   D 3.0×10^8 kg

2. Based on Figure 1, which ocean appears to have experienced the largest decline in species density between 1960 and 2000?

   A Atlantic Ocean
   B Indian Ocean
   C Pacific Ocean
   D The decline for all three oceans is quite similar.

3. Which ocean experienced the largest percentage increase in total catch of tuna and billfish between 1960 and 2000?

   A Atlantic Ocean
   B Indian Ocean
   C Pacific Ocean
   D The increase for all three oceans is quite similar.

Question 1: Clearly the issue is to follow the correct curve, read from the correct axis label, and interpret your findings carefully: No assumed knowledge.

We read the points for 1980 and 1987 from the red graph (since we are asked for "total catch") for the Indian Ocean, and read from the *y*-axis on the right (total catch).

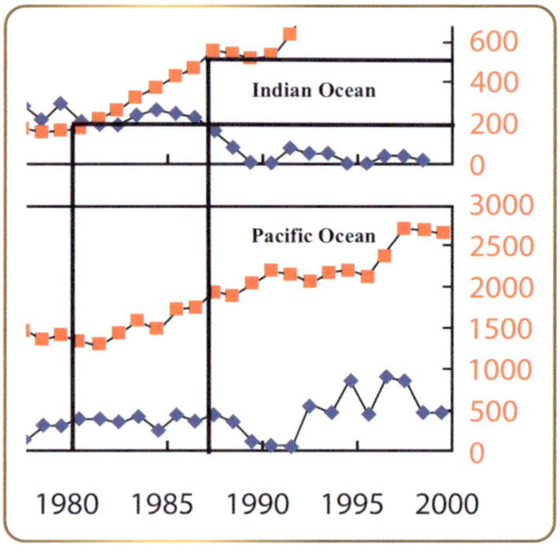

The difference is approximately 500 – 200 = 300. If you determined a response anywhere within the 150-450 range (or worse!), it simply would not matter because the answers are *orders of magnitude* different (e.g., at least 10 times different). OK, but 300 what? Check Figure 1, the units are "1000 tonnes," so we must have 300 000 tonnes, but the answers are in kg so we need a conversion factor (dimensional analysis; GAMSAT Maths Masters Series, GM 2.2). Note the "Note that" in bold below the diagram: 1 tonne = 1000 kilograms. And so, we have 300 000 000 kg, or 3.0×10^8 kg, answer choice D is correct.

The dimensional analysis: 300 000 tonnes x (1000 kilograms/tonne) = 300 000 000 kg.

For those of you thinking that this is some type of trick question, from the British Medical Journal (2020): "More than 237 million medication errors are made every year in England, the avoidable consequences of which cost the NHS upwards of £98 million and more than 1700 lives every year..." The figures in Australia, Ireland and other countries worldwide may be different but the numbers remain significant and avoidable. Always pay careful attention to units.

Question 2: We can see that species density is in blue and we can reasonably infer that it refers to "Proportion of species (%)" along the left *y*-axis. Again, the answers are so far apart that you will be able to easily estimate numbers even if the graph is on a computer monitor because, as long as you are reading the correct graphs, you can poorly estimate (relatively!) and still get the answer correct.

We have placed black lines on the graph but there really is no need for that, you can 'eyeball' the results: **1)** Atlantic Ocean, 90% - 50% = 40%; **2)** Indian Ocean, 80% - 50% = 30%; **3)** Pacific Ocean, 90% - 75% = 15%. Thus, answer choice A, the Atlantic Ocean, is correct.

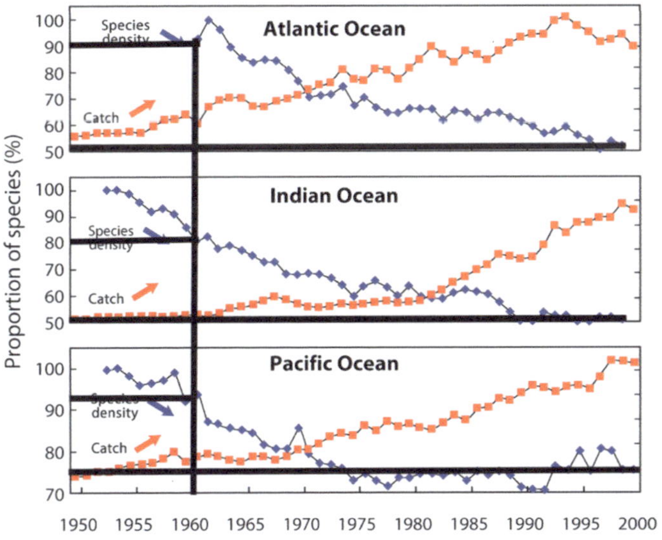

Note that, from afar, the graphs in Figure 1 all look like they have similar trends but it is important to notice that the scales from each ocean along the *y*-axes are not identical (i.e. the range of numbers differs).

Question 3: Back to "total catch" and so it is the red graph and the red-labelled, *y*-axis on the right side. We are comparing results for 1960 vs 2000; the latter lines up exactly with the *y*-axis on the right side.

Reasonable estimates derived from Figure 1: **1)** Atlantic Ocean, from approx. 100 to 500, an increase to a number that is 5 times (5 fold) greater (note: since percentage relates to proportion, GM 1.4.3, as a shortcut, we will follow the multiplier as being proportional to the percentage); **2)** Indian Ocean, from approx. 50 to 1000, an increase of a breathtaking 20 times; **3)** Pacific Ocean, from somewhere between 500 and 1000 to 2500, an increase between 5 times and 2.5 times. Thus, answer choice B, the Indian Ocean, is substantially correct.

Note: This image is upside down because the question is on a page facing the worked solution.

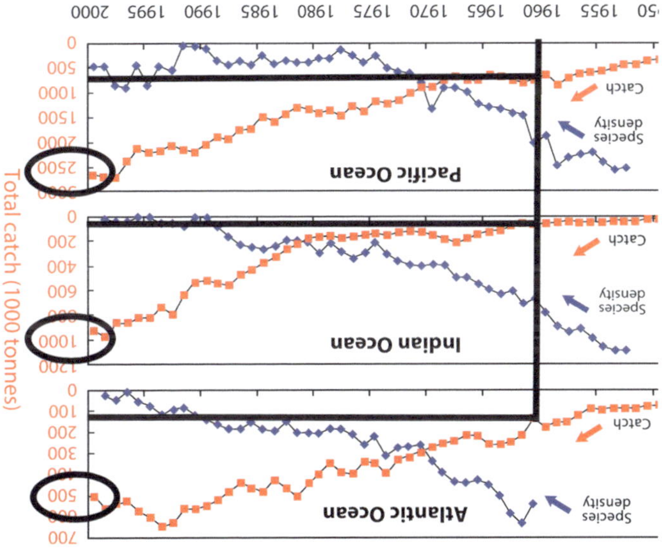

Unit 2, Question 4

The tarpon is among the world's most prized game fish. Adult tarpon are four to eight feet long and weigh 60 to 280 pounds. A graph (Figure 1) has been designed to provide a means to estimate the weight of a tarpon without killing and weighing the fish, using measurements of fork length and dorsal girth.

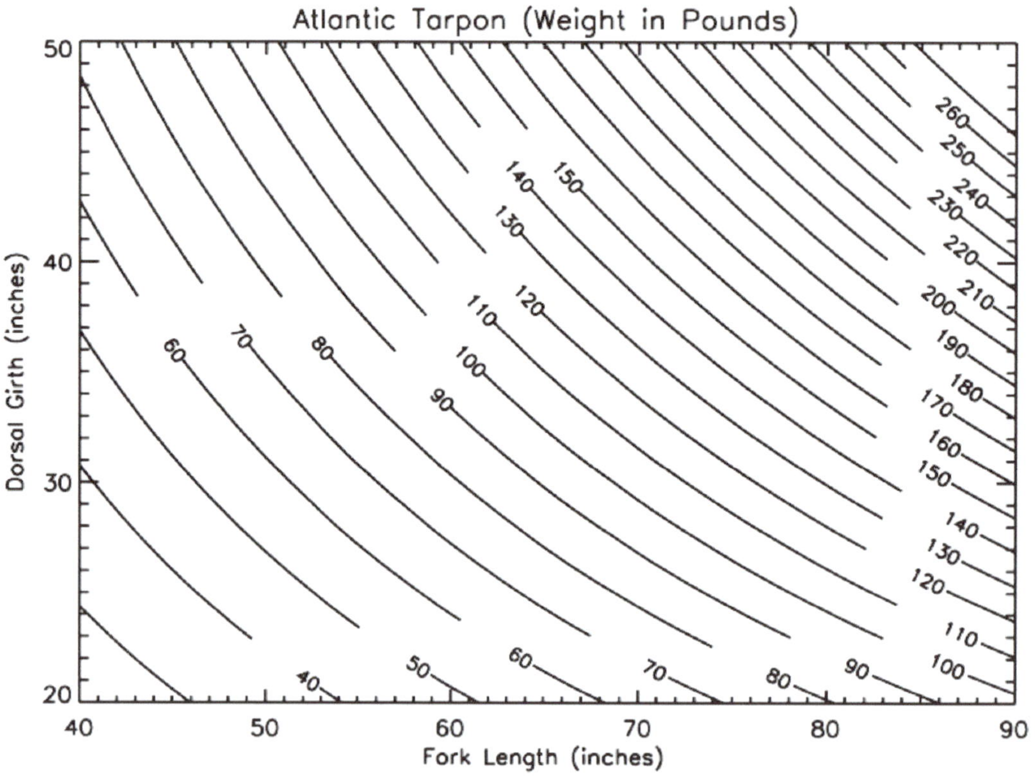

Figure 1: Estimating the weight of tarpon.
Jerald S Ault, PhD; University of Miami

Note that: Drawing a straight line from a fork length of 61 inches and then from a dorsal girth of 30 inches intersects the curvilinear line consistent with a weight of approximately 80 pounds.

4. According to Figure 1, which of the following is the best estimate of the dorsal girth in inches of a 210-pound tarpon with a fork length of 83 inches?

A Less than 39
B 39
C 40
D Over 40

Expect the unexpected! The real GAMSAT will certainly have some graph types that you are not expected to have seen before. In the case of this particular unit, it is a type of nomogram (GM 3.9), which is a diagram showing the relations between three or more variables using a number of scales arranged so that the value of one variable can be found by, for example, drawing a straight line intersecting the other scales. Note that even during the real exam, ACER will typically provide an example as to how to interpret a graph if they expect that they are presenting a graph that is likely novel to you. Pay careful attention when they say: “Note that”!

Some students will use their exam ID (e.g. driver’s license) or hold their writing implement towards the computer monitor to assess straight lines. Of course, a ruler is not permitted during the real exam.

Using the example provided, drawing a line from a fork length of 61 inches and dorsal girth of 30 inches, results in an intersection at the weight (curvilinear/curved line) of 80 pounds. That brings our attention to the curved lines, how they are continuous and numbered every 10 pounds with varying intervals. In particular, notice the curved line that says ‘80’ has 3 segments: a middle segment that intersects the data points that we evaluated, and the curved line extends to the bottom right and to the top left of the graph. Thus the example helps us interpret the curved lines. You can see our annotation of Figure 1 of the preceding reasoning in green on the next page (*au verso*).

Now when we assess the weight of 210, we must follow that curve upwards until it intersects the vertical line from 83 inches (fork length) and then we can read the dorsal girth, which is 42 inches. Since it is greater than 40 inches, answer choice D is correct.

There is some human biology on the GAMSAT, but fish, birds, bats, and insects are also quite popular!

Notice that Questions 1 to 4 are typically placed in the ‘Biology’ category but you would be hard pressed to find an introductory-level university course (or any uni. BIO course) that would ask such questions. That is just one of the many reasons that GAMSAT preparation has its own unique path to success.

Please keep in mind: Since some pharmaceutical companies may try to influence the prescribing patterns of doctors by presenting data in complex graphs, tables and/or diagrams, developing a skill for graph analysis will serve both you and your future patients well.

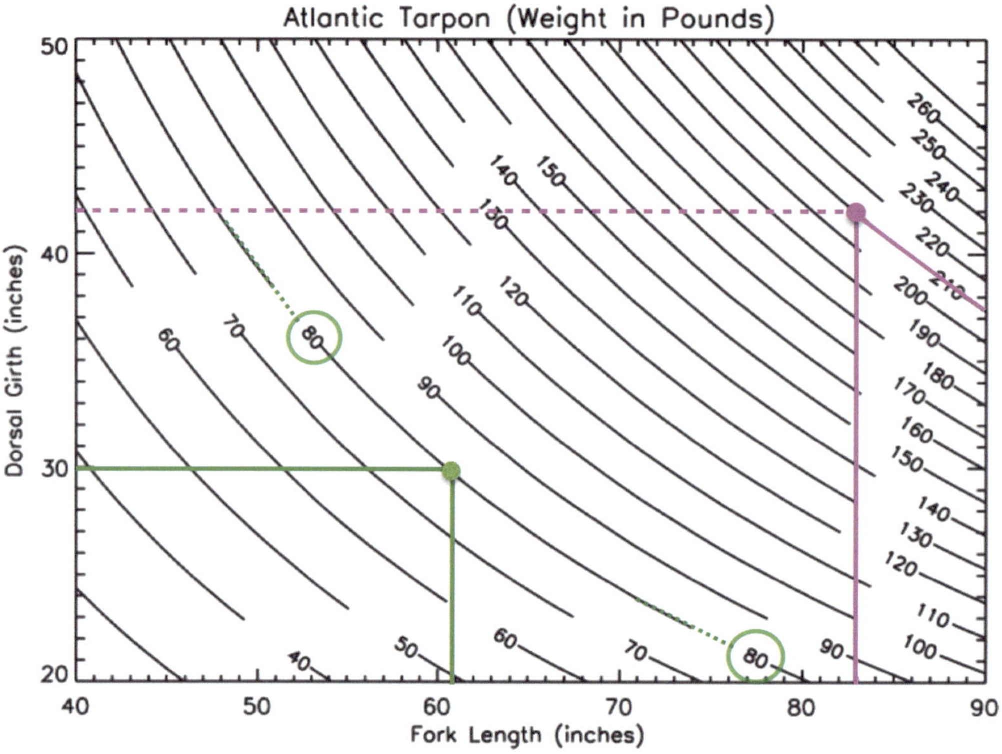

Unit 3, Questions 5-7

The chorioallantois is a highly vascularised membrane found in the eggs of certain amniotes like birds. It is the avian homologue of the mammalian placenta. It is the outermost extra-embryonic membrane which lines the non-vascular egg shell membrane. The chorioallantois functions as the site of gaseous exchange for oxygen and carbon dioxide between the growing embryo and the environment, eventually that role is supplanted by the lung as the chick's needs for oxygen grows. Consider Figure 1.

5. According to Figure 1, the rate of change of oxygen uptake of the bird embryo is zero at some time during which of the following?

   A Day 16
   B Day 20
   C Day 21
   D Day 22

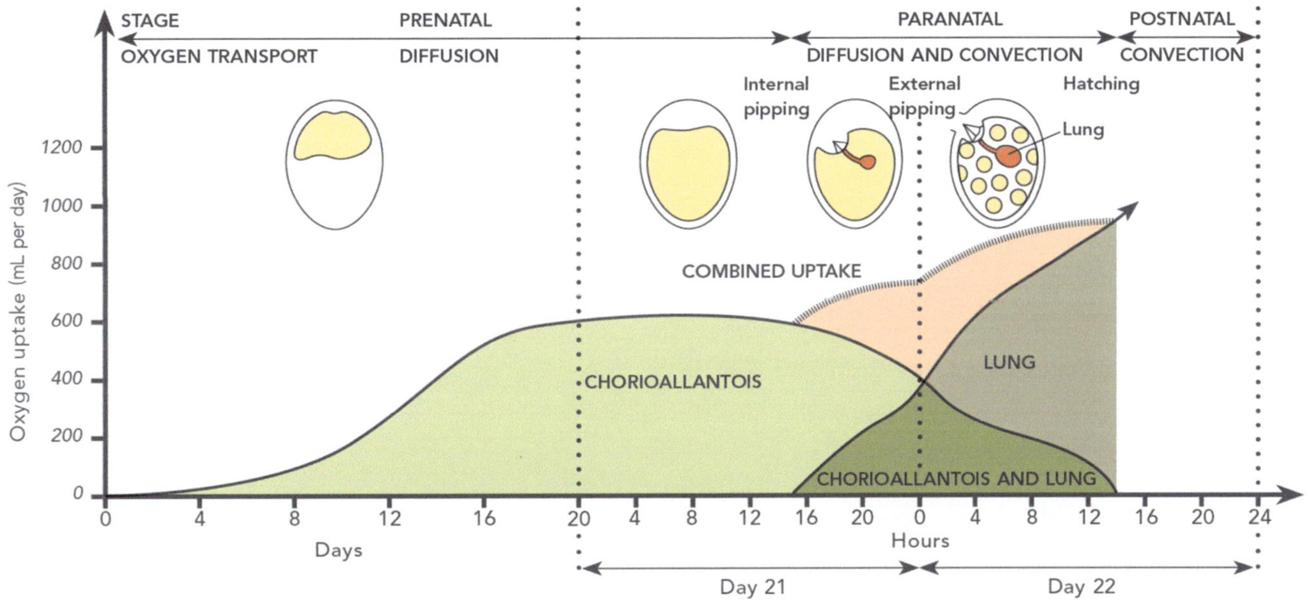

Figure 1: Transition from the chorioallantois to pulmonary (lung) respiration. Note that the "combined uptake" represents the sum total of both chorioallantois and lung during a period of time when both systems are functional. (Adapted from Petersime nv, 2020; originally from Rahn, Ar, and Paganelli, "*How Bird Eggs Breathe,*" Scientific American, 1979)

6. Based on Figure 1, estimate the total oxygen uptake in the first 20 days of incubation within the egg.

   A 0.12 L
   B 2.5 L
   C 4.2 L
   D 4.8 L

7. If the graph in Figure 1 continues as projected after the second half of Day 22, as compared to Days 1-20, the total oxygen uptake in Days 21 and 22 would be expected to be which of the following?

   A More than twice
   B More, but less than twice
   C Less, but more than half
   D Less than half

Question 5: Let's break down the expression "rate of change of oxygen uptake." Rate, in science, often refers to an event occurring over time (i.e. per unit time, thus mathematically, time is in the denominator). Of course, the slope of a line is the change in *y* over the change in *x* (GM 3.5), and so if *x* is time (which is clearly the case in Figure 1), the slope provides the rate. Since the label on the *y*-axis is "Oxygen uptake" then the slope of the graph in Figure 1 will provide us with the rate of change of oxygen uptake required to answer the question.

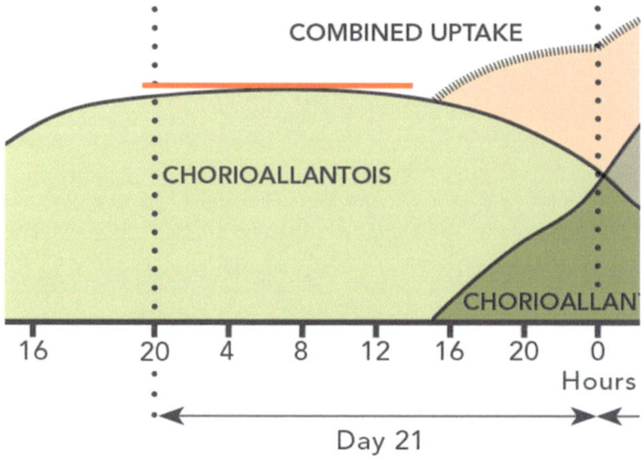

The question wants to know where the slope is zero, which can occur when the numerator for the slope, the change in *y*, is zero, which means the line (slope) must be horizontal. The slope of the curve keeps changing but it is possible to assess the slope at a particular point on the curve (assess a line *tangential* to the curve; GM 3.5.4) just by holding your writing implement horizontally up to the computer monitor (or, the page in this case) with slight movements. By doing so, one can determine that all answer choices have positive slopes at some point. Only Day 21 also has a slope of zero which is followed by a negative slope, and then a positive peach slope – all on the same day. We have placed a red line to identify the slope of zero revealing that C is the correct answer.

Side note: Figure 1 is a famous graph. Just how famous? It was used in a past GAMSAT (preserved in ACER's GAMSAT Practice Test 2), used by the Medical College Admission Test (MCAT; US and Canada), and used by various other standardised science exams. Of course, the questions are always different but the graph itself has many wonderful elements including the change in scale which we will explore next.

Question 6: We are looking for the total oxygen uptake which would be a bewildering question if not for one fact: All of the answers are in litres (L). This is plain dimensional analysis (GM 2.2), which refers to paying close attention to units in order to travel, mathematically, from where you are to where you want to go. The *y*-axis has mL/day and the *x*-axis has days, and if we multiply:

mL/day × days = mL, which can be converted into L.

The beauty of dimensional analysis is that you do not need to memorise if division (as we did in the previous question), or multiplication (as we will do for this question), or some other mathematical manipulation is needed, just follow the units.

If you have not considered this before, try the question again before continuing with the worked solution.

Of course, one side multiplied by the other side gives area (GM 4.2), so we want the area under the curve. We can't just multiply the highest number of *x* by the highest number of *y* because that is a rectangle which is clearly not the shape that we are looking at. We could use calculus but that's useless for GAMSAT! Perhaps the shape of the curve within the first 20 days resembles a triangle. Let's choose where to start and end that triangle so that it seems to encompass as much of the area in light green as possible, but not too much in terms of unneeded bits: Perhaps something that seems to balance the area missing in the triangle with bits outside of the triangle. See the annotated graph.

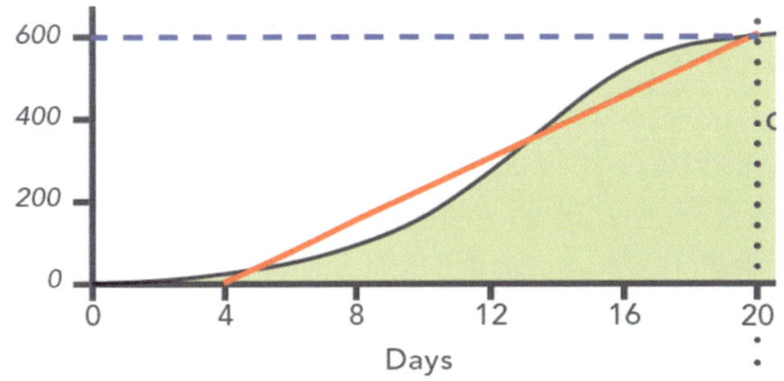

Now we take the area of the triangle (GM 4.2.2) which is ½(base)(height). The base of the triangle stretches from 4 days to 20 days, thus 16 days. And the height appears to be 600 mL/day. Thus, ½(16)(600) = (8)(600) = 4800 mL = 4.8 L, answer choice D is correct.

Question 7: During the real exam, ACER may have 1-3 questions wherein to proceed logically, one would have needed to understand the preceding question and choose the correct answer. Alas, question 7!

We have already determined that the area under the curve can get us the volume and we know that the first 20 days is equivalent to a total volume of 4.8 L. So, we just need to calculate the volume for the last 2 days, considering the projection (extrapolation = extend to the unknown, i.e. the direction of the arrow of Figure 1 on the far right leaving LUNG).

Well, that looks like many different shapes! Days 21 and 22 have the chorioallantois graph, the peach-flavoured combined uptake (which is clearly additive, taking into account both organs), and then on the 14th hour of Day 22, oxygen uptake due to 'lung' takes off. What to do? Calculate all of the areas separately and finish GAMSAT after 24 hours? No, let's exaggerate the situation and see if our exaggeration brings us to a reasonable answer. Let's create a rectangle 2 days at the base (Day 21, 22) and as high as 1000 mL/day, which is 1 L/day. That rectangle seems like an exaggeration of the actual area even if we take into account that in the last 10 hours of Day 22, a part of the graph will be above our rectangle (but that is not more area than the empty white space inside our rectangle).

Dimensional analysis: 2 days × 1 L/day = 2 L (not the most difficult equation you will ever see!). We exaggerated the volume from the last 2 days and it is still less than half of 4.8 L. The answer is clearly D.

Do not let your lying eyes fool you! ACER has a stable of graphs that may give a certain first impression but careful analysis proves otherwise. With just a glance, the area under the curve after Day 20 seems more than before Day 20. That is because there was a change in the scale along the *x*-axis so we were comparing the oxygen needs for 20 days vs. the needs for just 2 days. The uptake went up in those 2 days but over such a short period of time that it is still less than half of the volume of the first 20 days.

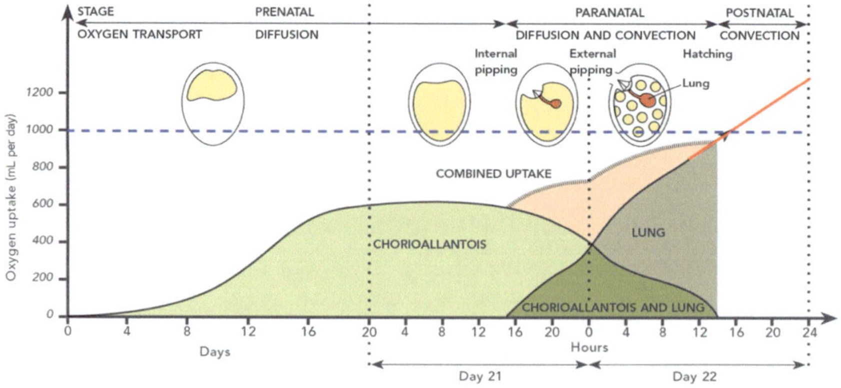

Unit 4, Question 8

In the following branched metabolic pathway, a blue dashed arrow with a minus sign represents the inhibition of a metabolic step by an end product: {*This is a bellwether question: If you struggle with this one, it would be better not to try the next unit yet; rather, return to both of these units after you have completed Chapter 4.*}

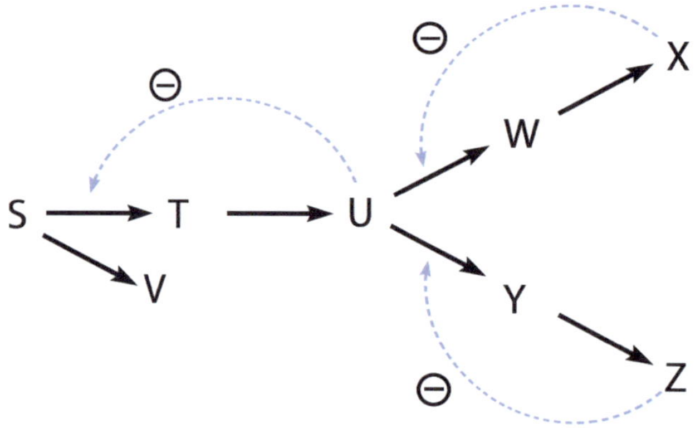

8. Identify the process(es) that would be dominant in the metabolic pathway provided if the 2 end products X and Z were both in relatively high concentrations.

A T → U
B S → V
C U → Y
D Both W → X and Y → Z

On the Surface: If X and Y are present in high concentrations then, according to the diagram, they will inhibit (i.e. negative feedback) the reactions U → W and U → Y (making answer choice C incorrect). This creates a blockage along the highway so U begins to accumulate. Now U will feedback to block (inhibit) the conversion of S → T (which means less T → U will take place, thus answer choice A is incorrect). Now S accumulates and has only one release valve: S → V (like taking the exit from a highway with loads of traffic; thus B is correct).

Going Deeper: Note that answer choice D is not consistent with negative feedback ("inhibition of a metabolic step by an end product" consistent with the diagram). If high concentrations of X and Z resulted in reactions that will make even more X and Z, then that is consistent with positive feedback and is analogous to a runaway, accelerating freight train. It is very important to understand, even if you are just following the arrows in the pathway, the moment that X and Z are elevated, the reaction that makes them is inhibited and therefore cannot be dominant. Potentially, answer choice D would usually be correct when X and Z are in relatively low concentrations.

We will later see classic examples of positive feedback including blood clotting (in the next unit) and contractions in childbirth (BIO 6.3.7). When uterine contraction occurs, the hormone 'oxytocin' is released into the body which stimulates even more contractions. Thus, the result is an increased amplitude and frequency of contractions. The loop is only broken once the baby leaves the uterus.

Side note: There are many different ways to symbolise positive/negative feedback. They may use + or - symbols which may or may not be enclosed in a circle (like the previous image). Or they could use solid or dashed lines with arrow heads, or in the case of negative feedback, it could end with a "T" (for example, the pathway in the next unit). You do not need to commit the various options to memory since a 'key' or legend will be provided or, alternatively, a description will be given as to the meaning of the arrows or connections in the pathway provided.

Side note #2! When is an arrow an arrow? This is not a philosophical question and, in fact, ACER designed different types of questions related to this one point. In Physics, an arrow typically represents the magnitude and direction of a vector (e.g. acceleration). In Chemistry (General and Organic) and Biochemistry (represented by the metabolic pathway in the preceding question), an arrow means that reactant(s) is (are) converted into product(s), S → T. Biology includes all of the above and presents many new, testable meanings for an arrow.

Perhaps it is a hormone that stimulates another organ to mass produce a different hormone that is completely unrelated chemically to the first hormone. No arrow in Chemistry would be acceptable in that situation since they are not related! Perhaps an arrow refers to a complex interplay between molecules (again, nothing to do with vectors, nor reactants/products), such as the central dogma of Biology: DNA → RNA → protein (Chapter 3). The latter is NOT saying that DNA becomes RNA! The irony is that ACER normally defines the meaning of the arrow in the passage but a substantial number of students miss the definition and choose the answer based on instinct. Practice arrows are on the way...

Unit 5, Questions 9-14

Coagulation (i.e. *clotting*) is the process by which blood changes from a liquid to a cross-linked fibrin gel referred to as a 'blood clot'. This process may stop blood loss from a damaged vessel (*haemostasis*). For normal coagulation to occur, the necessary clotting factors must be present in the blood. There are a number of diseases that arise from disorders of coagulation which can range from bleeding (haemorrhage, bruising) to obstructive clotting (thrombosis).

The coagulation cascade (Figure 1) has two initial pathways which lead to fibrin formation. These are the contact activation (intrinsic) pathway, and the tissue factor (extrinsic) pathway, which both lead to the final 'common pathway' of factor X, thrombin and fibrin. The pathways are a series of reactions in which an inactive protein enzyme precursor, and sometimes its co-factor, are altered to become active components that then catalyse the next reaction in the cascade. Coagulation factors are generally indicated by Roman numerals, with a lowercase 'a' appended to indicate an active form.

9. According to Figure 1, thrombin is directly converted to which of the following?

A Thrombomodulin
B Factor VIII
C Both **A** and **B**
D Neither **A** nor **B**

10. Vitamin K is required to synthesise factors II, VII, IX and X. A person with a significant deficiency in vitamin K may have:

A thrombosis due to the activation of both the intrinsic pathway and extrinsic pathway.
B thrombosis due to the lack of reaction progress in both the intrinsic pathway and extrinsic pathway.
C haemorrhage due to the lack of reaction progress in either the intrinsic pathway or extrinsic pathway.
D haemorrhage due to the lack of reaction progress in both the intrinsic pathway and extrinsic pathway.

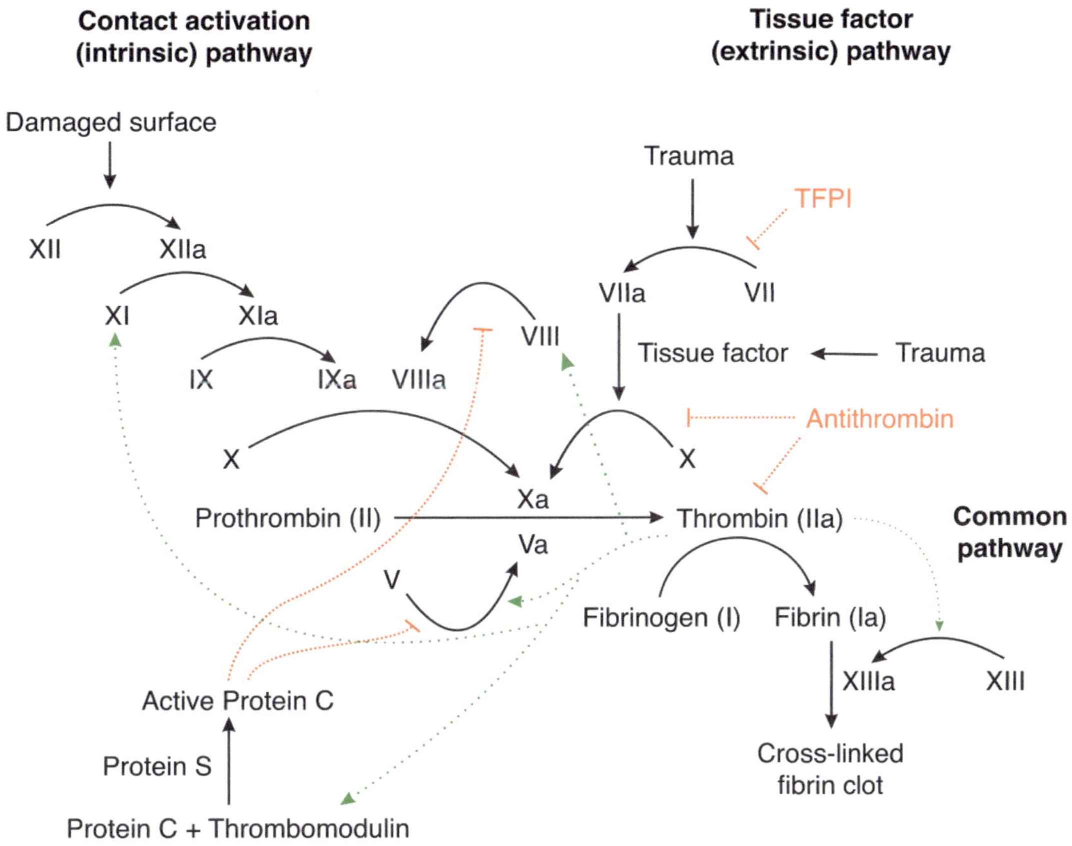

Figure 1: Coagulation cascade. Red dotted lines ending in "T" indicate negative (inhibitory) feedback; green dotted lines ending with an arrow head indicate positive (stimulatory) feedback; curvilinear black arrows indicate 'conversion to'; a factor (or factors) written above and/or below an arrow indicate(s) a catalytic function. For example, factor XIIa catalyses the reaction that converts factor XI to factor XIa. Wikimedia; Joe D, 2007.

11. According to the information provided, the final common pathway is most directly activated by:

A tissue factor and factor VIIa.
B a blood clot.
C the activated form of factor XII.
D antithrombin.

12. In biochemical regulatory mechanisms, negative feedback:

A is the process of maintaining steady change in one direction.
B occurs rarely and only in the presence of positive feedback.
C can operate to maintain a substance's concentration nearly constant.
D helps to amplify the body's response to a stimulus.

13. A blood clot, formally a 'thrombus', has 2 components: aggregated platelets and red blood cells that form a plug, and a mesh of cross-linked protein. The protein component is largely composed of a more or less equal quantity of factors:

A from I to XIII.
B in the common pathway.
C Ia and XIIIa.
D neither **A** nor **B** nor **C**.

14. Which of the following is likely the best treatment option for a person with severe protein S deficiency?

A Factor VIIIa
B Factor Xa inhibitors
C Fibrinogen
D Factor XIII activators

Question 9: The caption to Figure 1 states that "curvilinear black arrows indicate 'conversion to'". And so, since there is no curvilinear arrow beginning with thrombin, we have no information as to what thrombin is converted to. Thus answer choice D is correct.

Going Deeper: The caption also states that "a factor (or factors) written above and/or below an arrow indicate(s) a catalytic function" and so we can conclude from Figure 1 that thrombin is the enzyme that catalyses the reaction that produces fibrin. And since the caption states "green dotted lines ending with an arrow head indicate positive (stimulatory) feedback," thus thrombin must stimulate the production of factors VIII and XI, as well as the conversions of V to Va, and XIII to XIIIa, and some stimulatory role with respect to thrombomodulin. To stimulate or catalyse a reaction is wholly different from being the chemical (or substrate/reactant) converted into another chemical (product). We can see from Figure 1 that thrombin is a very important and central component to the coagulation cascade.

Question 10: According to Figure 1, prothrombin (factor II) produces thrombin in the presence of activated factor X and V as part of the final common pathway. If only factors II and X were deficient, that would be enough to retard the normal progress of both the intrinsic and extrinsic pathways, independently, because the common pathway cannot proceed as usual (like a traffic jam along the highway!). A lack of the factors involved in coagulation, as alluded to in the opening paragraph, would reasonably result in bleeding (haemorrhage). Thus answer choice D is correct.

Question 11: The second paragraph of the preamble states "the final 'common pathway' of factor X, thrombin and fibrin." Taking that information, we can see that Figure 1 shows 2 different ways that factor X can be activated to produce Xa which then activates prothrombin. And now we can see exactly how 2 different pathways come together for the final common pathway (note the placement of the words 'Common pathway' in bold on the same line with factor Xa). We can see that in the extrinsic pathway, factor VIIa works with tissue factor to activate the conversion of factor X to factor Xa which is needed for the common pathway. Thus answer choice A is correct.

Regarding the other answer choices: (B) we do not see an arrow in Figure 1 coming from the end product, 'clot', to suggest positive or negative feedback. However, the objective of the pathway is to make a blood clot so it seems suspicious, once the objective is met, that the clot would feedback to activate the forming of yet more clot. At any rate, we do not have sufficient "information provided" to conclude that the clot most directly activates the common pathway; (C) the activated form of factor XII, which is XIIa, begins a cascade activating several steps which finally produces Xa. Answer choice A is the better answer since it accomplishes the same task in fewer steps ("most directly"); (D) antithrombin clearly inhibits the common pathway making it the least plausible of the options.

Going Deeper: You may have noticed and/or you could be asked about examples in the cascade where a factor needs some help to accomplish its task. Answer choice A is such a situation where an activated factor (VIIa) needs help (tissue factor) in order to activate another factor (X). So tissue factor is called the 'cofactor' of factor VIIa. Using Figure 1 and its caption, can you identify other cofactors with Roman numerals? Also, given that tissue factor is actually factor III, can you identify which Roman numerals are missing from the sequence in the cascade?

The caption states that "a factor (or factors) written above and/or below an arrow indicate(s) a catalytic function." There are 2 instances where 2 factors are clearly written in association with an arrow: factor IXa and its cofactor VIIIa; and factor Xa and its cofactor Va.

The 2 factors missing from the sequence shown in Figure 1, from I to XIII, include Factor IV which is calcium, and factor VI which does not exist!

Question 12: A positive feedback loop causes a self-amplifying cycle where a physiological change leads to even greater change in the same direction (thus answer choices A and D are incorrect). A negative feedback loop is a process in which the body senses a change, and activates mechanisms to reverse that change. Of course, such a process is essential for homeostasis (steady state, thus answer choice C is correct).

Although positive feedback in unlikely to occur in the absence of negative feedback (such as in Figure 1), the reverse is not true (answer choice B is incorrect). In fact, negative feedback is far more common than positive feedback. Throughout the BIO chapters, we will be exploring many pathways governed by negative feedback.

Going Deeper: Positive feedback responds to a perturbation in the same direction as the perturbation. In so doing, there is amplification or growth of the output signal which typically occurs to a point until a negative feedback response takes over and restores order. In other words, we can see the example in Figure 1 that positive feedback occurs first, it is most urgent, the person is bleeding. Negative feedback takes longer but you want it to occur at some point because you do not want blood clots forming uncontrollably since they can block the circulation of blood, and thus result in a lack of oxygenated blood to parts of your body with potential consequences including stroke, gangrene, etc. Thus positive feedback can lead to the rapid loss of internal stability (homeostasis) and is therefore the source of many diseases.

You can deduce the answer to Question 12 just by having considered the events in Figure 1; however, this is one of the less common GAMSAT-style questions where having specific background knowledge is disproportionately beneficial. Later, we will explore metabolic pathways (BIO 4.4-4.10), hormones (BIO Chapter 6), positive and negative feedback (BIO 6.3.6, 6.3.7), blood clotting (BIO 7.5), etc. We will continually try to remind you not to get lost in details, like trying to commit the names and actions of each hormone to memory. Rather, it is the understanding of the big picture and key interactions which will then permit you to more quickly assess flow charts like Figure 1.

Question 13, On the Surface: The end product of the cascade, mentioned in the preamble and shown in the diagram, is fibrin which forms the blood clot. The factors are referred to as proteins in paragraph 2 of the preamble suggesting that fibrin, factor Ia, is a protein and is clearly an integral component of the 'cross-linked fibrin clot' in Figure 1. You might be tempted to believe that factor XIIIa might be part of the clot but recall from the second paragraph of the preamble: "an inactive protein enzyme precursor, and sometimes its co-factor, are altered to become active components that then **catalyse** the next reaction in the cascade."

Thus factor XIIIa, being an enzyme that catalyses the reaction that converts fibrin to a clot ('crosslinks fibrin'), like all enzymes, is not consumed by the reaction (thus does not become part of the product). Thus the protein component of the clot is mainly fibrin and we have no information about any other possible component, thus the correct answer is D.

Going Deeper: Almost all metabolic processes in the cell need enzymes in order to occur at rates fast enough to sustain life. The set of enzymes produced in a cell determines which metabolic pathways occur in that cell. Like all catalysts, enzymes increase the reaction rate by lowering the activation energy but they do not alter the equilibrium of a reaction. Some enzymes can make their conversion of substrate to product occur many millions of times faster. In practical terms, this means that reactions that would normally take years, occur in fractions of a second. Many therapeutic drugs are enzyme inhibitors which aim to correct an aberrant cellular pathway.

Question 14: According to Figure 1, Protein S appears to assist in the production of active protein C which inhibits (negative feedback, mentioned in the caption of Figure 1) the reaction that produces Va (which is a cofactor for Xa) and VIIIa (which is a cofactor for IXa that results in the production of Xa). Thus in both instances, the production of thrombin is inhibited and thus the common pathway which leads to a blood clot (*thrombosis*, alluded to in paragraph 2 in the preamble) is inhibited. And so, we can conclude that a protein S deficiency means that the common pathway is NOT blocked and therefore proceeds uninhibited. For blood, this suggests uninhibited thrombosis.

Thus the solution would be to treat the patient with something that imitates the natural role of protein S. Since we want to inhibit the common pathway, the best answer choice is B. The other answer choices promote the coagulation cascade and thus worsen the condition of blood clotting (thrombosis).

More Fun Awaits!

If you feel like you are on a roll, and you are yearning for another complex pathway flow chart, go to gamsat-prep.com and try the test GS-Free. The first unit has heaps of pathway questions. If you are an NSB candidate, try GS-Free after you have completed BIO Chapter 1 so you will have some basic background to make the unit a little easier. Despite the latter suggestion, please notice how little assumed GAMSAT Biology knowledge was necessary to answer the questions in the last few units of this Introduction.

If it is the first time that you have seen problems like the ones that you have just experienced, then of course it can be quite a challenge. But please remember: There are hundreds of practice questions in this book ranging from simple to GAMSAT level. It is probably not accurate to say 'practice makes perfect' but certainly targeted and efficient practice can help you optimise your GAMSAT score; ultimately, with the objective being to get you beyond the requirement for the medical or dental school that you wish to attend.

A Word About Your Online Access . . .

The GS Online Access has saved thousands of trees and has reduced the cost of this book to you. It is not just the hundreds of online answers and worked solutions that you get access to with your gamsat-prep.com/gamsat-biology account, it is the fact that we do not have to limit the length of our worked solutions because of printing cost restrictions. It permits this textbook to sell for less than most with the same production value, while at the same time, providing you with more detailed worked solutions than any other GAMSAT publication, ever. You will also be able to access dozens of hours of topical videos with clear teaching which help to convert a static book into a dynamic multimedia experience.

Cross-references...

Wherever possible, we will identify another chapter, section or subsection of the book where you can find more information regarding a particular topic. For the most part, each book is self-contained but there are some exceptional cases where we cross-reference between different Masters Series books. The following table contains a summary of the abbreviations used throughout the Masters Series.

Cross-references to the Masters Series books, videos, apps, etc.

Abbreviation	Subject	Theme, Book
RHSS	Reasoning in Humanities & Social Sciences	Section 1, Book 1
WC	Written Communication	Section 2, Book 2
GM	GAMSAT Maths	Physical Sciences, Book 3
PHY	Physics	Physical Sciences, Book 3
CHM	General Chemistry	Physical Sciences, Book 4
ORG	Organic Chemistry	Biological Sciences, Book 5
BIO	Biology	Biological Sciences, Book 6

For example, BIO 6.3.7 means that you will find more information by looking at your Masters Series textbook, Chapter 6 Biology, in the subsection 6.3.7. After a few chapters, you will find the system to be quite straightforward and, often, helpful.

Note: Despite the many new additions throughout this textbook, it remains 99% error-free. Should you have any doubts, join us at gamsat-prep.com/forum.

The Natural Order for the Study of Science

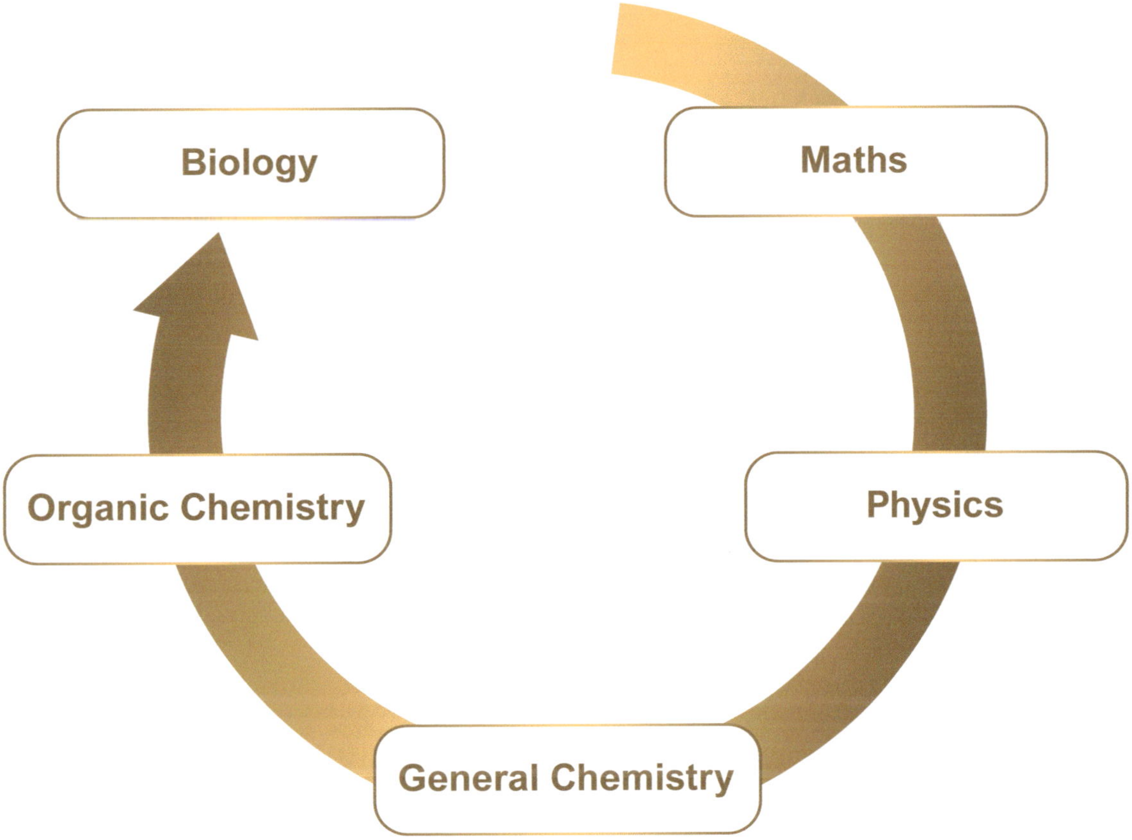

Keeping to this natural order of learning is particularly helpful for GAMSAT, since most GAMSAT Biology, General Chemistry and Physics questions have mathematics as a foundation.

The only logical reason to start your studies with GAMSAT Biology would be if you have an academic background specific to maths, physics, chemistry and/or engineering. Even if you previously sat the real GAMSAT and struggled with GAMSAT Biology, the problem is more likely attributable to an issue with GAMSAT Maths skills: Graph analysis, dimensional analysis, equation manipulation, and the assessment of tables and diagrams. If you have already laid the foundation, then you are ready to build upon those skills for the final installment of the sciences . . .

A Quote with a Dual Purpose

Here is a beauty that you can use for GAMSAT Section 2 (Written Communication) and, hopefully, it will provide some exhortation as you face the Masters Series GAMSAT Book 6!

> *Now this is not the end. It is not even the beginning of the end. But it is, perhaps, the end of the beginning.*
>
> Winston Churchill

Good luck!

- BF, MD

GAMSAT BIOLOGY

5 Sections • 16 Chapters

01 The Cell and Metabolism

Chapter 1: Generalized Eukaryotic Cell
Chapter 2: Microbiology
Chapter 3: Protein Synthesis
Chapter 4: Enzymes and Cellular Respiration

02 Systems Biology Part 1

Chapter 5: Specialized Eukaryotic Cells and Tissues
Chapter 6: Nervous and Endocrine Systems
Chapter 7: The Circulatory System
Chapter 8: The Immune System
Chapter 9: The Digestive System

03 Systems Biology Part 2

Chapter 10: The Excretory System
Chapter 11: The Musculoskeletal System
Chapter 12: The Respiratory System
Chapter 13: The Skin as an Organ System

04 Multiply and Grow

Chapter 14: Reproduction and Development

05 Genes and How Genes Change with Time

Chapter 15: Genetics
Chapter 16: Evolution

GAMSAT-prep.com

GENERALISED EUKARYOTIC CELL
Chapter 1

Memorise

* Structure/function: cell/components
* Components and function: cytoskeleton
* DNA structure and function
* Transmission of genetic information
* Mitosis, events of the cell cycle

Understand

* 1st year university level info*
* Membrane transport
* Hyper/hypotonic solutions
* Saturation kinetics: graphs
* Unique features of eukaryotes
* Basics: Cell junctions, microscopy

Importance

High level: 15% of GAMSAT Biology questions released by ACER are related to content in this chapter (in our estimation).
* Note that approximately 75% of the questions in GAMSAT Biology are related to just 7 chapters: 1, 2, 3, 4, 7, 12, and 15.

GAMSAT-Prep.com

Introduction

Cells are the basic organisational unit of living organisms. They are contained by a plasma membrane and/or cell wall. Eukaryotic cells (*eu* = true; *karyote* refers to nucleus) are cells with a true nucleus found in all multicellular and nonbacterial unicellular organisms including animal, fungal and plant cells. The nucleus contains genetic information, DNA, which can divide into 2 cells by mitosis.

Get ready to waste some time! Glad to have your attention! Our experience is that most students 'overstudy' Biology and underperform in Biology when they see the types of questions that are asked on the GAMSAT. Please do not get trapped in details. We'll guide you as much as we can but in the end, it's up to you: colour-coded table of contents, yellow highlighter, underline, foundational and GAMSAT-level practice questions at the end of the chapter, etc. For now, enjoy the story that you are expected to be exposed to for the GAMSAT, but generally the content will likely be more helpful to you in medical school.

Multimedia Resources at GAMSAT-Prep.com

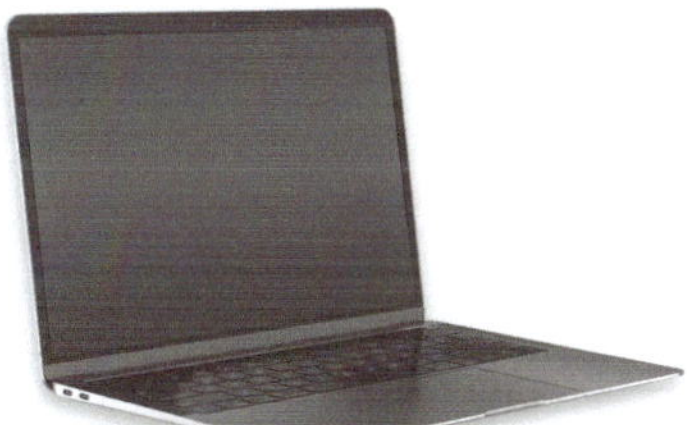

Open Discussion Boards
(*gamsat-prep.com/forum*)

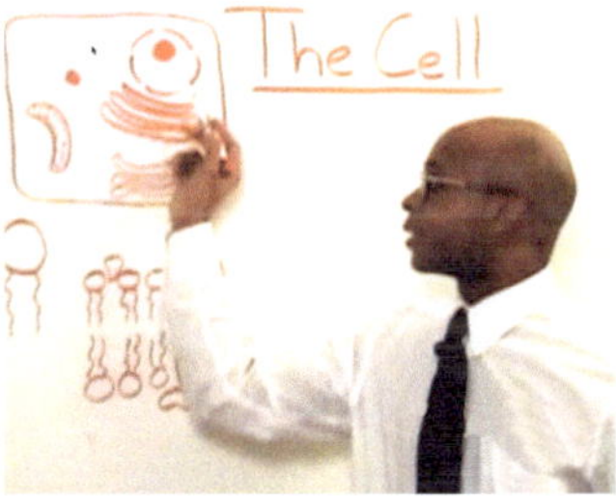

Foundational Videos

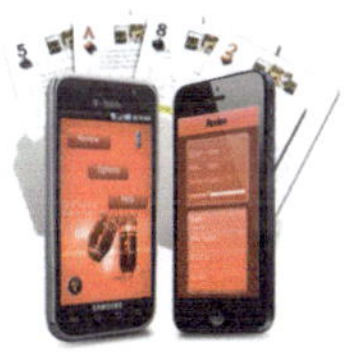

Flashcards

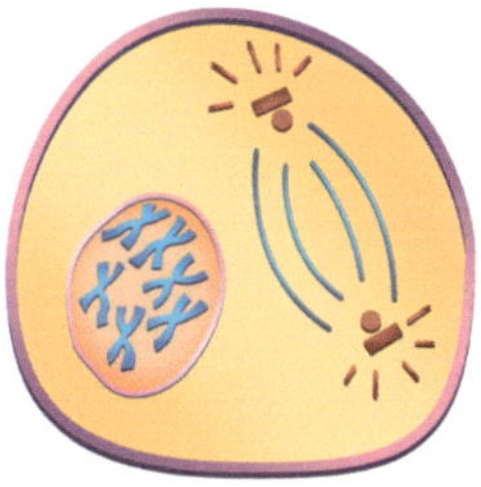

Special Guest

* The real GAMSAT may have advanced-level information presented (i.e. in a passage) but previous knowledge of said information is not required to answer the questions that would follow. Practice questions at the end of this chapter, as well as ACER and GS (HEAPS) practice GAMSATs can help you clarify this point.

1.1 Plasma Membrane: Structure and Functions

The plasma membrane is a semipermeable barrier that defines the outer perimeter of the cell. It is composed of lipids (fats) and protein. The membrane is dynamic, selective, active, and fluid. It contains phospholipids which are amphipathic molecules. They are amphipathic because their tail end contains fatty acids which are insoluble in water (*hydrophobic)*, the opposite end contains a charged phosphate head which is soluble in water (*hydrophilic*). The plasma membrane contains two layers or "leaflets" of phospholipids thus it is called a bilipid layer. Unlike eukaryotic membranes, prokaryotic membranes do not contain steroids such as cholesterol.

The Fluid Mosaic Model tells us that the hydrophilic heads project to the outside and the hydrophobic tails project towards the inside of the membrane. Further, these phospholipids are fluid - thus they move freely from place to place in the membrane. Fluidity of the membrane increases with increased temperature and with decreased saturation of fatty acyl tails. Fluidity of the membrane decreases with decreased temperature, increased saturation of fatty acyl tails and increase in the membrane's cholesterol content. The structures of these and other biological molecules were discussed in Organic Chemistry Chapter 12.

Glycolipids are limited to the extracellular aspect of the membrane or outer leaflet. The carbohydrate portion of glycolipids extends from the outer leaflet into the extracellular space and forms part of the glycocalyx. "Glycocalyx" is the sugar coat on the outer surface of the outer leaflet of plasma membrane. It consists of oligosaccharide linked to

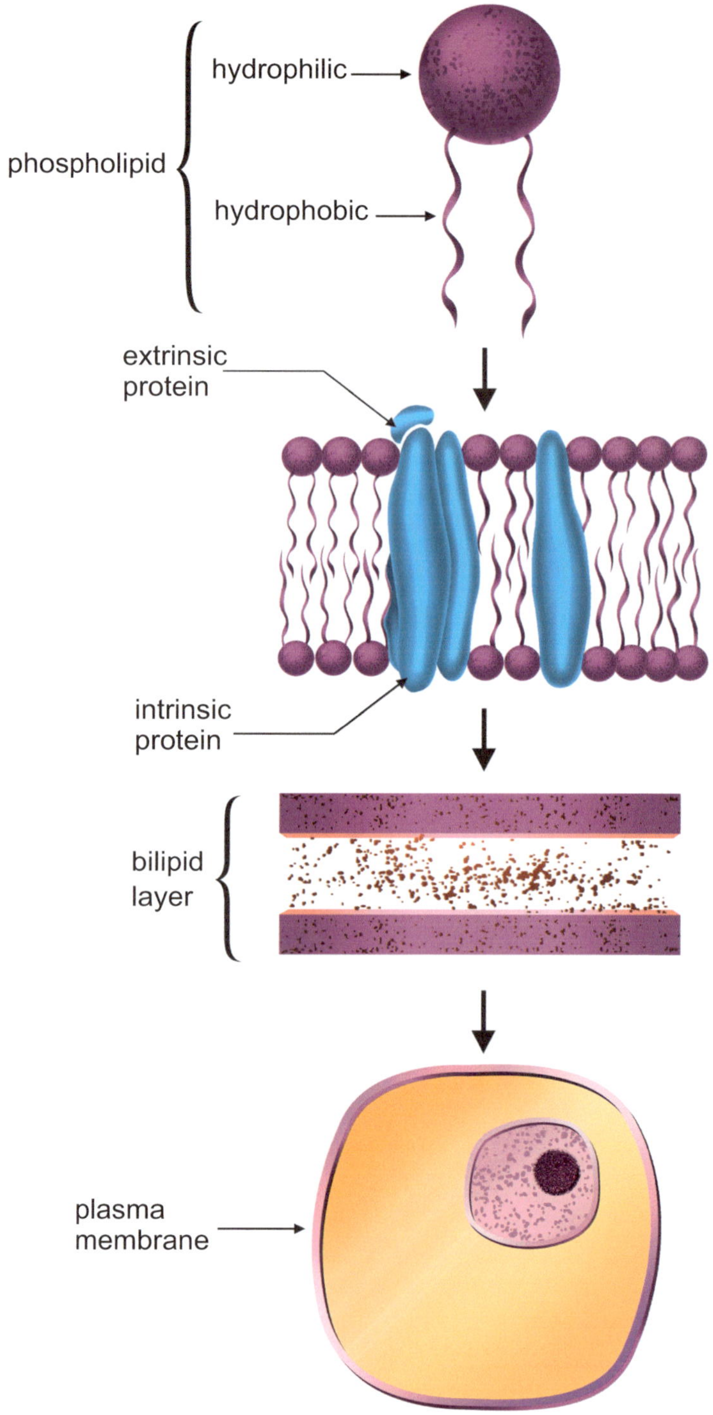

Figure IV.A.1.1: Structure of the plasma membrane. Note that: hydro = water, phobic = fearing, philic = loving

protein or lipids of the plasma membrane. The glycocalyx aids in attachment of some cells, facilitates cell recognition, helps bind antigen and antigen-presenting cells to the cell surface. Distributed throughout the membrane is a <u>mosaic</u> of proteins with limited mobility.

Proteins can be found associated with the outside of the membrane (<u>ex</u>trinsic or peripheral) or may be found spanning the membrane (<u>in</u>trinsic or integral). Integral proteins are dissolved in the lipid bilayer. Transmembrane proteins contain hydrophilic and hydrophobic amino acids and cross the entire plasma membrane. Most transmembrane proteins are glycoproteins. They usually function as membrane receptors and transport proteins.

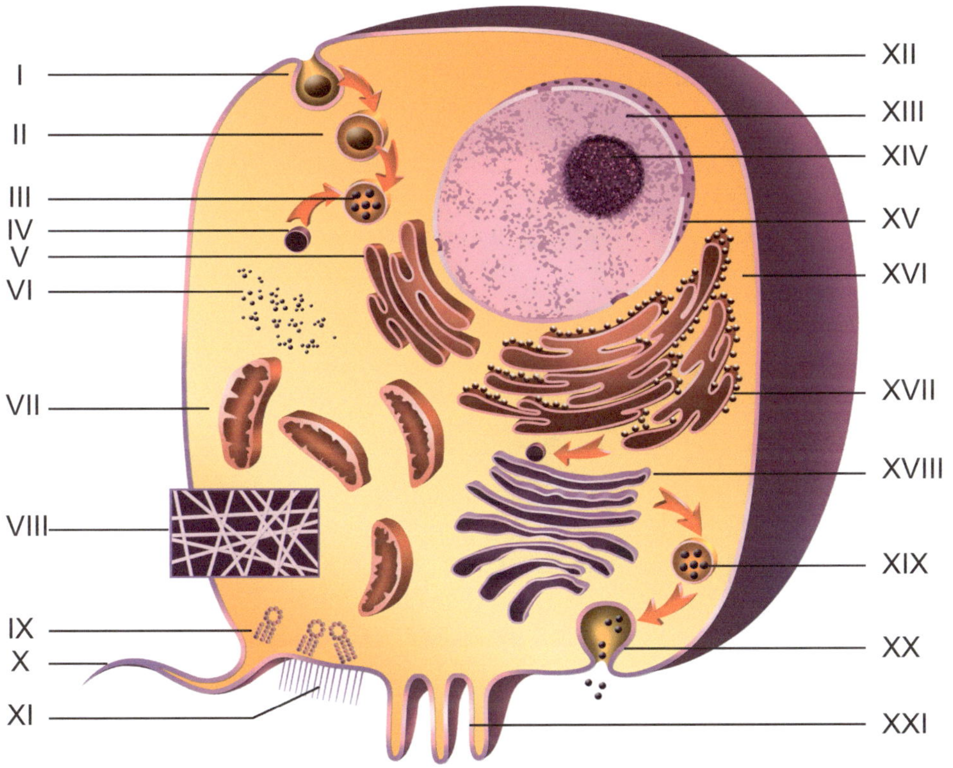

Figure IV.A.1.2: The generalised eukaryotic cell

I	endocytosis	VIII	cytoskeleton (further magnified)	XV	nuclear envelope
II	endocytotic vesicle	IX	basal body (magnified)	XVI	cytosol
III	secondary lysosome	X	flagellum	XVII	rough endoplasmic reticulum
IV	primary lysosome	XI	cilia	XVIII	Golgi apparatus
V	smooth endoplasmic reticulum	XII	plasma membrane	XIX	exocytotic vesicle
VI	free ribosomes	XIII	nucleus	XX	exocytosis
VII	mitochondrion	XIV	nucleolus	XXI	microvillus

Peripheral proteins do not extend into the lipid bilayer but can temporarily adhere to either side of the plasma membrane. They bond to phospholipid groups or integral proteins of the membrane via noncovalent interactions. Common functions include regulatory protein subunits of ion channels or transmembrane receptors, associations with the cytoskeleton and extracellular matrix, and as part of the intracellular second messenger system.

The plasma membrane is semipermeable. In other words, it is permeable to small uncharged substances which can freely diffuse across the membrane (i.e. O_2, CO_2, urea). The eukaryotic plasma membrane does not have pores, as pores would destroy the barrier function. On the other hand, it is relatively impermeable to charged or large substances which may require transport proteins to cross the membrane (i.e. ions, amino acids, sugars) or cannot cross the membrane at all (i.e. protein hormones, intracellular enzymes). Substances which can cross the membrane may do so by simple diffusion, carrier-mediated transport, or by endo/exocytosis.

1.1.1 Simple Diffusion

Simple diffusion is the spontaneous spreading of a substance going from an area of higher concentration to an area of lower concentration (i.e. a concentration gradient exists). Gradients can be of a chemical or electrical nature. A chemical gradient arises as a result of an unequal distribution of molecules and is often called a concentration gradient. In a chemical (or concentration) gradient, there is a higher concentration of molecules in one area than there is in another area, and molecules tend to diffuse from areas of high concentration to areas of lower concentration.

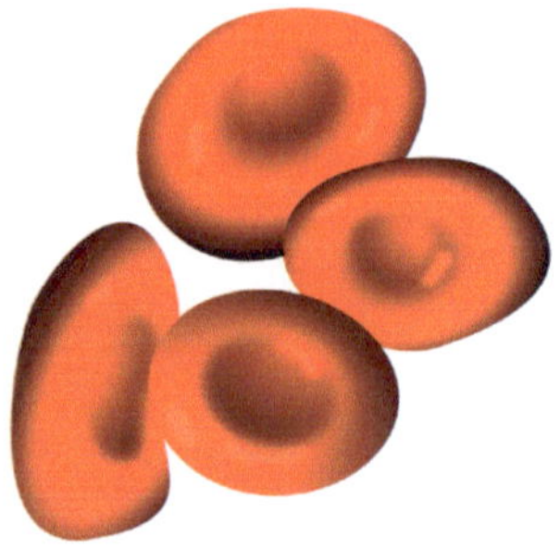

Figure IV.A.1.2.1a: Isotonic Solution.
The fluid bathing the cell (i.e. red blood cell or RBC in this case; *see* BIO 7.5) contains the same concentration of solute as the cell's inside or cytoplasm. When a cell is placed in an isotonic solution, the water diffuses into and out of the cell at the same rate.

An electrical gradient arises as a result of an unequal distribution of charge. In an electrical gradient, there is a higher concentration of charged molecules in one area than in another (this is independent of the concentration of all molecules in the area). Molecules tend to move from areas of higher concentration of charge to areas of lower concentration of charge.

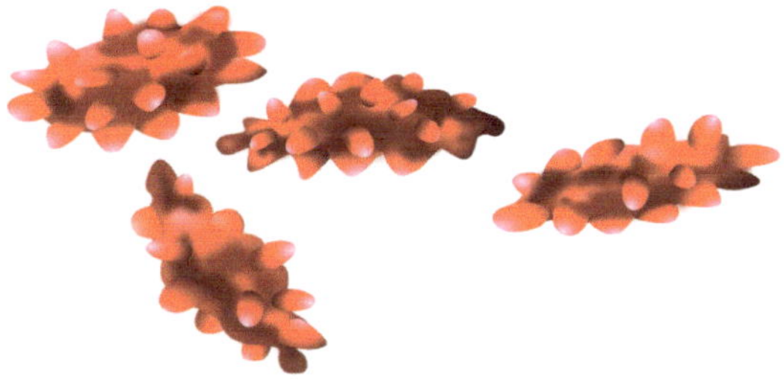

Figure IV.A.1.2.1b: Hypertonic Solution. Here the fluid bathing the RBC contains a high concentration of solute relative to the cell's cytoplasm. When a cell is placed in a hypertonic solution, the water diffuses out of the cell, causing the cell to shrivel (crenation).

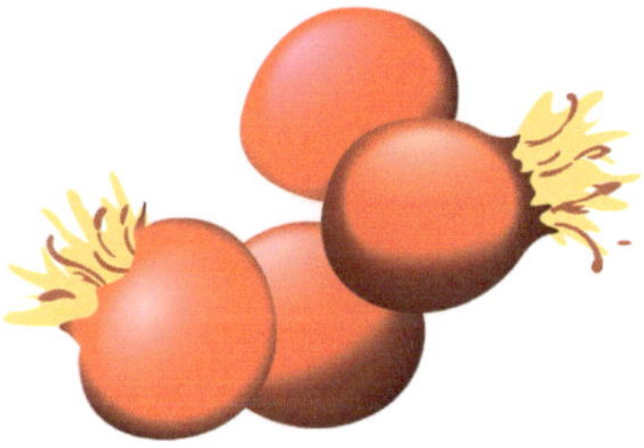

Figure IV.A.1.2.1c: Hypotonic Solution. Here the surrounding fluid has a low concentration of solute relative to the cell's cytoplasm. When a cell is placed in a hypotonic solution, the water diffuses into the cell, causing the cell to swell and possibly rupture (lyse).

Osmosis is the diffusion of water across a semipermeable membrane moving from an area of higher water concentration (i.e. lower solute concentration = hypotonic) to an area of lower water concentration (i.e. higher solute concentration = hypertonic). The hydrostatic pressure needed to oppose the movement of water is called the osmotic pressure. Thus, an isotonic solution (i.e. the concentration of solute on both sides of the membrane is equal), would have an osmotic pressure of zero.

{Memory guide: notice that the "O" in hyp-O-tonic looks like a swollen cell. The O is also a circle which makes you think of the word "around." So IF the environment is hypOtonic AROUND the cell, then fluid rushes in and the cell swells like the letter O}.

1.1.2 Carrier-mediated Transport

Amino acids, sugars and other solutes need to reversibly bind to proteins (carriers) in the membrane in order to get across. Because there are a limited amount of carriers, if the concentration of solute is too high, the carriers would be saturated, thus the rate of crossing the membrane would level off (= saturation kinetics).

The two carrier-mediated transport systems are:

(i) <u>facilitated transport</u> where the carrier helps a solute diffuse across a membrane it could not otherwise penetrate. Facilitated diffusion occurs via ion channels or carrier proteins and transport molecules down a concentration of electrochemical gradient. Ions and large molecules are therefore able to cross the membrane that would otherwise be impermeable to them.

(ii) <u>active transport</u> where energy (i.e. ATP) is used to transport solutes <u>against</u> their concentration gradients. The Na^+-K^+ exchange pump uses ATP to actively pump Na^+ to where its concentration

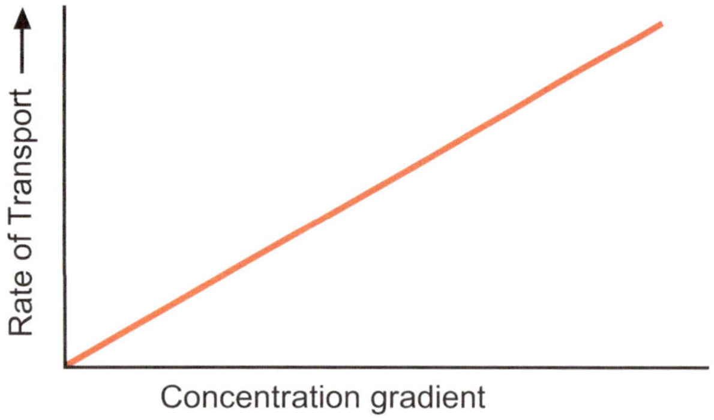

Simple Diffusion: the greater the concentration gradient, the greater the rate of transport across the plasma membrane.

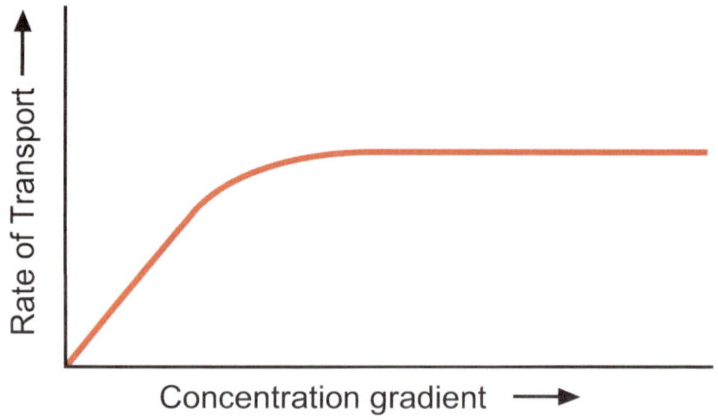

Carrier-mediated Transport: increasing the concentration gradient increases the rate of transport up to a maximum rate, at which point all membrane carriers are saturated.

Figure IV.A.1.3: Simple diffusion versus Carrier-mediated transport.

is highest (outside the cell) and K^+ is brought within the cell where its concentration is highest (*see* Neural Cells and Tissues, BIO 5.1.1).

1.1.3 Endo/Exocytosis

Endocytosis is the process by which the cell membrane actually invaginates, pinches off and is released intracellularly (endocytotic *vesicle*). If a solid particle was ingested by the cell (i.e. a bacterium), it is called *phagocytosis*. If fluid was ingested, it is *pinocytosis*.

Clathrin is a protein that plays a major role in the formation of coated vesicles. The receptor-mediated endocytosis of ligands (e.g. low density lipoprotein, growth factors, antibodies, etc.) is due to clathrin-coated vesicles (CCVs). CCVs are found in virtually all cells and form areas in the plasma membrane termed clathrin-coated pits. Caveolae are the most common reported non-clathrin-coated plasma membrane buds, which exist on the surface of many, but not all cell types. They consist of the cholesterol-binding protein caveolin with a bilayer enriched in cholesterol and glycolipids.

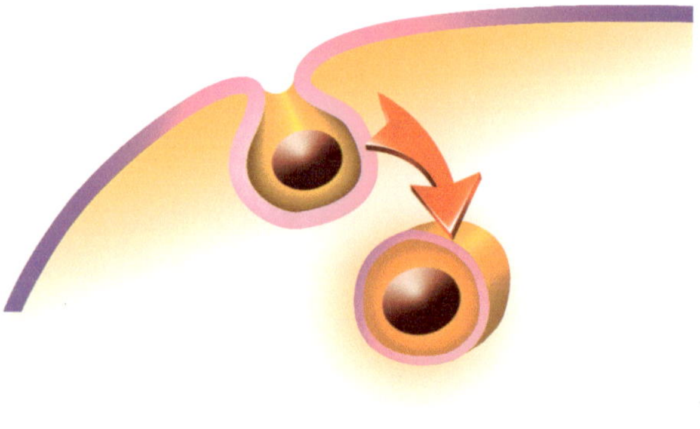

Figure IV.A.1.4: Endocytosis.

Exocytosis is, essentially, the reverse process. The cell directs an intracellular vesicle to fuse with the plasma membrane thus releasing its contents to the exterior (i.e. neurotransmitters, pancreatic enzymes, cell membrane proteins/lipids, etc.).

The transient vesicle fusion with the cell membrane forms a structure shaped like a pore (= *porosome*). Thus porosomes are cup-shaped structures where vesicles dock in the process of fusion and secretion. Porosomes contain many different types of protein including chloride and calcium channels, actin, and SNARE proteins that mediate the docking and fusion of vesicles with the cell membrane. The primary role of SNARE proteins is to mediate vesicle fusion through full fusion exocytosis or open and close

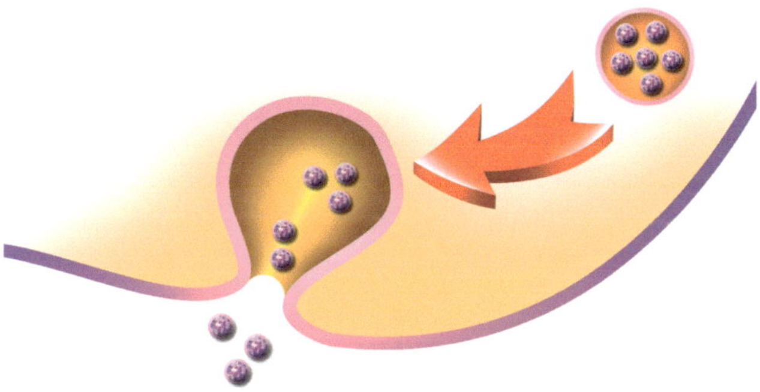

Figure IV.A.1.5: Exocytosis.

exocytosis. The former is where the vesicle collapses fully into the plasma membrane; in the latter, the vesicle docks transiently with the membrane (= “kiss-and-run”) and is recycled (i.e. in the synaptic terminal; BIO 1.5.1, 5.1).

1.2 The Interior of a Eukaryotic Cell

Cytoplasm is the interior of the cell. It refers to all cell components enclosed by the cell's membrane which includes the cytosol, the cytoskeleton, and the membrane bound organelles. Transport within the cytoplasm occurs by cyclosis (circular motion of cytoplasm around the cell).

Cytosol is the solution which bathes the organelles and contains numerous solutes like amino acids, sugars, proteins, etc.

Cytoskeleton extends throughout the entire cell and has particular importance in shape and intracellular transportation. The cytoskeleton also makes extracellular complexes with other proteins forming a matrix so that cells can "stick" together. This is called cellular adhesion.

The components of the cytoskeleton in increasing order of size are: microfilaments, intermediate filaments, and microtubules. Microfilaments are important for cell movement and contraction (i.e. actin and myosin. *See* Contractile Cells and Tissues, BIO 5.2). Microfilaments, also known as actin filaments, are composed of actin monomer (G actin) linked into a double helix. They display polarity (= having distinct and opposite poles), with polymerisation and depolymerisation occuring preferentially at the barbed end [also called the plus (+) end which is where ATP is bound to G actin; BIO 5.2]. Microfilaments squeeze the membrane together in phagocytosis and cytokinesis. They are also important for muscle contraction and microvilli movement.

High-level Importance

Intermediate filaments and microtubules extend along axons and dendrites of neurons acting like railroad tracks, so organelles or protein particles can shuttle to or from the cell body. Microtubules also form:

(i) the core of cilia and flagella (*see* the 9 doublet + 2 structure in BIO 1.5);
(ii) the mitotic spindles which we shall soon discuss; and
(iii) centrioles.

A flagellum is an organelle of locomotion found in sperm and bacteria. Eukaryotic flagella are made from microtubule configurations while prokaryotic flagella are thin strands of a single protein called flagellin. Thus, eukaryotic flagella move in a whip-like motion while prokaryotic flagella rotate. Cilia are hair-like vibrating organelles which can be used to move particles along the surface of the cell (e.g., in the fallopian tubes cilia can help the egg move toward the uterus). Microtubules are composed of tubulin subunits. They display polarity, with polymerisation and depolymerisation occuring preferentially at the plus end where GTP is bound to the tubulin subunit. Microtubules are involved in flagella and cilia construction, and the spindle apparatus. Centrioles are cylinder-shaped complexes of microtubules associated with the mitotic spindle (MTOC, *see* later). At the base of flagella and cilia, two centrioles can be found at right angles to each other: this is called a basal body.

A pseudopod (i.e. pseudopodium) is a *temporary* arm-like projection of a eukaryotic plasma membrane involved in movement and ingestion. Filled with cytoplasm, pseudopodia primarily consist of actin filaments, as well as microtubules and intermediate filaments.

Microvilli are regularly arranged finger-like projections with a core of cytoplasm (*see* BIO 9.5). They are commonly found in the small intestine where they help to increase the absorptive and digestive surfaces (= brush border).

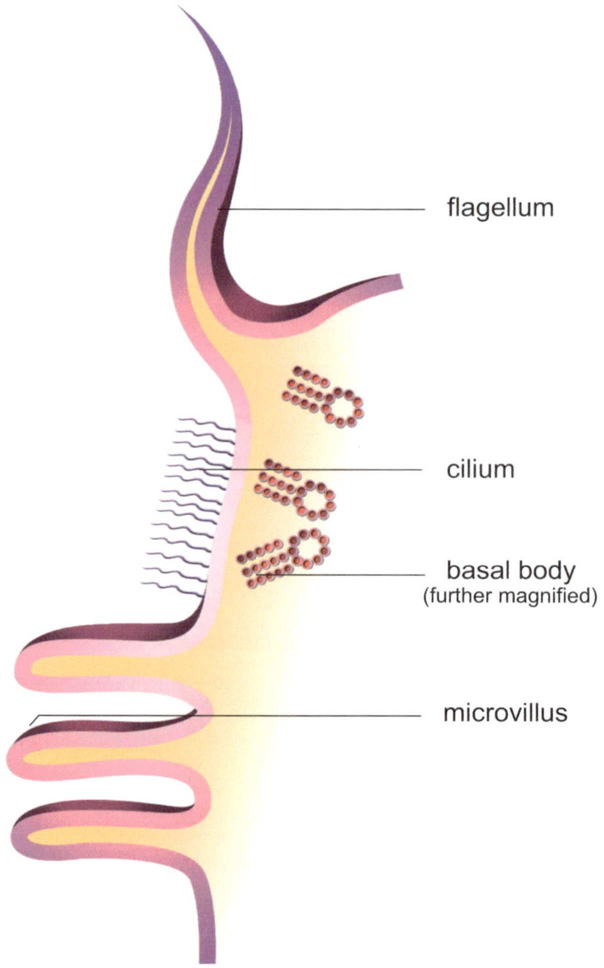

Figure IV.A.1.6: Cytoskeletal elements and the plasma membrane. The core of cilia and flagella is composed of 9 doublet or pairs of microtubules with another *doublet* in the centre (= *axoneme*; *see* BIO 1.5).

Mitochondrion: The Power House

Mitochondria produce most of the chemical energy for the cell - stored in the molecule ATP - via aerobic respiration (BIO 4.4). It is a double-membraned organelle whose inner membrane has shelf-like folds which are called *cristae*. The matrix, the fluid within the inner membrane, contains the enzymes for the Krebs cycle (BIO 4.7) and circular DNA. The latter is the only cellular DNA found outside of the nucleus with the exception of chloroplasts (= the organelle capable of photosynthesis, the conversion of light into chemical energy, in plant cells). There are numerous mitochondria in muscle cells. The Krebs cycle can oxidise glucose, amino acids or fatty acids. Using the enzyme ATP *synthase*, mitochondria *synthesise* ATP ('high energy') from ADP and inorganic phosphate (BIO 4.7, 4.8, 4.9).

Mitochondria have their own DNA and ribosomes and replicate independently from eukaryotic cells. However, most proteins used in mitochondria are coded by nuclear DNA, not mitochondrial DNA (mtDNA). In most species, including humans, mtDNA is inherited solely from the mother (BIO 15.6.1).

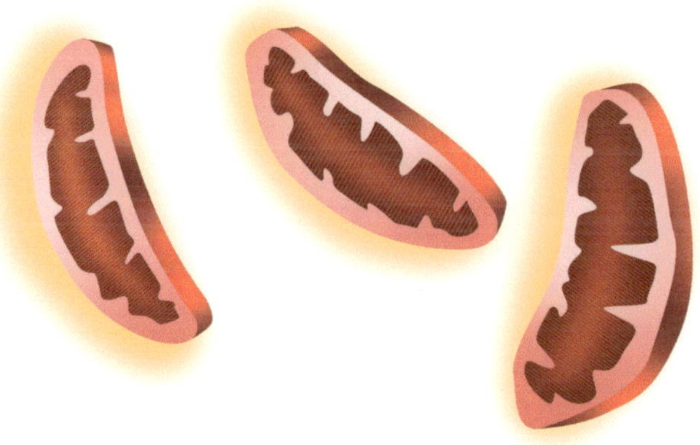

Figure IV.A.1.7: Mitochondria.

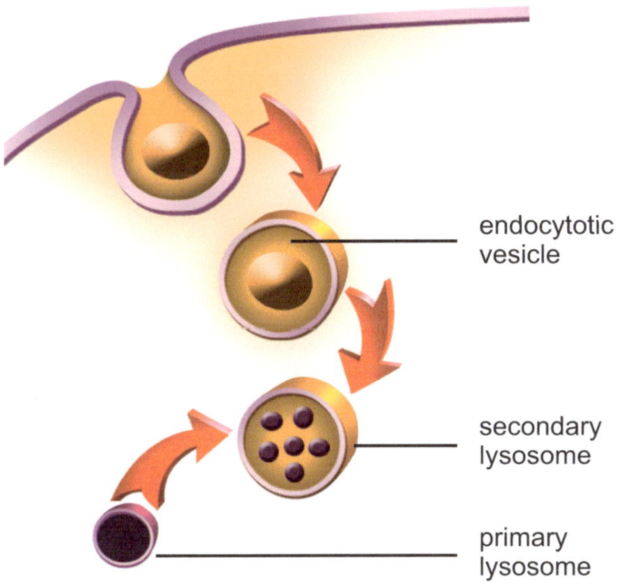

Figure IV.A.1.8: Heterolysis.

Lysosomes: Suicide Sacs

In a diseased cell, lysosomes may release their powerful acid hydrolases to digest away the cell (autolysis). In normal cells, a primary (normal) lysosome can fuse with an endocytotic vesicle to form a secondary lysosome where the phagocytosed particle (i.e. a bacterium) can be digested. This is called heterolysis. There are numerous lysosomes in phagocytic cells of the immune system (i.e. macrophages, neutrophils; BIO 7.5).

Endoplasmic Reticulum: Synthesis Centre

The endoplasmic reticulum (ER) is an interconnected membraned system resembling flattened sacs and extends from the cell membrane to the nuclear membrane.

High-level Importance

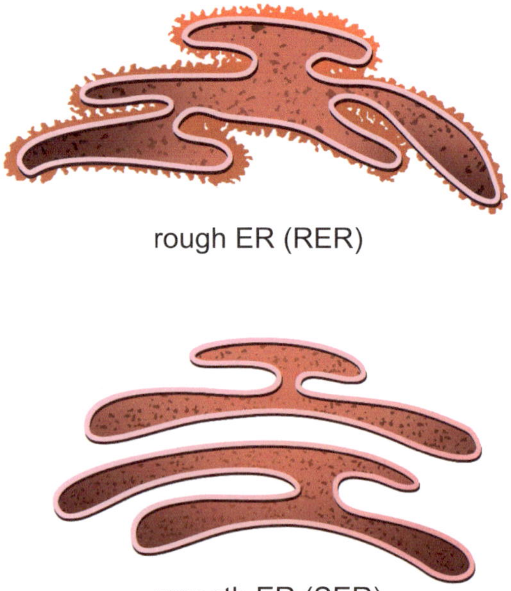

Figure IV.A.1.9: The endoplasmic reticulum.

There are two kinds: **(i)** dotted with ribosomes on its surface which is called rough ER and **(ii)** without ribosomes which is smooth ER.

The ribosomes are composed of ribosomal RNA (rRNA) and numerous proteins. It may exist freely in the cytosol or bound to the rough ER or outer nuclear membrane. The ribosome is a site where mRNA is translated into protein.

Rough ER is important in protein synthesis and is abundant in cells synthesising secretory proteins. It is associated with the synthesis of secretory protein, plasma membrane protein, and lysosomal protein. Smooth ER is abundant in cells synthesising steroids, triglycerides and cholesterol. It is associated with the synthesis and transport of lipids such as steroid hormone and detoxification of a variety of chemicals. It is also common in skeletal muscle cells involving muscle contraction and relaxation. It is a factor in phospholipid and fatty acid synthesis and metabolism.

Golgi Apparatus: The Export Department

The Golgi apparatus forms a stack of smooth membranous sacs or *cisternae* that function in protein modification, such as the addition of polysaccharides (i.e. glycosylation). The Golgi also packages secretory proteins in membrane bound vesicles which can be exocytosed.

The Golgi apparatus has a distinct polarity with one end being the "cis" face and the other being "trans". The cis face lies close to a separate vesicular-tubular cluster (VTC) also referred to as the ER-Golgi intermediate compartment (ERGIC) which is an organelle. The ERGIC mediates trafficking between the ER and Golgi complex, facilitating the sorting of 'cargo'. The medial (middle) compartment of the Golgi lies between the cis and trans faces.

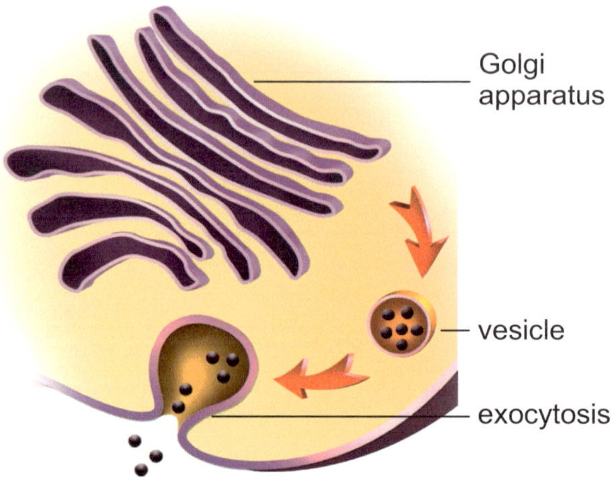

Figure IV.A.1.10: Golgi apparatus.

The trans face is oriented towards vacuoles and secretory granules. The trans Golgi network separates from the trans face and sorts proteins for their final destination.

An abundant amount of RER and Golgi is found in cells which produce and secrete protein. For example, *B-cells* of the immune system which secrete antibodies, *acinar cells* in the pancreas which secrete digestive enzymes into the intestines, and *goblet cells* of the intestine which secrete mucus into the lumen.

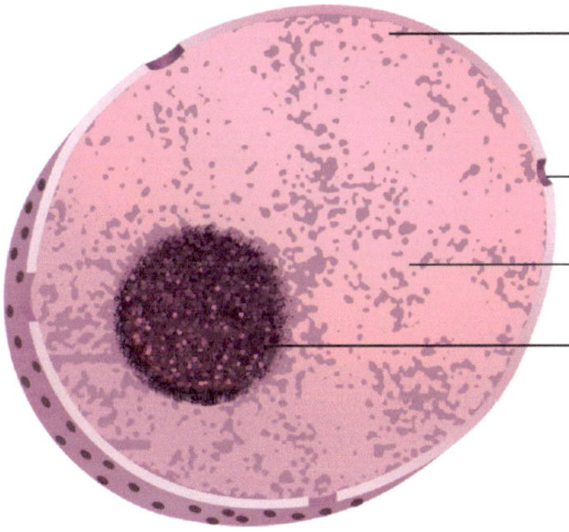

Figure IV.A.1.11: The nucleus.

Peroxisomes (Microbodies)

Peroxisomes are membrane bound organelles that contain enzymes whose functions include oxidative deamination of amino acids, oxidation of long chain fatty acids and synthesis of cholesterol.

The name "*perox*isome" comes from the fact that it is an organelle with enzymes that can transfer hydrogen from various substrates to oxygen, producing and then degrading hydrogen *perox*ide (H_2O_2).

The Nucleus

The nucleus is surrounded by a double membrane called the nuclear envelope. Throughout the membrane are nuclear pores which selectively allow the transportation of large particles to and from the nucleus. The nucleus is responsible for protein synthesis in the cytoplasm via ribosomal RNA (rRNA), messenger RNA (mRNA), and transfer RNA (tRNA).

DNA can be found within the nucleus as chromatin (DNA complexed to proteins like *histones*) or as chromosomes which are more clearly visible in a light microscope. The nucleolus is not membrane bound. It contains mostly ribosomal RNA and protein as well as the DNA necessary to synthesise ribosomal RNA.

The nucleolus is associated with the synthesis of ribosomal RNA (rRNA) and its assembly into ribosome precursors.

Chromosomes are basically extensively folded chromatin maintained by histone proteins. Each chromosome is composed of DNA and associated proteins, forming a nucleosome, the basic structural unit of chromatin. Chromatin exists as heterochromatin and euchromatin. Heterochromatin is a transcriptionally inactive form of chromatin while euchromatin is a transcriptionally active form of chromatin. Chromatin is responsible for RNA synthesis.

High-level Importance

1.2.2 DNA: The Cell's Architect

High-level Importance

Deoxyribonucleic acid (DNA) and ribonucleic acid (RNA) are essential components in constructing the proteins which act as the cytoskeleton, enzymes, membrane channels, antibodies, etc. It is the DNA which contains the genetic information of the cell.

DNA and RNA are both important nucleic acids. Nucleotides are the subunits which attach in sequence or in other words polymerise via phosphodiester bonds to form nucleic acids. A nucleotide (also called a *nucleoside phosphate*) is composed of a five-carbon sugar (*pentose*), a nitrogen base, and an inorganic phosphate.

The sugar in RNA is ribose but for DNA an oxygen atom is missing in the second position of the sugar thus it is 2-deoxyribose.

There are two categories of nitrogen bases: *purines* and *pyrimidines*. The purines have two rings and include adenine (A) and guanine (G). The pyrimidines contain one ring and include thymine (T), cytosine (C), and uracil (U).

DNA contains the following four bases: adenine, guanine, thymine, and cytosine. RNA contains the same bases except uracil is substituted for thymine.

Watson and Crick's model of DNA has allowed us to get insight into what takes shape as the nucleotides polymerise to form this special nucleic acid. The result is a double *helical* or *stranded* structure.

The DNA double helix is composed of two complementary and anti-parallel DNA strands held together by hydrogen bonds between base pairing A-T and G-C.

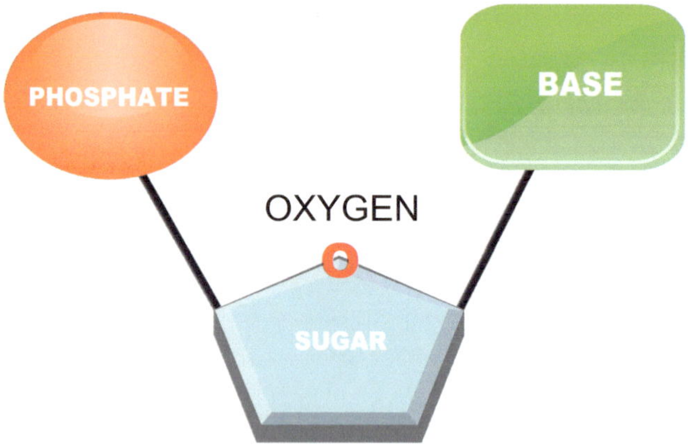

Figure IV.A.1.12a: A nucleotide: schematic. Details in Organic Chemistry Chapter 12.

DNA is made from deoxyribose while RNA is made from ribose. DNA is double stranded while RNA is single stranded. DNA contains thymine while RNA contains uracil.

The backbone of each helix is the 2-deoxyribose phosphates. The nitrogen bases project to the centre of the double helix in order to hydrogen bond with each other (imagine the double helix as a winding staircase: each stair would represent a pair of bases binding to keep the shape of the double helix intact).

There is specificity in the binding of the bases: one purine binds one pyrimidine. In fact, adenine only binds thymine (through two hydrogen bonds) and guanine only binds cytosine (through three hydrogen bonds). The more the H-bonds (i.e. the more G-C), the more stable the helix will be.

The *replication* (duplication) of DNA is semi-conservative: each strand of the double helix can serve as a template to generate a complementary strand. Thus for each

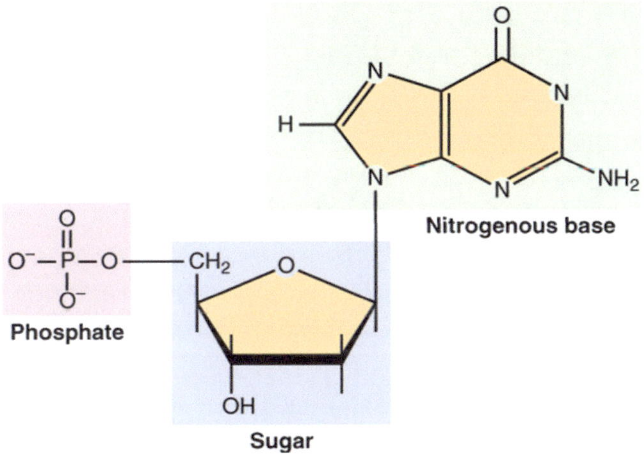

Figure IV.A.1.12b: A nucleotide: basic molecular structure.

double helix there is one parent strand (*old*) and one daughter strand (*new*). The latter is synthesised using one nucleotide at a time, enzymes including DNA polymerase, and the parent strand as a template. The preceding is termed "DNA S̲ynthesis" and occurs in the S̲ stage of interphase during the cell cycle.

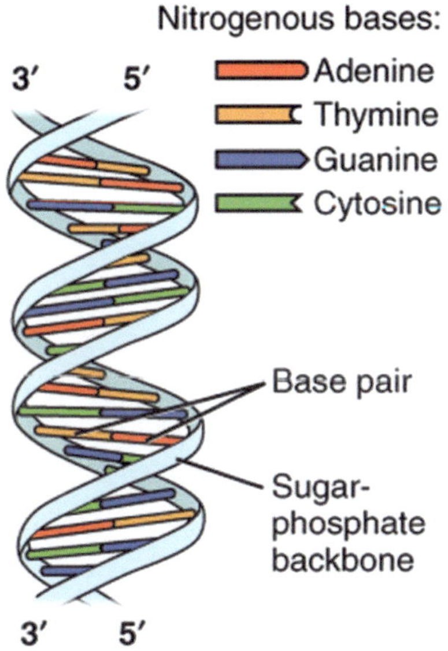

Figure IV.A.1.12d: Antiparallel DNA.

Each nucleotide has a hydroxyl or phosphate group at the 3rd and 5th carbons designated the 3′ and 5′ positions (*see* ORG 12.3.2, 12.5). Phosphodiester bonds can be formed between a free 3′ hydroxyl group and a free 5′

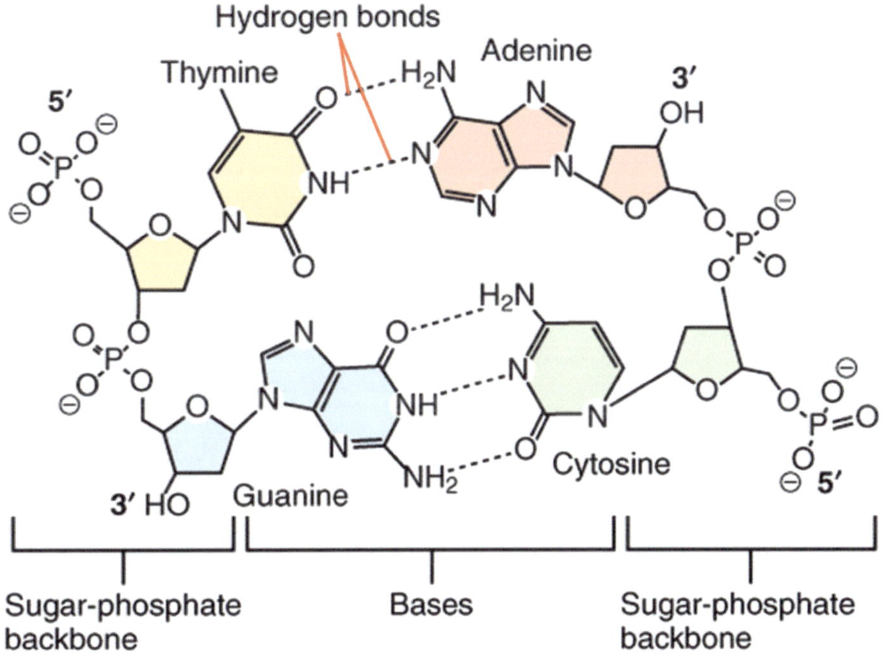

Figure IV.A.1.12c: Nucleotides join together: T and G on the left are bound by a phosphate group (*phosphodiester bond*), and likewise A and C on the right. Left and right molecules are bound by H-bonds: famously, A:T, G:C. Note that the 2 molecules lie parallel to each other, but one orientation is 5′ to 3′, and the other is 3′ to 5′: thus *antiparallel*.

High-level Importance

phosphate group. Thus the DNA strand has *polarity* since one end of the molecule will have a free 3′ hydroxyl while the other terminal nucleotide will have a free 5′ phosphate group. Polymerisation of the two strands occurs in opposite directions (= *antiparallel*). In other words, one strand runs in the 5′ - 3′ direction, while its partner runs in the 3′ - 5′ direction.

DNA replication is semi-discontinuous. DNA polymerase can only synthesise DNA in the 5′ to 3′ direction. As a result of the antiparallel nature of DNA, the 5′ - 3′ strand is replicated continuously (the *leading strand*), while the 3′ - 5′ strand is replicated discontinuously (the *lagging strand*) in the reverse direction. The short, newly synthesised DNA fragments that are formed on the lagging strand are called *Okazaki fragments*. DNA synthesis begins at a specific site called the replication origin (*replicon*) and proceeds in both directions. Eukaryotic chromosomes contain multiple origins while prokaryotic chromosomes contain a single origin. The parental strand is always read in the 3′ - 5′ direction and the daughter strand is always synthesised in the 5′ - 3′ direction.

Previous knowledge of recombinant DNA techniques, restriction enzymes, hybridisation, DNA repair mechanisms, etc., is not normally required for the GAMSAT. However, because

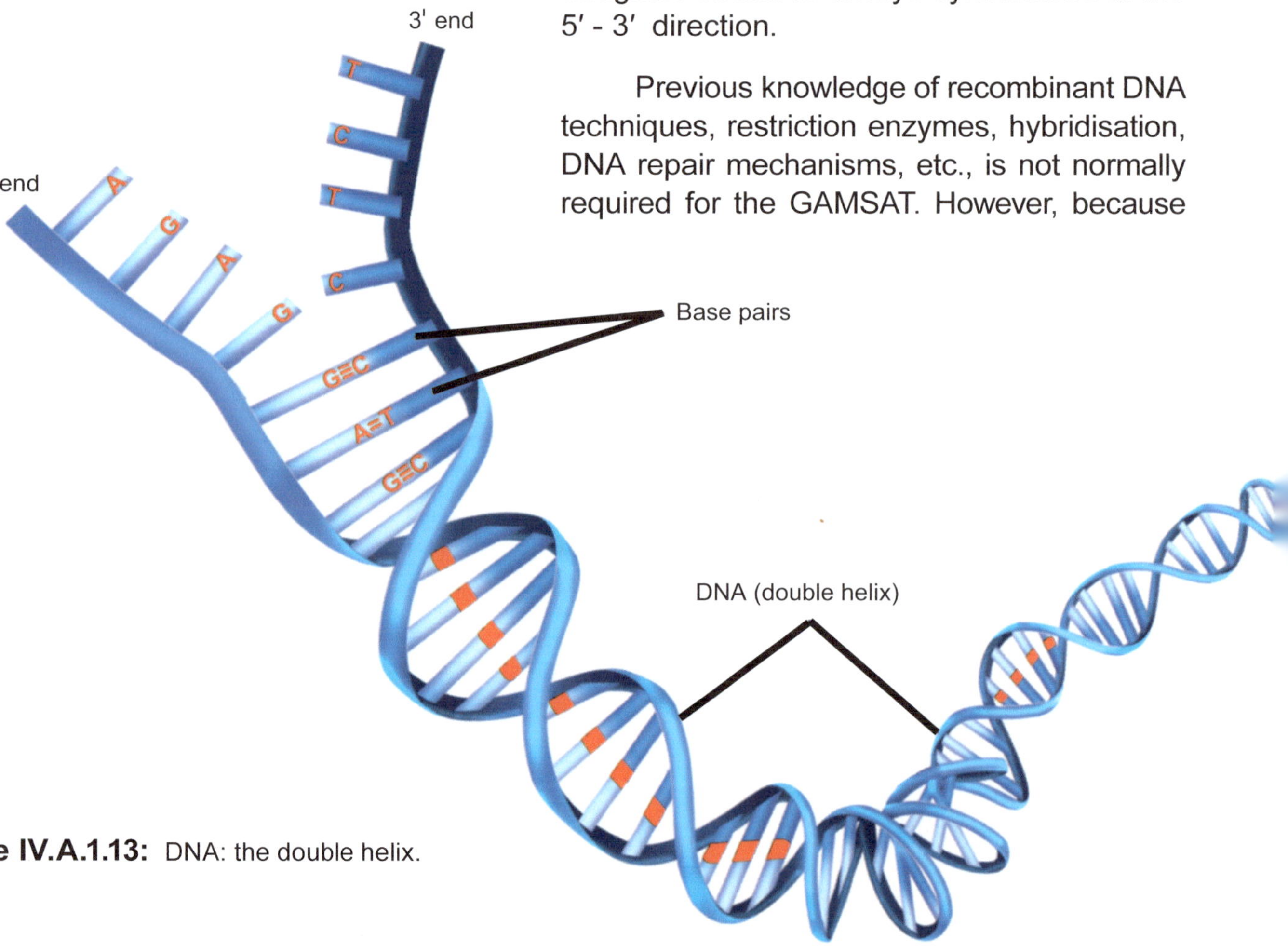

Figure IV.A.1.13: DNA: the double helix.

these topics do occasionally show up on the exam, they are discussed here and in BIO 2.2.1 and BIO 15.7. The following is an overview regarding DNA repair.

Because of environmental factors including chemicals and UV radiation, any one of the trillions of cells in our bodies may undergo as many as 1 million individual molecular "injuries" per day. Structural damage to DNA may result and could have many effects such as inducing mutation. Thus our DNA repair system is constantly active as it responds to damage in DNA structure.

A cell that has accumulated a large amount of DNA damage, or one that no longer effectively repairs damage to its DNA, can: **(1)** become permanently dormant; **(2)** exhibit unregulated cell division which could lead to cancer; **(3)** succumb to cell suicide, also known as *apoptosis* or programmed cell death.

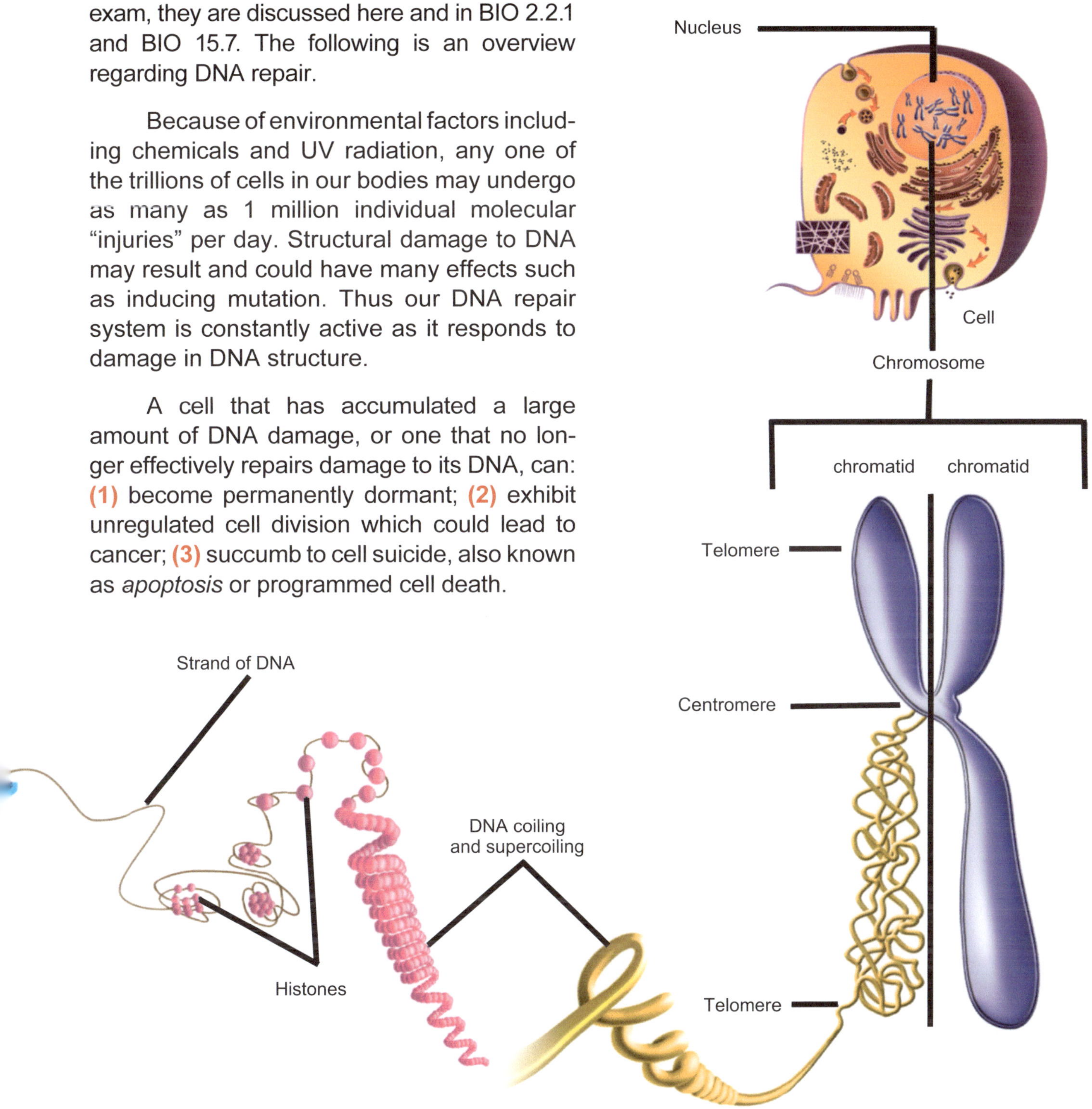

1.3 The Cell Cycle

High-level Importance

The cell cycle is a period of approximately 18 - 22 hours during which the cell can synthesise new DNA and partition the DNA equally; thus the cell can divide. Mitosis involves nuclear division (*karyokinesis*) which is usually followed by cell division (*cytokinesis*). Mitosis and cytokinesis together define the mitotic (M) phase of the cell cycle - the division of the mother cell into two daughter cells, genetically identical to each other and to their parent cell. The cell cycle is divided into a number of phases: interphase (G_1, S, G_2) and mitosis (prophase, metaphase, anaphase and telophase).

The cell cycle is temporarily suspended in resting cells. These cells stay in the G_0 state but may reenter the cell cycle and start to divide again. The cell cycle is permanently suspended in non-dividing differentiated cells such as cardiac muscle cells.

Interphase occupies about 90% of the cell cycle. During interphase, the cell prepares for DNA synthesis (G_1), synthesises or replicates DNA (S) resulting in duplication of chromosomes, and ultimately begins preparing for mitosis (G_2). During interphase, the DNA is not folded and the individual chromosomes are not visible. Also, centrioles grow to maturity; RNA and protein for mitosis are synthesised. Mitosis begins with prophase.

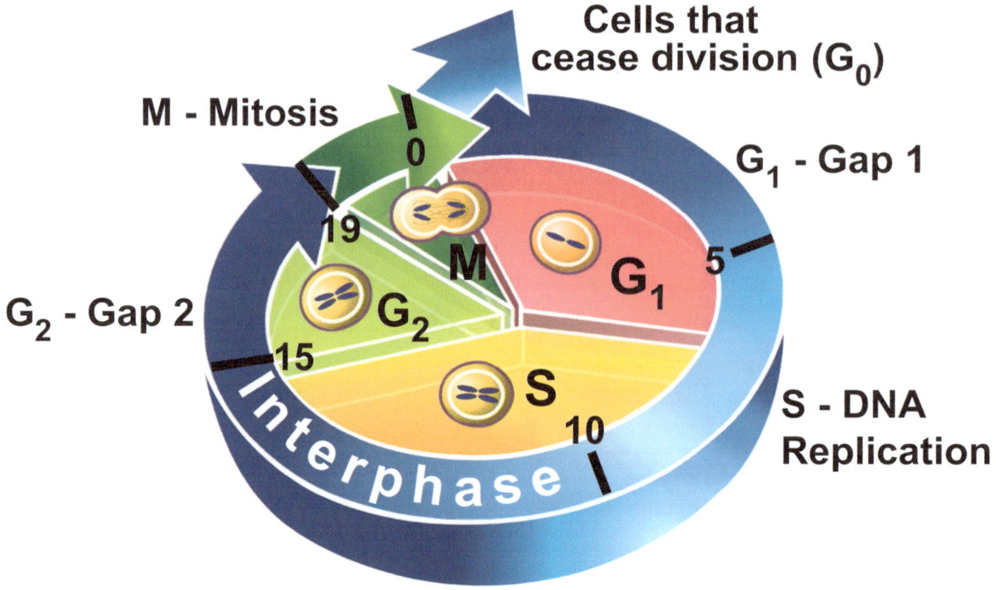

Figure IV.A.1.14: The cell cycle.
The numbers represent time in hours. Note how mitosis (M) represents the shortest period of the cycle.

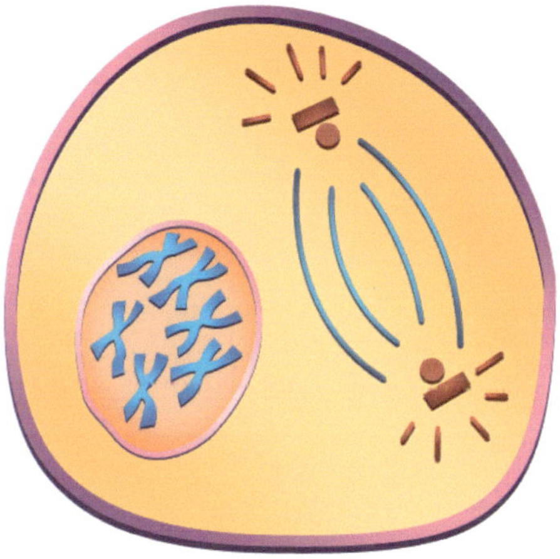

Figure IV.A.1.15: Prophase.

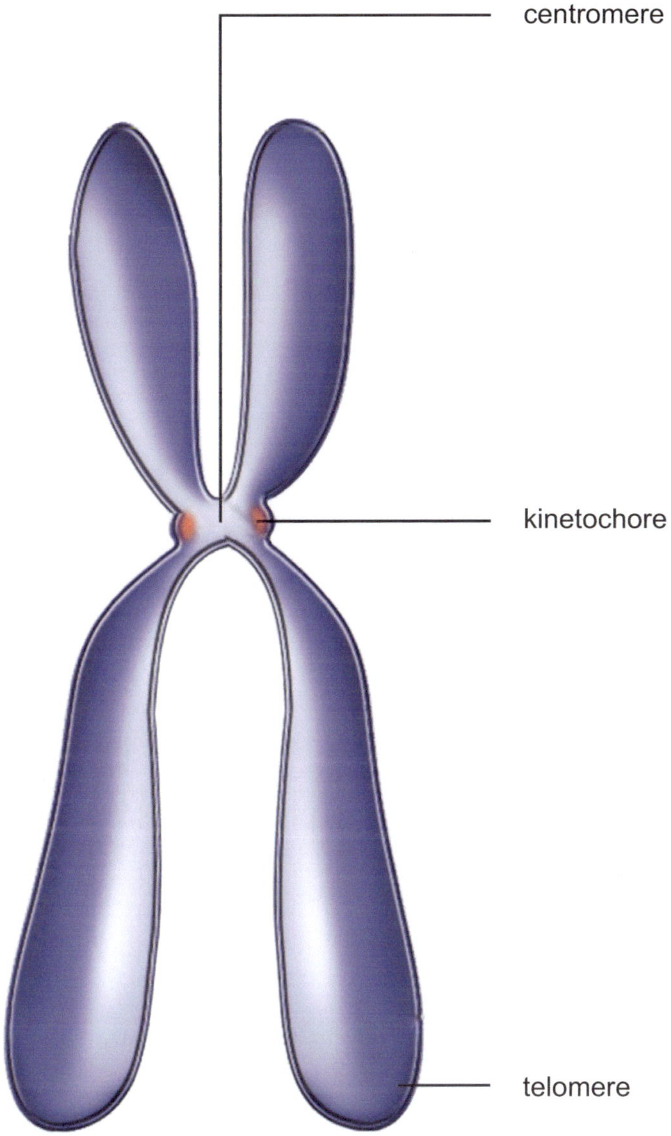

Figure IV.A.1.16: Chromosome Anatomy. Each chromosome has two arms separated by the centromere, labeled p (the shorter, named for 'petit' meaning 'small') and q (the longer of the two). The telomeres contain repetitive nucleotide sequences which protect the end of the chromosome. Over time, due to each cell division, the telomeres become shorter.

Prophase: pairs of centrioles migrate away from each other while microtubules appear in between forming a spindle. Other microtubules emanating from the centrioles give a radiating star-like appearance; thus they are called asters. Therefore, centrioles form the core of the Microtubule Organising Centres (MTOC). The MTOC is a structure found in eukaryotic cells from which microtubules emerge and associate with the protein tubulin.

Simultaneously, the diffuse nuclear chromatin condenses into the visible chromosomes which consist of two sister chromatids - each being identical copies of each other. Each chromatid consists of a complete double stranded DNA helix. The area of constriction where the two chromatids are attached is the *centromere*. Kinetochores develop at the centromere region and function as MTOC. Just as centromere refers to the centre, *telomere* refers to the ends of the chromosome (note: as cells divide and we age, telomeres progressively shorten). Ultimately, the nuclear envelope disappears at the end of prophase.

High-level Importance

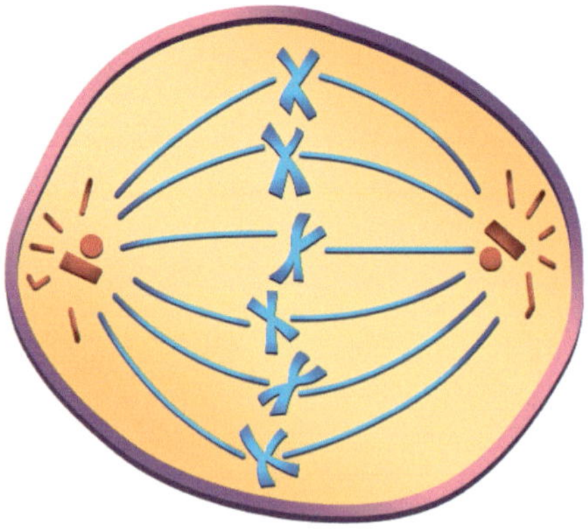

Figure IV.A.1.17: Metaphase.

<u>Metaphase</u>: centromeres line up along the equatorial plate. At or near the centromeres are the *kinetochores* which are proteins that face the spindle poles (asters). Microtubules, from the spindle, attach to the kinetochores of each chromosome.

<u>Anaphase</u>: sister chromatids are pulled apart such that each migrates to opposite poles being guided by spindle microtubules. At the end of anaphase, a cleavage furrow forms around the cell due to contraction of actin filaments called the contractile ring.

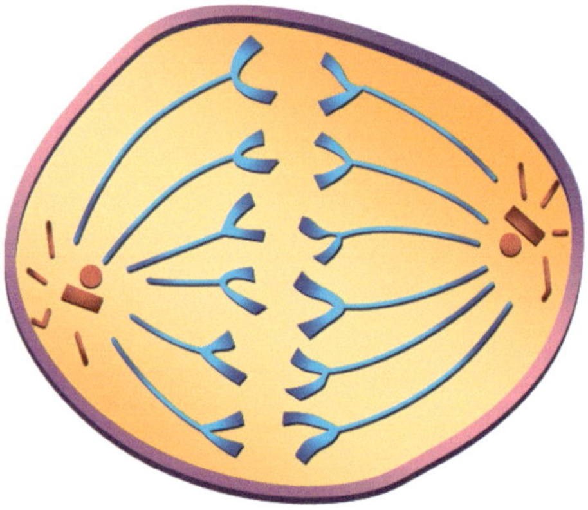

Figure IV.A.1.18: Anaphase.

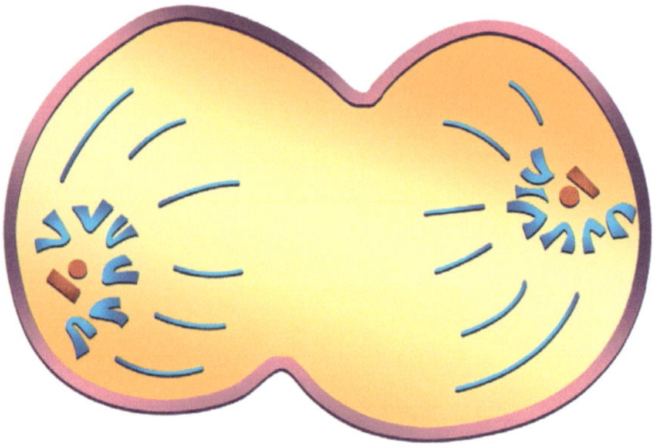

Figure IV.A.1.19: Telophase.

<u>Telophase</u>: new membranes form around the daughter nuclei; nucleoli reappear; the chromosomes uncoil and become less distinct (decondense). At the end of telophase, the cleavage furrow becomes deepened, facilitating the division of cytoplasm into two new daughter cells - each with a nucleus and organelles.

Finally, *cytokinesis* (cell separation) occurs. The cell cycle continues with the next interphase. {Mnemonic for the sequence of phases: P. MATI}

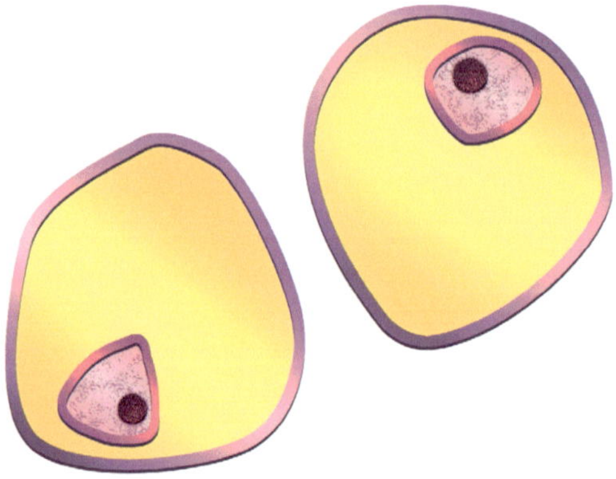

Figure IV.A.1.20: Interphase.

1.4 Cell Junctions

Multicellular organisms (i.e. animals) have cell junctions or intercellular bridges. They are especially abundant in epithelial tissues and serve as points of contact between cells and/or the extracellular matrix (BIO 4.3, 4.4). The multiprotein complex that comprise cell junctions can also build up the barrier around epithelial cells (*paracellular*) and control paracellular transport.

The molecules responsible for creating cell junctions include various cell adhesion molecules (CAMs). CAMs help cells stick to each other and to their surroundings. There are four main types: selectins, cadherins, integrins, and the immunoglobulin superfamily.

You are expected to have been exposed to these topics but please do not try to memorise details: BIO 1.4.1, 1.5, 1.5.1.

1.4.1 Types of Cell Junctions

There are three major types of cell junctions in vertebrates:

1. **Anchoring junctions**: (note: "adherens" means "to adhere to"): **(i)** Adherens junctions, AKA "belt desmosome" because they can appear as bands encircling the cell (= zonula adherens); they link to the actin cytoskeleton; **(ii)** desmosomes, AKA macula (= "spot") adherens analogous to spot welding. Desmosomes include cell adhesion proteins like cadherins which can bind intermediate filaments and provide mechanical support and stability; and **(iii)** hemidesmosomes ("hemi" = "half"), whereas desmosomes link two cells together, hemidesmosomes attach one cell to the extracellular matrix (usually anchoring the 'bottom' or basal aspect of the epithelial cell or keratinocyte to the basement membrane; *see* Fig. IV.A.1.21 and BIO 5.3).
2. **Communicating junctions**: Gap junctions which are narrow tunnels which allow the free passage of small molecules and ions. One gap junction channel is composed of two connexons (or hemichannels) which connect across the intercellular space.
3. **Occluding junctions**: Tight junctions, AKA zonula occludens, as suggested by the name, are a junctional complex that join together forming a virtually impermeable barrier to fluid. These associate with different peripheral membrane proteins located on the intracellular side of the plasma membrane which anchor the strands to the actin component of the cytoskeleton. Thus, tight junctions join together the cytoskeletons of adjacent cells. Often tight junctions form narrow belts that circumferentially surround the upper part of the lateral (i.e. "side") surfaces of adjacent epithelial cells.

Invertebrates have several other types of specific junctions; for example, the septate junction which is analogous to the tight junction in vertebrates.

In multicellular plants, the structural functions of cell junctions are instead provided for by cell walls. The analogues of communicating cell junctions in plants are called plasmodesmata.

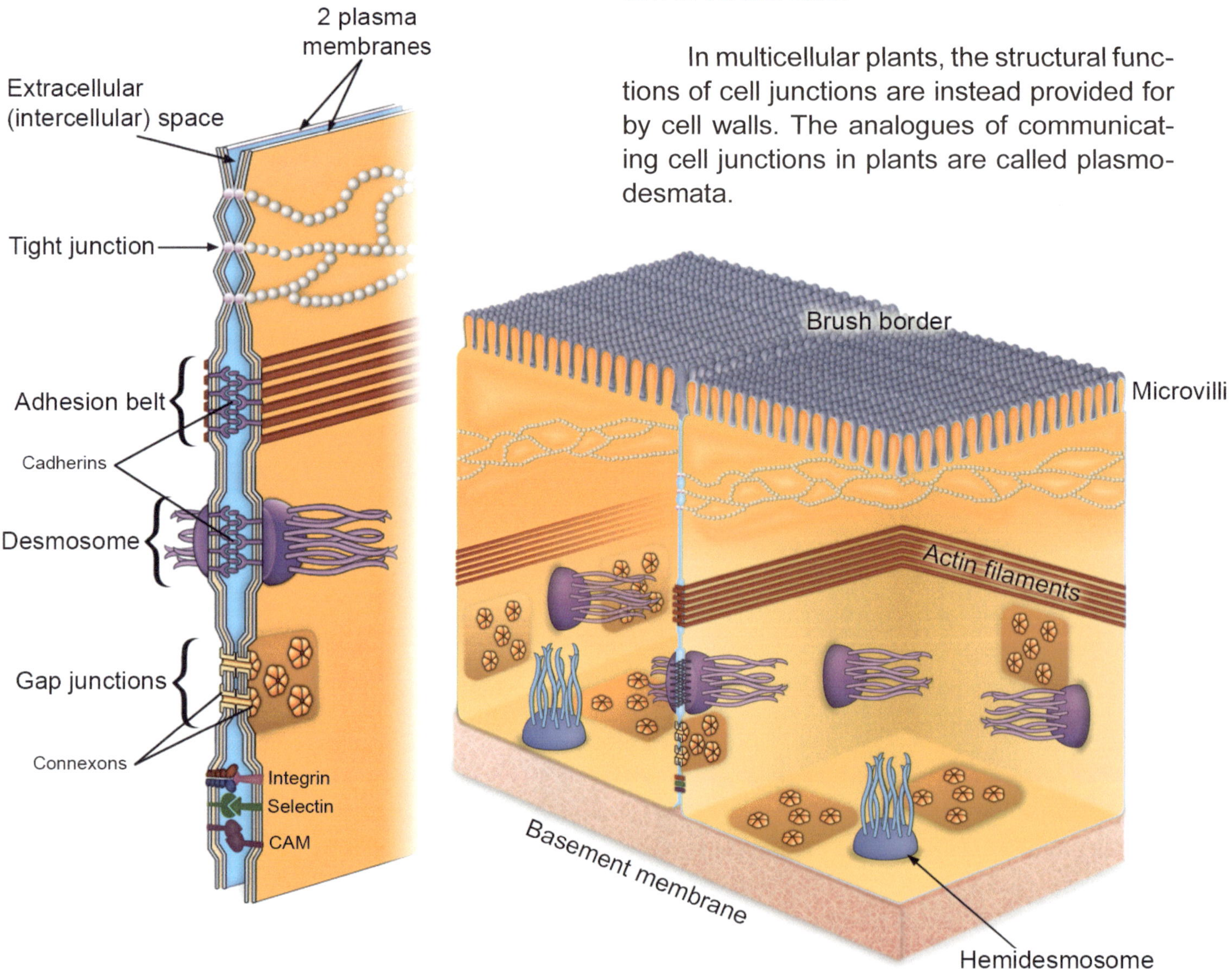

Figure IV.A.1.21: Various cell junctions in epithelia with microvilli at the surface (brush border, BIO 9.5).

1.5 Microscopy

A natural question about cells would be: if they are so small, how do we know what the inside of a cell really looks like? The story begins with the instrument used to produce magnified images of objects too small to be seen by the naked eye: the microscope.

Let us compare the basic principles of two popular methods of microscopy utilised by the vast majority of molecular biology research scientists: **(1)** the optical or light microscope; and **(2)** the electron microscope (the transmission electron microscope or TEM and the scanning electron microscope or SEM).

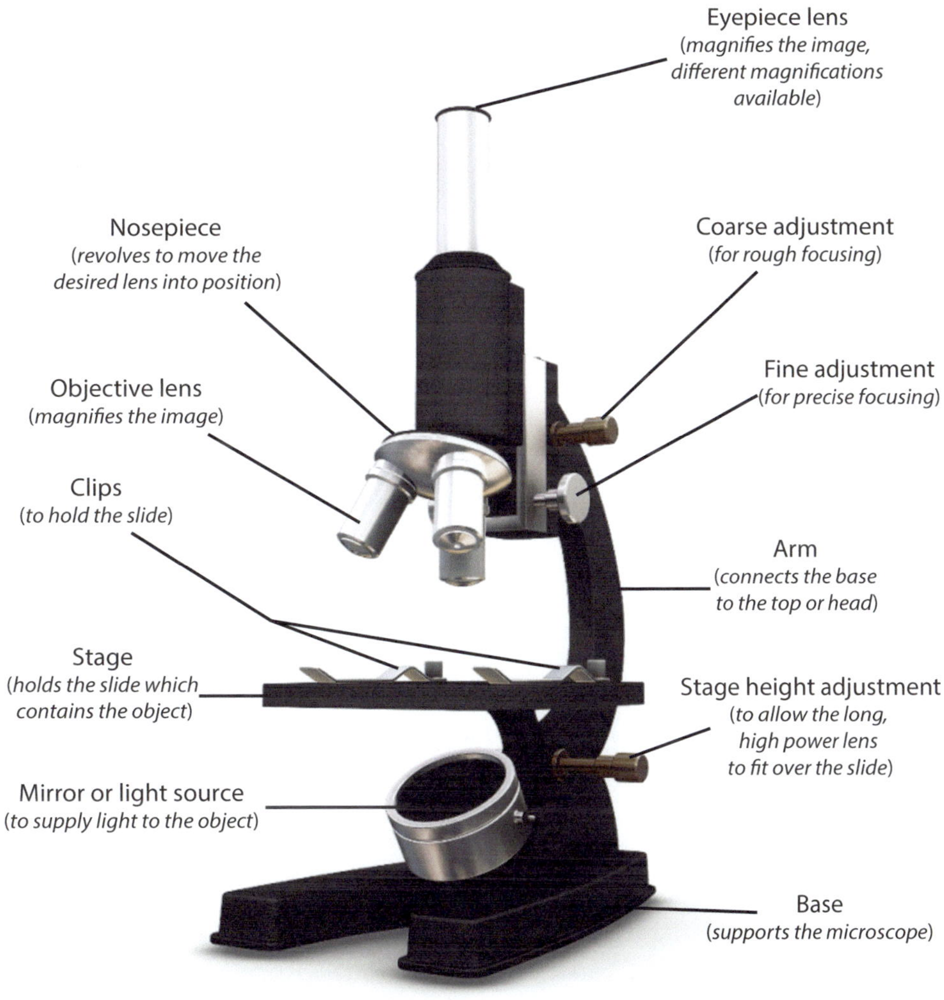

Figure IV.A.1.22: Compound light microscope. Typical magnification for the eyepiece is 10x and for the objective: 10x, 40x or 100x.

High-level Importance

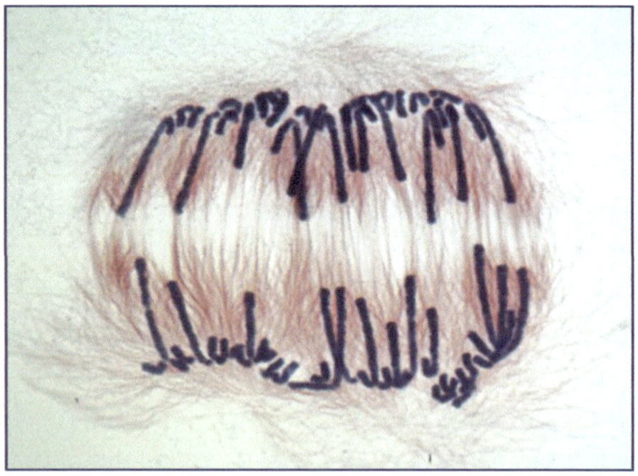
(Bajer, CIL: 197)

Figure IV.A.1.23: Light microscope image of a cell from the endosperm (= tissue in the seed) of an African lily. Staining shows microtubules in red and chromosomes in blue during late anaphase (BIO 1.3).

Light microscopy involves the use of an external or internal light source. The light first passes through the *iris* which controls the amount of light reaching the specimen. The light then passes through a *condenser* which is a lens that focuses the light beam through the specimen before it ultimately meets the *objective lens* which magnifies the image depending on your chosen magnification factor. Two terms you should be familiar with are *magnification* (how much bigger the image appears) and *resolution* (the ability to distinguish between two points on an image).

Magnification (PHY 11.3, 11.5) is the ratio between the apparent size of an object (or its size in an image) and its true size, and thus it is a dimensionless number usually followed by the letter “x”. A compound microscope uses multiple lenses to collect light from the sample or specimen (this lens is the objective with a magnification of up to 100x), and then a separate set of lenses to focus the light into the eye or camera (the eyepiece, magnification up to 10x). So the total magnification can be 100 x 10 = 1000 times the size of the specimen (1000x makes a 100 nanometre object visible).

Light microscopes enjoy their popularity thanks to their relative low cost and ease of use. A very important feature is that they can be used to view live specimens. Their shortfall is that the magnification is limited.

Common Units of Length in Biology
For details on units, see GM 2.1.2, 2.1.3

- m = metre(s)
- cm = centimetre(s) (1 cm = 10^{-2} m)
- mm = millimetre(s) (1 mm = 10^{-3} m)
- μm = micrometre(s) (1 μm = 10^{-6} m) NOT micron or μ
- nm = nanometre(s) (1 nm = 10^{-9} m)
- Å = angstrom(s) (1 Å = 10^{-10} m)
- pm = picometre(s) (1 pm = 10^{-12} m)

The term "micron" is no longer in technical use.

Electron microscopy is less commonly used due to its high price and associated scarcity. It also cannot observe live organisms as a vacuum is required and the specimen is flooded with electrons. All images being produced are in black and white though colour is sometimes added to the raw images. Its primary advantage lies in the fact that it is possible to achieve a magnification up to 10,000,000x and it is the obvious choice when a high level of detail is required using an extremely small specimen. In fact, an object as tiny as a small fraction of a nanometre becomes visible with an incredible 50 picometre resolution. TEM shows the interior of the cell while SEM shows the surface of the specimen.

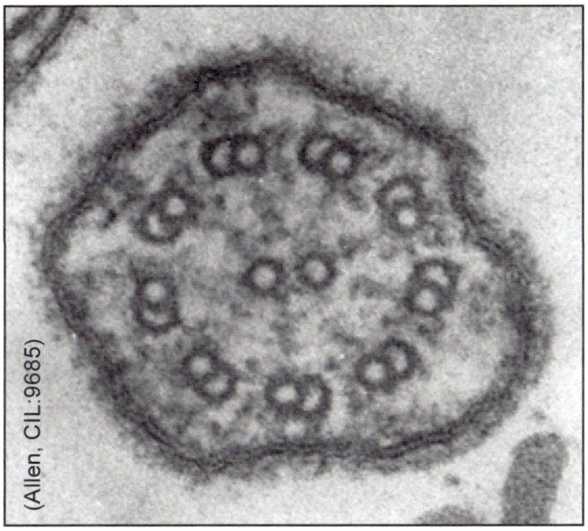

Figure IV.A.1.24: TEM of the cross section of a cilium (BIO 1.2) showing an axoneme consisting of 9 doublet and 2 central microtubules (= 9x2 + 2). Each doublet is composed of 2 subfibers: a complete A subfiber with dynein and an attached B subfiber. Eukaryotic flagella are also 9x2 + 2.

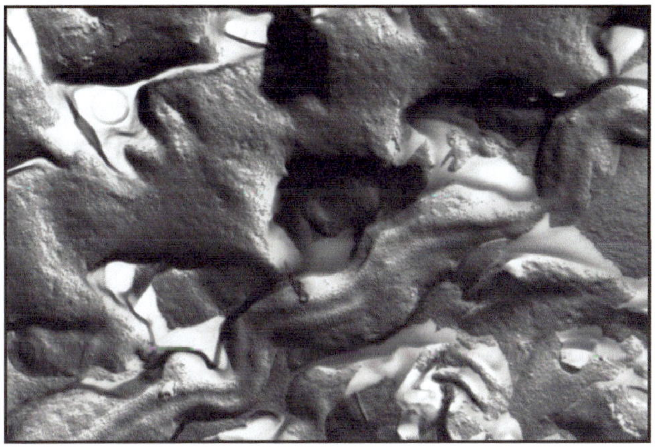

Figure IV.A.1.25: TEM freeze fracture of the plasma membrane which is cleaved between the acyl tails of membrane phospholipids (BIO 1.1; ORG 12.4), leaving a monolayer on each half of the specimen. The "E" face is the inner face of the outer lipid monolayer. The complementary surface is the "P" face (the inner surface of the inner leaflet of the bilayer shown above). The 2 large ribbons are intrinsic proteins.

1.5.1 Fluorescent Microscopy and Immunofluorescence

Lastly, you should be familiar with fluorescent microscopy which is commonly used to identify cellular components (organelles, cytoskeleton, etc.) and microbes with a high degree of specificity and colour. The fluorescent microscope makes use of a special filter that only permits certain radiation wavelengths that matches the fluorescing material being analysed. It is an optical microscope and very similar to the light microscope except that a highly intensive light source is used to excite a fluorescent species in the sample of interest.

Immunofluorescence is a technique that uses the specificity of the antibody-antigen interaction (BIO 8.2) to target fluorescent dyes to specific molecules in a cell. Immunofluorescence can be used on tissue sections, cultured cell lines or individual cells. This can be called *immunostaining*, or specifically, *immunohistochemistry* where the location of the antibodies can be seen using fluorophores (= a fluorescent chemical that can re-emit light upon light excitation; PHY 12.5, 12.6).

There are two classes of immunofluorescence: direct (= primary) and indirect (= secondary).

Direct immunofluorescence uses a single antibody linked to a fluorophore. The antibody binds to the target molecule (antigen), and the fluorophore attached to the antibody can be detected with a microscope. This technique is cheaper, faster but less sensitive than indirect immunofluorescence.

Indirect immunofluorescence uses two antibodies: **(1)** the unlabeled first, or primary, antibody binds the antigen; and **(2)** the secondary antibody, which carries the fluorophore and recognises the primary antibody and binds to it.

Photobleaching is the photochemical destruction of a dye or a fluorophore. Thus the fluorescent molecules are sometimes destroyed by the light exposure necessary to stimulate them into fluorescing. On the other hand, photobleaching can be fine tuned to improve the signal-to-noise ratio (like seeing the tree from the forest). Photobleaching can also be used to study the motion of molecules (i.e. FRAP).

Immunofluorescence samples can be seen through a simple fluorescent microscope (*epifluorescence*) or through the more complex *confocal* microscope.

A confocal microscope is a state-of-the-art fluorescent microscope which uses a laser as the light source. The confocal microscope is used in FRAP, fluorescence recovery after photobleaching, which is an optical technique used to "view" the movement of proteins or molecules. FRAP is capable of quantifying the 2D diffusion of a thin film of molecules containing fluorescently labeled probes, or to examine single cells. FRAP has had many uses including: studies of cell membrane diffusion and protein binding; determining if axonal transport is retrograde or anterograde, meaning towards or away from the neuron's cell body (*soma*), respectively.

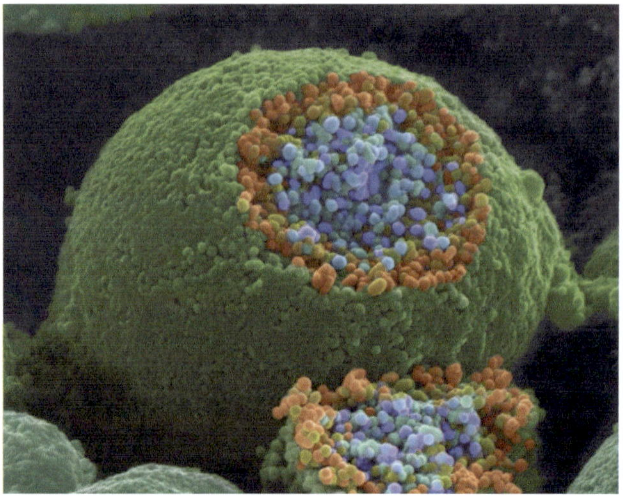

(Carvalho, CIL: 214)

Figure IV.A.1.26: SEM colourised image of a neuron's presynaptic terminal (BIO 5.1) that has been broken open to reveal the synaptic vesicles (orange and blue) beneath the cell membrane.

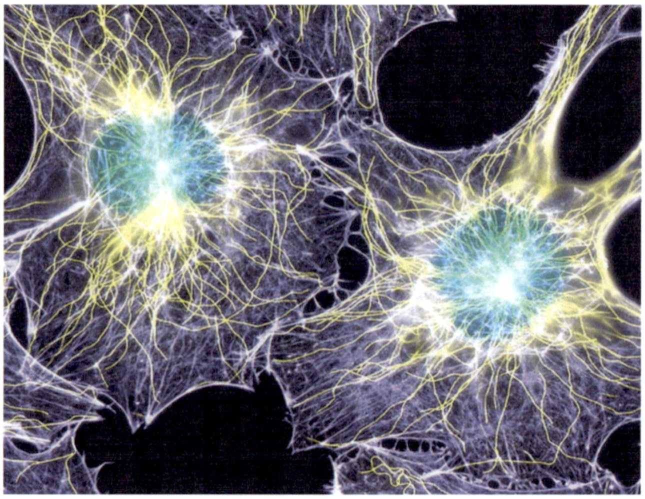

(Wittmann, CIL: 240)

Figure IV.A.1.27: Fluorescence microscopy of two interphase cells with immunofluorescence labeling of actin filaments (purple), microtubules (yellow), and nuclei (green).

CHAPTER 1: Generalised Eukaryotic Cell

GOLD STANDARD FOUNDATIONAL GAMSAT PRACTICE QUESTIONS

Foundational practice questions are meant to underline some basic assumed knowledge. Students with little or no background in this subject can treat the questions as open-book practice questions. Expect mistakes! Remember: This is not a traditional exam. Practice is a process.

And finally, our Foundational GAMSAT Practice Questions are followed by GAMSAT-level Practice Questions. Only students with a solid background in this subject should consider using a timer when completing any multiple-choice questions (maximum: *average 2 minutes per question*). For others, take your time and try your best before consulting the online answers and worked solutions. Good luck!

1) If increasing the concentration gradient across the plasma membrane increases the rate of transport until a maximum rate is reached, this would be convincing evidence for:

A. simple diffusion.
B. carrier-mediated transport.
C. osmosis.
D. the Fluid Mosaic model.

2) Fas/APO-1 is a transmembrane receptor which, when stimulated, may activate intra-cellular mechanisms leading to cell death. Fas/APO-1 is likely:

A. a phospholipid.
B. a complex carbohydrate.
C. synthesised in the nucleus.
D. synthesised by rough endoplasmic reticulum.

3) In mammals, a cancer cell loses its ability to divide in a normal fashion. The source of this abnormality is likely in the cell's:

A. lysosomes.
B. Golgi apparatus.
C. DNA.
D. tRNA.

4) When the base composition of *E. coli* DNA was determined, 16% of the bases were found to be adenine. Since A binds to T, and G binds to C, what is the G + C content of the *E. coli* DNA?

A. 16%
B. 32%
C. 34%
D. 68%

5) A mistake in DNA replication, causing the substitution of a cytosine by an adenine in one strand, will result in the changing of the complementary base in the other strand to:

A. adenine.
B. guanine.
C. cytosine.
D. thymine.

6) In a small portion of one DNA molecule, the sequence of nucleotide bases is 5′ TACTTG 3′. The sequence of the corresponding portion of the complementary strand would be:

A. 3′ TACTTG 5′.
B. 3′ ATGAAC 5′.
C. 3′ AUGAAC 5′.
D. 3′ UACUUG 5′.

High-level Importance

GOLD STANDARD GAMSAT-LEVEL PRACTICE QUESTIONS

7) Four dialysis bags, constructed from a semi-permeable membrane that is impermeable to sucrose, were filled with various concentrations of sucrose and then placed in separate beakers containing an initial concentration of 0.85 M sucrose solution. At 10-minute intervals, the bags were massed (weighed) and the percent change in mass of each bag was expressed in Figure 1.

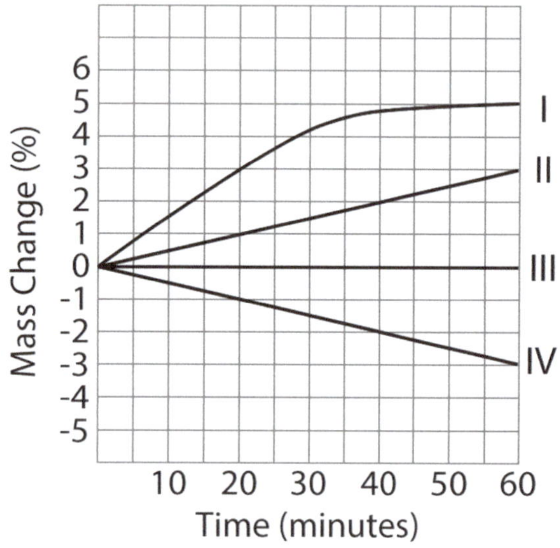

Figure 1

Which of the following labels from Figure 1 is most consistent with a bag that contained a solution that is hypotonic to the 0.85 molar solution at the beginning of the experiment?

A. I only
B. I and II only
C. III only
D. IV only

Questions 8–10

The method of DNA replication proposed by James Watson and Francis Crick is known as semi-conservative replication since each new double helix retains one strand of the original DNA double helix. The evidence for this mechanism was provided by a series of classic experiments carried out by Meselson and Stahl in 1958 which proceeded as follows:

1. Cultures of the bacterium *E. coli*, which has a single circular chromosome, were grown for many generations in a medium containing the heavy isotope of nitrogen ^{15}N.

2. The cells containing the DNA labelled with ^{15}N were transferred to a culture medium containing the normal isotope of nitrogen (^{14}N).

3. After periods of time corresponding to the generation time for *E. coli* (50 min at 3 °C) samples were removed and the DNA extracted.

4. The DNA was then centrifuged at 40 000 times gravity for 20 h in a solution of cesium chloride (CsCl).

During centrifugation the heavy CsCl molecules began to sediment at the bottom of the centrifuge tubes producing an increasing density gradient from the top of the tube to the bottom. The DNA settled out where its density equalled that of the CsCl solution. When examined under ultraviolet light the DNA appeared in the centrifuge tube as a narrow band.

Two other hypotheses were advanced to explain the process of DNA replication. One is known as conservative replication and the other as dispersive replication. These hypotheses are summarised in Figure 1.

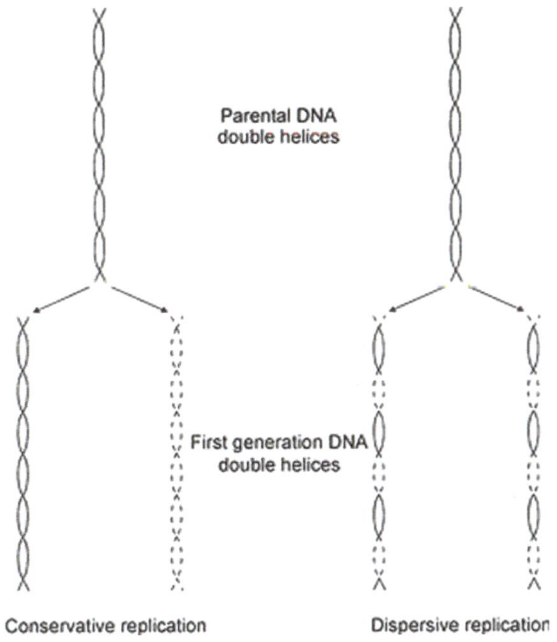

Figure 1

8) Based on the passage, which of the following represents the appearance of the tubes after the cells had been allowed to grow in the ^{14}N for two generations?

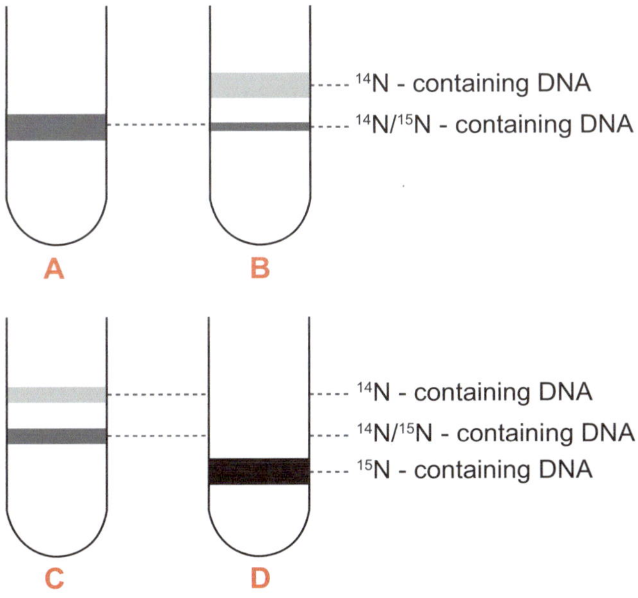

9) Had conservative replication been the correct hypothesis, which of the following would represent the appearance of the tubes after the cells had been allowed to grow in the ^{14}N for one generation?

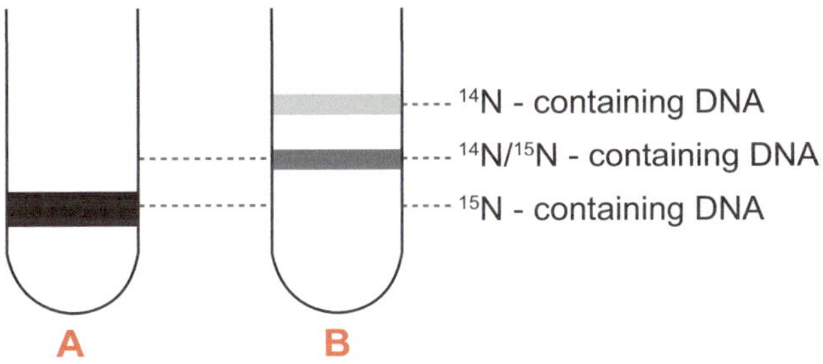

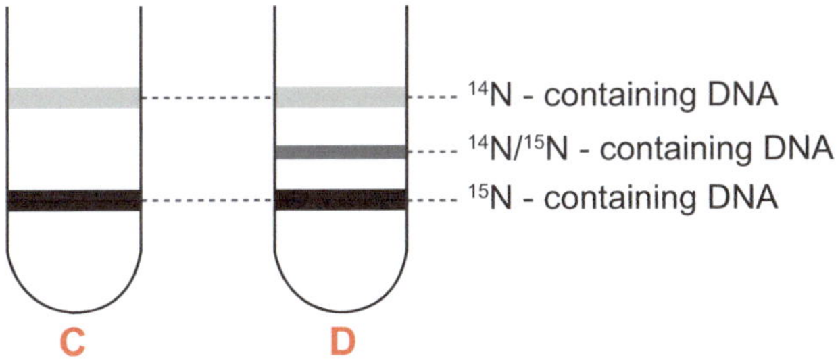

10) Had dispersive replication been the correct hypothesis, which of the following would represent the appearance of the tubes after the cells had been allowed to grow in the ^{14}N for one generation?

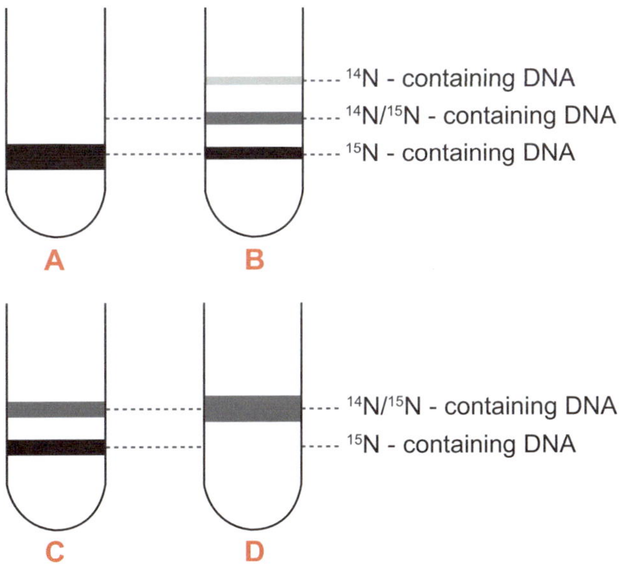

High-level Importance

11) The degree of sensitivity to ionising radiation (measured in grays, Gy) varies with the different cell cycle phases. Consider Figure 1.

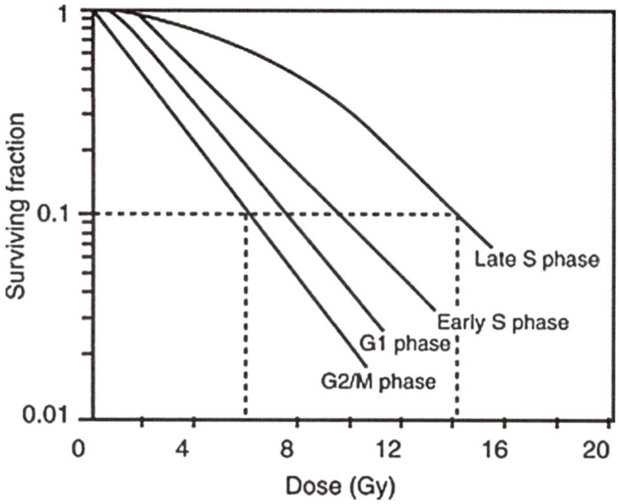

Figure 1

Given a radiation dose of 10 Gy, late S phase cells show a greater survival than G1 phase cells. According to Figure 1, late S phase cells' survival is approximately how much greater?

A. Less than twice
B. 2-3 times
C. 7-8 times
D. More than 10 times

12) If the rate of DNA replication is one thousand nucleotides per second, approximately how long would it take a one-million base-pair segment of DNA to replicate?

A. 1000 minutes
B. 500 minutes
C. 100 minutes
D. 20 minutes

13) Consider the base-pair binding pattern of DNA (A:T, G:C). Which of the following would be the expected result of a DNA nucleotide analysis?

A. A = G
B. A + G = C + T
C. A + C = G + T
D. More than one of the above is correct.

14) Consider the binding pattern of DNA (A:T, G:C) and its antiparallel nature. Which of the following pairs of DNA base sequences could form a short, normal double helix?

A. 5′-A-T-G-C-3′ with 5′-G-C-A-T-3′
B. 5′-A-G-C-T-3′ with 5′-T-C-G-A-3′
C. 5′-G-C-G-C-3′ with 5′-T-A-T-A-3′
D. Neither **A** nor **B** nor **C**

15) A "DNA sequence" refers to the order of nucleotides in DNA. During an experiment, a single ten-base DNA sequence yielded 2 five-base fragments: GATTG and TGGAT. The 2 five-base fragments might represent what length of the original ten-base DNA sequence by percent, at a minimum and maximum, respectively?

A. 70%, 80%
B. 70%, 100%
C. 80%, 100%
D. 90%, 100%

Answers and worked solutions? Online! Go to www.gamsat-prep.com/gamsat-biology to register your book. Having solutions online reduces the risk of annoying typos in a printed answer grid; allows us to provide more details in the solutions including images; permits us to embed free discussion boards for each chapter; and finally, we provide dozens of hours of free topical videos with clear teaching. We look forward to seeing you online!

SPOILER ALERT

Gold Standard has cross-referenced the content in this chapter to examples from ACER's official GAMSAT practice materials (*only ACER sells their eBooks brand new*). It is for you to decide when you want to explore these questions since you may want to preserve some of ACER's materials for timed mock-exam practice.

Number	1	2	3	4	5
Title	GAMSAT Practice Questions	GAMSAT Sample Questions	GAMSAT Practice Test 1	GAMSAT Practice Test 2	GAMSAT Practice Test 3

Examples – Osmosis (BIO 1.2.2) Q9 of 1, and Q31 of 2; cell Q12-16 of 4; cell cycle Q11-13 of 5; DNA sequence overlap Q52 of 5; DNA puzzle Q90-93 of 5. Note that "Q" is followed by the question number, and, for example, "of 1" refers to booklet number 1 in the table above. Also note that your gamsat-prep.com Masters Series online account has direct links to the step-by-step worked solutions for all of ACER's Section 3 practice questions (the solutions can also be found in the Gold Standard GAMSAT YouTube Channel). The 15 full-length GAMSAT practice tests by Gold Standard, HEAPS-1 through HEAPS-15, contain specific cross-references to this chapter within the worked solutions. Note that Questions 8-10 of the GAMSAT-level practice questions in this chapter come from HEAPS-5.

Chapter Checklist

- ☐ Access your free online account at www.gamsat-prep.com/gamsat-biology to view answers, worked solutions and discussion boards for chapter-ending practice questions.
- ☐ Reassess your 'learning objectives' for this chapter: Go back to the first page of this chapter and re-evaluate the top 3 boxes and the Introduction.
- ☐ Complete a maximum of 1 page of notes using symbols/abbreviations to represent the entire chapter based on your learning objectives. These are your Gold Notes.
- ☐ Consider your multimedia options based on your optimal way of learning:
  - ☐ Download the free Gold Standard GAMSAT app for your Android device or iPhone.
  - ☐ Create your own, tangible study cards or try the free app: Anki.
  - ☐ Record your voice reading your Gold Notes onto your smartphone (audio files, e.g., *memo* or MP3s) and listen during exercise, transportation, etc.
  - ☐ Try out the Gold Standard GAMSAT online videos at gamsat-prep.com, or you can try other options on YouTube like Khan Academy or Crash Course Biology.
- ☐ Schedule your full-length GAMSAT practice tests: ACER and/or HEAPS exams. Schedule one full day to complete a practice test and 1-2 days for a thorough assessment of worked solutions while adding to your abbreviated Gold Notes.
- ☐ Schedule and/or evaluate stress reduction techniques such as regular exercise (sports), yoga, meditation and/or mindfulness exercises (*see* YouTube for suggestions).

MICROBIOLOGY

Chapter 2

Memorise	Understand	Importance
* Equation for bacterial doubling * Differences, similarities: viruses vs. cells	* Viruses vs. eukaryotes vs. prokaryotes * General aspects of life cycles * Gen. aspects of genetics/reproduction * Calculation of exponential growth * Basics: the lac operon * Scientific method	**Medium level: 8% of GAMSAT Biology** questions released by ACER are related to content in this chapter (in our estimation). * Note that approximately 75% of the questions in GAMSAT Biology are related to just 7 chapters: 1, 2, 3, 4, 7, 12, and 15.

GAMSAT-Prep.com

Introduction

Microbiology is the study of microscopic organisms including viruses, bacteria and fungi. It is important to be able to focus on the differences and similarities between these microorganisms and the generalised eukaryotic cell you have just studied. The exponential growth of bacteria can be the source of challenging GAMSAT questions for students with poor skills in basic algebra and logs (GM Chapter 2, 3). Please be sure that you have completed a basic GAMSAT Maths revision before attempting the questions at the end of this chapter.

Gene expression in viruses, prokaryotes and even eukaryotes can be regulated, in part, via *operons*. An operon is a group of genes that have a single starting point (a *promoter*) to begin its activity (transcribe mRNA). The first operon to be understood comes from bacteria and it makes the milk sugar lactose (the *lac operon*). Understanding the basics of the scientific method will allow you to assess research-based questions in any of the GAMSAT sciences.

Multimedia Resources at GAMSAT-Prep.com

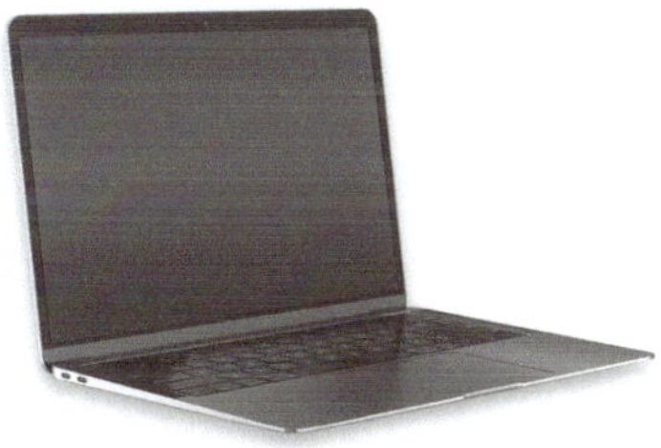

Open Discussion Boards
(*gamsat-prep.com/forum*)

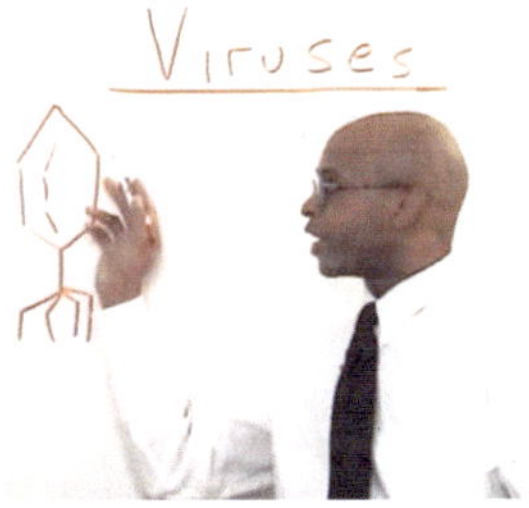

Foundational Videos

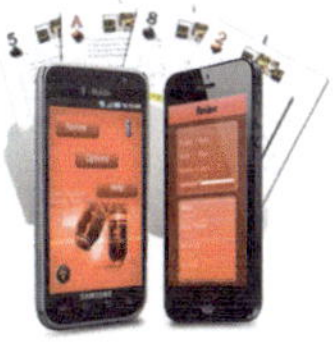

Flashcards

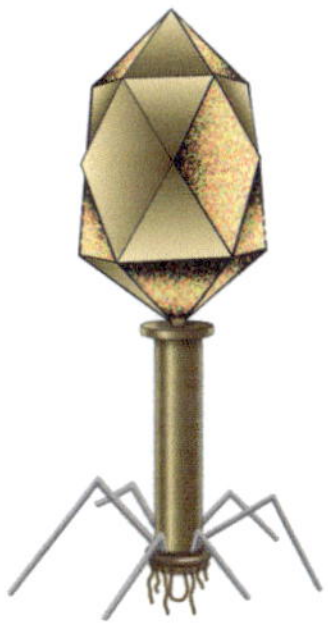

Special Guest

* The real GAMSAT may have advanced-level information presented (i.e. in a passage) but previous knowledge of said information is not required to answer the questions that would follow. Practice questions at the end of this chapter, as well as ACER and GS (HEAPS) practice GAMSATs can help you clarify this point.

2.1 Viruses

Unlike cells, viruses are too small to be seen directly with a light microscope. Viruses infect all types of organisms, from animals and plants to bacteria and archaea (BIO 2.2). Only a very basic and general understanding of viruses is required for the GAMSAT.

Viruses are obligate intracellular parasites; in other words, in order to replicate their genetic material and thus multiply, they must gain access to the inside of a cell. Replication of a virus takes place when the virus takes control of the host cell's synthetic machinery. Viruses are often considered non-living for several reasons:

(i) they do not grow by increasing in size
(ii) they cannot carry out independent metabolism
(iii) they do not respond to external stimuli
(iv) they have no cellular structure.

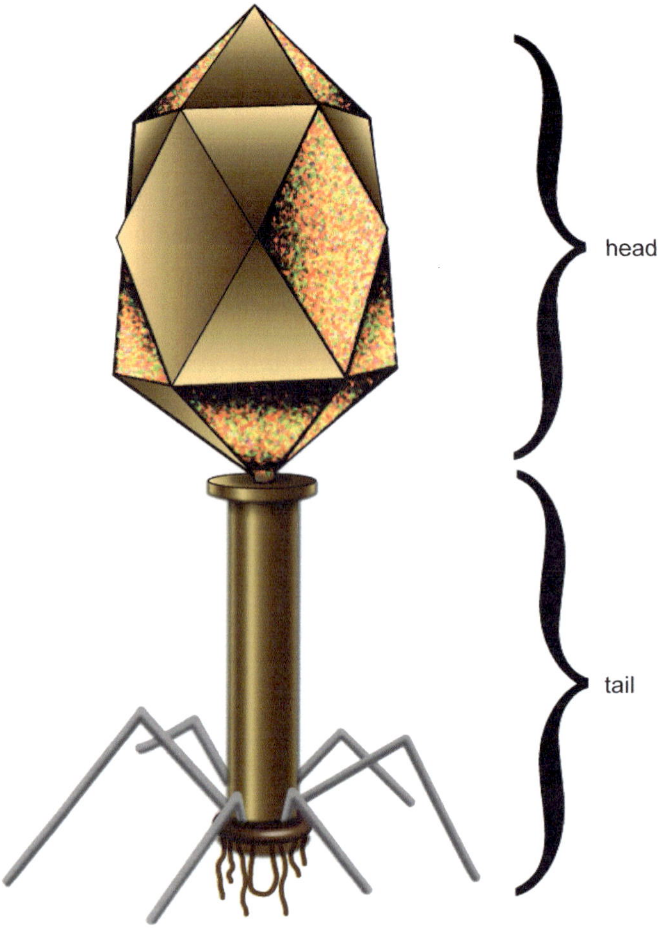

Figure IV.A.2.1: A virus.

The genetic material for viruses may be either DNA or RNA, never both. Viruses do not have organelles or ribosomes. The nucleic acid core is encapsulated by a protein coat (capsid) which together forms the head region in some viruses. The tail region helps to anchor the virus to a cell. An extracellular viral particle is called a *virion*.

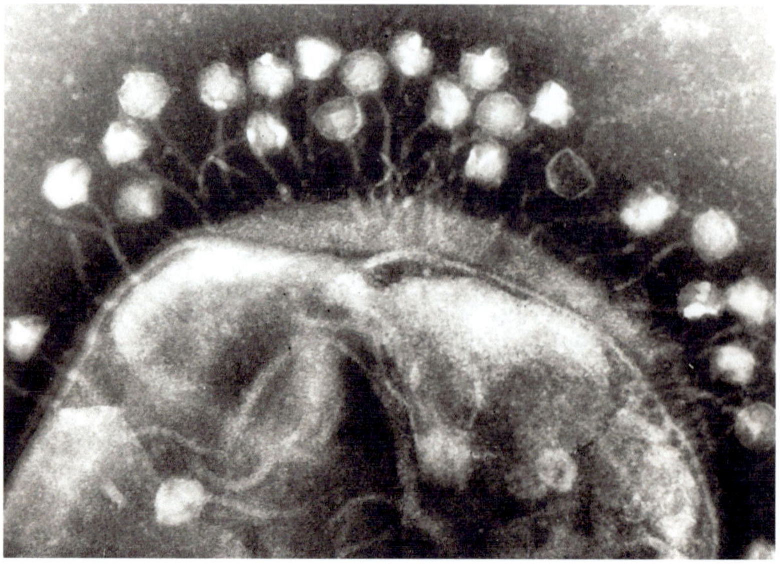

Figure IV.A.2.1.1: A relatively large bacterium (*below*) under attack by many smaller viruses (= *"bacteriophages" on the sides, above and particles within the bacterium*). TEM (BIO 1.5), 200,000x; Ref: α.

Medium-level Importance

Viruses are much smaller than prokaryotic cells (i.e. bacteria) which, in turn, are much smaller than eukaryotes (i.e. animals, fungi). A virus which infects bacteria is called a bacteriophage or simply a phage.

The life cycle of viruses has many variants; the following represents the main themes for GAMSAT purposes. A virus attaches to a specific receptor on a cell. Some viruses may now enter the cell; others, as in the diagram, will simply inject their nucleic acid. Either way, viral molecules induce the metabolic machinery of the host cell to produce more viruses.

The new viral particles may now exit the cell by lysing (bursting). This is also a feature of many bacteria. The preceding is deemed lytic or virulent. Some viruses lie latent for long periods of time without lysing the host and its genome becomes incorporated by genetic recombination into the host's chromosome. Therefore, whenever the host replicates, the viral genome is also replicated. These are called lysogenic or temperate viruses. Eventually, at some point, the virus may become activated and lyse the host cell.

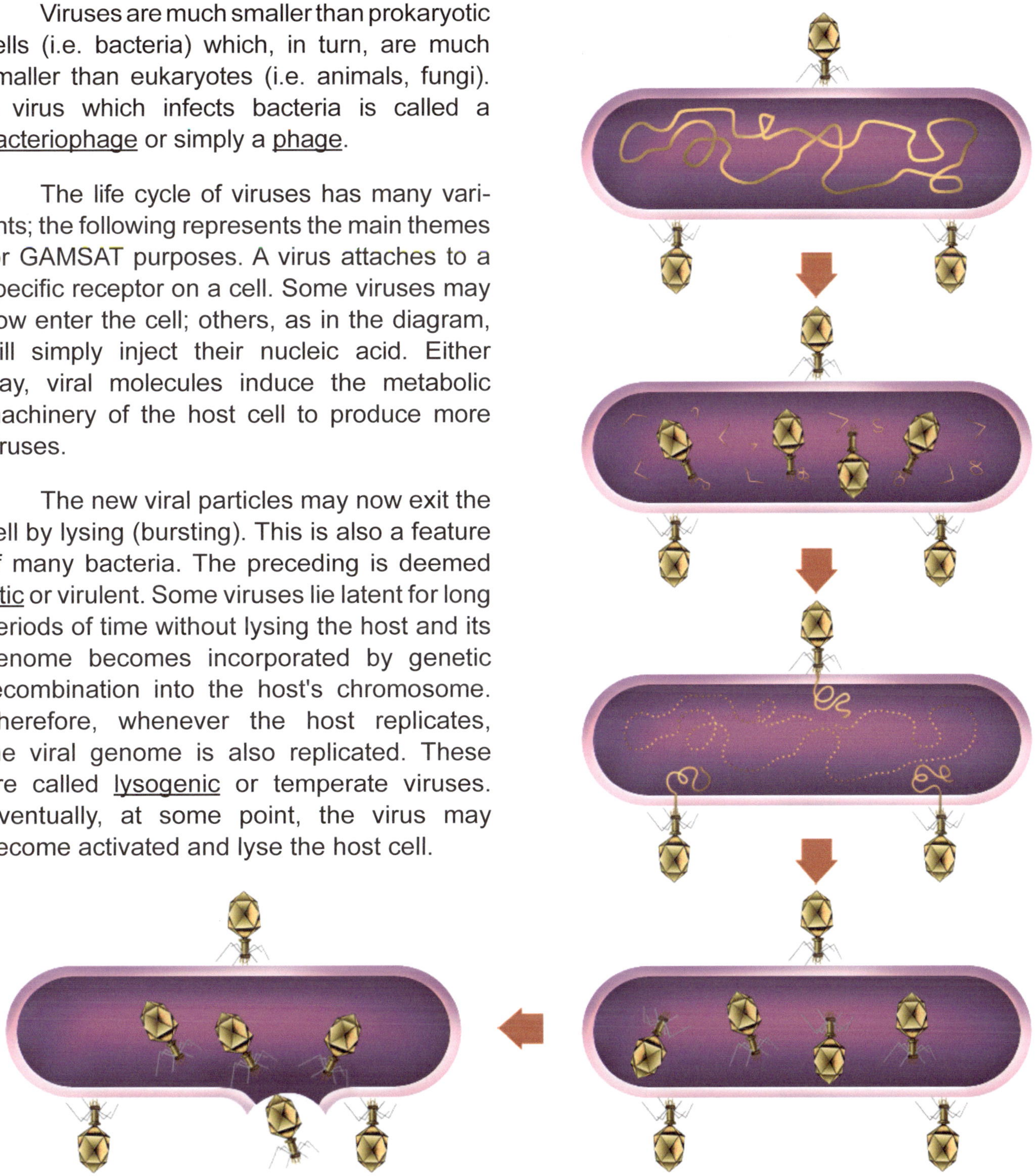

Figure IV.A.2.2: Lytic viral life cycle in a rod shaped bacterium (bacilli).

2.1.1 The Coronavirus Responsible for COVID-19

Medium-level Importance

Coronaviruses are a group of related RNA viruses that cause diseases in birds and mammals. In humans, they cause respiratory tract infections that can range from mild to deadly. Mild illnesses include some cases of the common cold (*which is also caused by other viruses, predominantly rhinoviruses*), while more lethal varieties can cause SARS, MERS and COVID-19. "**Coronavirus disease 2019**" (= COVID-19) is a contagious disease, responsible for the deaths of millions of people during a global pandemic, caused by the coronavirus: SARS-CoV-2.

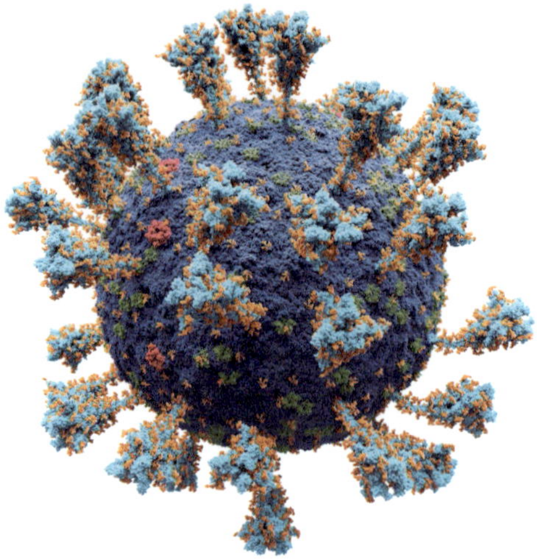

Figure IV.A.2.2.1: Accurate atomic model of the external structure of SARS-CoV-2. Ref: β.

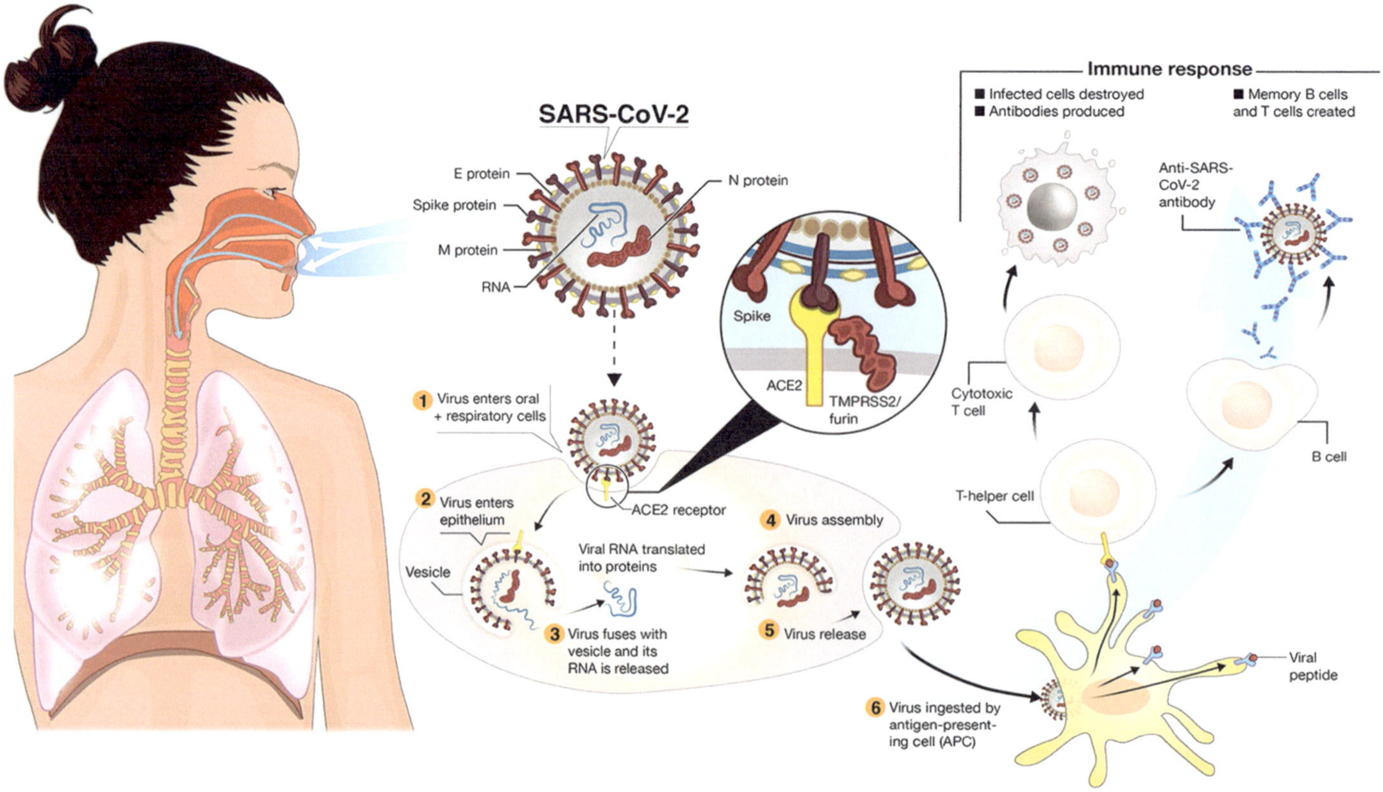

Figure IV.A.2.2.2: Transmission and life cycle of SARS-CoV-2 which causes COVID-19. SARS-CoV-2 is transmitted via respiratory droplets of infected individuals to oral and respiratory mucosal cells. The virus possesses a single-stranded RNA genome wrapped in a nucleocapsid (N) protein and three major surface proteins: membrane (M), envelope (E) and Spike. The virus replicates and passes to the lower airways potentially leading to severe pneumonia. The gateway to host cell entry (magnified view) is via a Spike-converting enzyme 2 (ACE2) interaction with the cleavage of Spike by proteases TMPRSS-2/furin. A simplified depiction of the life cycle of the virus is shown along with potential immune responses elicited (BIO 8.2). Ref: δ.

A retrovirus uses RNA as its genetic material. It is called a retrovirus because of an enzyme (reverse transcriptase) that gives these viruses the unique ability of transcribing RNA (their RNA) into DNA (*see* Biology Chapter 3 for the central dogma regarding protein synthesis). The retroviral DNA can then integrate into the chromosomal DNA of the host cell to be expressed there. The human immunodeficiency virus (HIV), the cause of AIDS, is a retrovirus.

Retroviruses are used, in genetics, to deliver DNA to a cell (= a vector); in medicine, they are used for gene therapy.

2.2 Prokaryotes

Prokaryotes (= pre-nucleus) are organisms without a membrane bound nucleus which includes 2 types of organisms: bacteria (= Eubacteria) and archaea (= bacteria-like organisms that live in extreme environments). For the purposes of the GAMSAT, we will focus on bacteria.

Bacteria are haploid and have a long circular strand of DNA within the *nucleoid*. The nucleoid is a region in a bacterium that contains DNA but is not surrounded by a nuclear membrane. Because bacterial DNA is not surrounded by a nuclear membrane, transcription and translation can occur at the same time, that is, protein synthesis can begin while mRNA is being produced. Bacteria also have smaller circular DNA called plasmid, which is an extra chromosomal genetic element that can replicate independently of the bacterial chromosome and helps to confer resistance to antibiotics.

Bacteria do not have mitochondria, Golgi apparatus, lysosomes, nor endoplasmic reticulum. Instead, metabolic processes

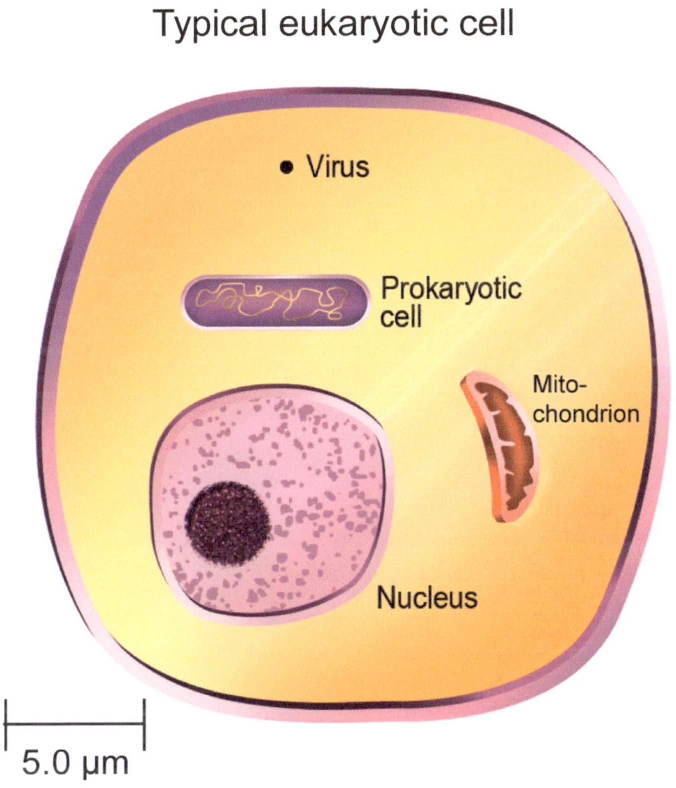

Figure IV.A.2.3
Comparing the size of a typical eukaryote, prokaryote and virus. Note that both the prokaryote and mitochondrion are similar in size and both contain circular DNA suggesting an evolutionary link.

Medium-level Importance

can be carried out in the cytoplasm or associated with bacterial membranes. Bacteria have ribosomes (smaller than eukaryotes), plasma membrane, and a cell wall. The cell wall, made of peptidoglycans, helps to prevent the hypertonic bacterium from bursting. Some bacteria have a slimy polysaccharide mucoid-like capsule on the outer surface for protection.

Bacteria can achieve movement with their flagella. Bacterial flagella are helical filaments, each with a rotary motor at its base which can turn clockwise or counterclockwise. The form and rotary engine of flagella are maintained by proteins (i.e. flagellin) which interact with the plasma membrane and the basal body (BIO 1.2). Power is generated by a proton motive force similar to the proton pump in metabolism (Biology, Chapter 4).

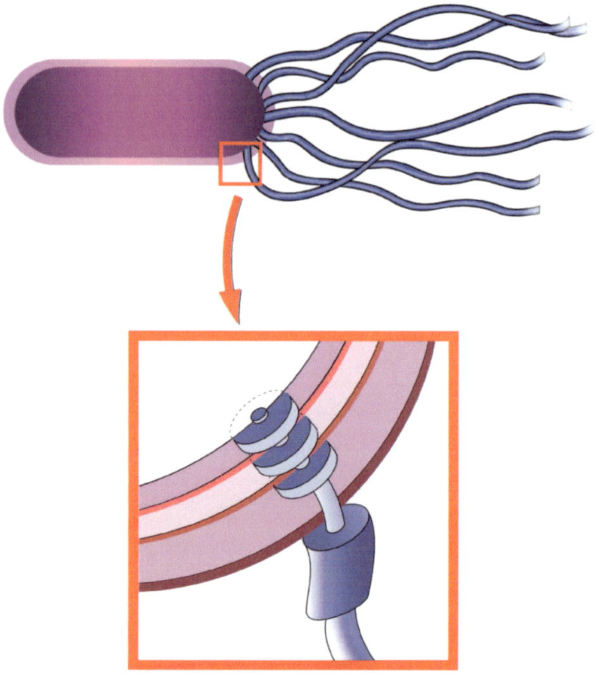

Figure IV.A.2.4

Schematic representation of the basis for flagellar propulsion. The flagellum, similar to a flexible hook, is anchored to the membrane and cell wall by a series of protein rings forming a motor. Powered by the flow of protons, the motor can rotate the flagellum more than 100 revolutions per second.

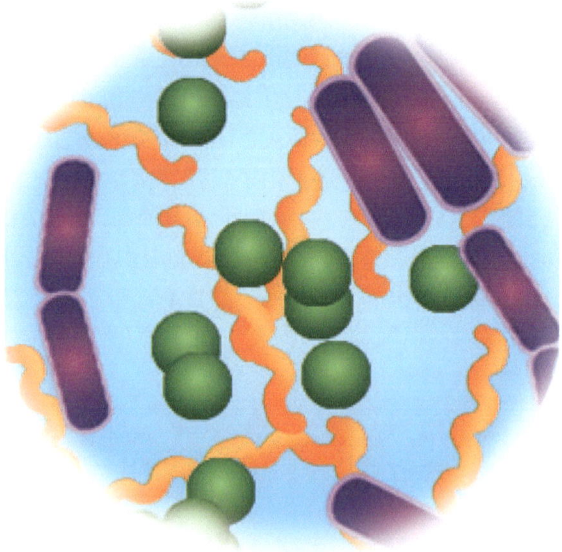

Figure IV.A.2.5

Schematic representation of bacteria coloured for the purpose of identification: cocci (spherical, green), bacilli (cylindrical, purple) and spirilla (helical, orange).

Bacteria also have short, hairlike filaments called pili (also called fimbriae) arising from the bacterial cell wall. These pili are much shorter than flagella. Common pili can serve as adherence factors which promote binding of bacteria to host cells. Sex pili, encoded by a self-transmissible plasmid, are involved in transferring of DNA from one bacterium to another via conjugation.

Bacteria are partially classified according to their shapes: <u>cocci</u> which are spherical or sometimes elliptical; <u>bacilli</u> which are rod shaped or cylindrical (Fig. IV.A.2.2 in BIO 2.1 showed phages attacking a bacillus

Prokaryotic Cells	Eukaryotic Cells
Small cells (1-10 μm)	Larger cells (10-100 μm)
Organisms are always unicellular	Organisms are often multicellular
No nuclei or any membrane-bound organelles, such as mitochondria	Always have nuclei and other membrane-bound organelles
DNA is circular, without proteins	DNA is linear and associated with proteins to form chromatin
Ribosomes are small (70S)	Ribosomes are large (80S)
No cytoskeleton	Always has a cytoskeleton
Motility by rigid rotating flagellum (made of flagellin)	Motility by flexible waving cilia or flagellae (made of tubulin)
Cell division is by binary fission	Cell division is by mitosis or meiosis
Reproduction is always asexual	Reproduction is asexual or sexual
Great variety of metabolic pathways	Common metabolic pathways

Table IV.A.2.1: Summary of the differences between prokaryotic and eukaryotic cells.

bacterium); spirilla which are helical or spiral. They are also classified according to whether or not their cell wall reacts to a special dye called a Gram stain; thus they are gram-positive if they retain the stain and gram-negative if they do not.

Most bacteria engage in a form of asexual reproduction called binary fission. Two identical DNA molecules migrate to opposite ends of a cell as a transverse wall forms, dividing the cell in two. The cells can now separate and enlarge to the original size. Under ideal conditions, a bacterium can undergo fission every 10-20 minutes producing over 10^{30} progeny in a day and a half. If resources are unlimited, exponential growth would be expected.

The doubling time of bacterial populations can be calculated as follows:

$$b = B \times 2^n$$

where b is the number of bacteria at the end of the time interval, B is the number of bacteria at the beginning of the time interval and n is the number of generations. Thus if we start with 2 bacteria and follow for 3 generations then we get:

$$b = B \times 2^n = 2 \times 2^3 = 2 \times 8 = 16$$

bacteria after 3 generations.

{Note: bacterial doubling time is a relatively popular question type.}

Medium-level Importance

Bacteria do not produce gametes nor zygotes, nor do they undergo meiosis; however, four forms of genetic recombination do occur: transduction, transformation, conjugation and transposon insertion.

In transduction, fragments of bacterial chromosomes accidentally become packaged into viruses during a viral infection. These viruses may then infect another bacterium. A piece of bacterial DNA that the virus is accidentally carrying will be injected and incorporated into the host chromosome if there is homology between the newly injected piece of DNA and the recipient bacterial genome.

In transformation, a foreign chromosome fragment (plasmid) is released from one bacterium during cell lysis and enters into another bacterium. The DNA can then become incorporated into the recipient's genome if there is homology between the newly incorporated genome and the recipient one.

In conjugation, DNA is transferred directly by cell-to-cell contact formed by a conjugation bridge called the sex pilus. For conjugation to occur, one bacterium must have the sex factor called F plasmid. Bacteria that carry F plasmids are called F^+ cells. During conjugation, a F^+ cell replicates its F factor and will pass its F plasmid to an F^- cell, converting it to an F^+ cell. This type of exchange is the major mechanism for transfer of antibiotic resistance.

In transposon insertion, mobile genetic elements called transposons move from one position to another in a bacterial chromosome or between different molecules of DNA without having DNA homology.

Most bacteria cannot synthesise their own food and thus depend on other organisms for it; such a bacterium is heterotrophic. Most heterotrophic bacteria obtain their food from dead organic matter; this is called saprophytic. Some bacteria are autotrophic meaning they can synthesise organic compounds from simple inorganic substances. Thus some are photosynthetic producing carbohydrate and releasing oxygen, while others are chemoautotrophic obtaining energy via chemical reactions including the oxidation of iron, sulfur, nitrogen, or hydrogen gas.

Bacteria can be either aerobic or anaerobic. The former refers to metabolism in the presence of oxygen and the latter in the absence of oxygen (i.e. fermentation).

Based on variations in the oxygen requirement, bacteria are divided into four types:

1) Obligate aerobes: require oxygen for growth
2) Facultative anaerobes: are aerobic; however, can grow in the absence of oxygen by undergoing fermentation
3) Aerotolerant anaerobes: use fermentation for energy; however, can tolerate low amounts of oxygen
4) Obligate anaerobes: are anaerobic, can be damaged by oxygen

Symbiosis generally refers to close and often long term interactions between different biological species. Bacteria have various symbiotic relationships with, for example, humans. These include mutualism (both benefit: GI tract bacteria, BIO 9.5), parasitism (parasite benefits over the host: tuberculosis, appendicitis) and commensalism (one benefits and the other is not significantly harmed or benefited: some skin bacteria).

2.2.1 Gene Expression: Operons

Gene expression is the process by which information from a gene is used in the synthesis of a functional gene product. The product is usually a protein, but in non-protein-coding genes such as transfer RNA (tRNA) and small nuclear RNA (snRNA), the product is a functional noncoding RNA.

Gene expression is the most fundamental level at which the genotype (*an individual's collection of genes*) gives rise to the phenotype (*the observable trait*). All steps in the gene expression process may be modulated (*regulated*), including the transcription, RNA splicing, translation, and post-translational modification of a protein. Regulation of gene expression gives control over the timing, location, and amount of a given gene product (protein or noncoding RNA) present in a cell and can have a profound effect on the cellular structure and function. Regulation of gene expression is the basis for cellular differentiation, development, morphogenesis (*the shaping of organs and tissues in the embryo*), and the versatility and adaptability of any organism.

We will now examine one aspect of gene expression (*operons*), and we will examine other aspects of gene expression in Chapters 3, 14, 15 and 16.

An operon is a functioning unit of DNA containing a cluster of genes under the control of a single promoter. Thus, the genes contained in the operon are either expressed together or not at all. Operons are composed of:

1. A repressor which can bind to an operator and prevent gene expression by blocking RNA polymerase. However, in the presence of an inducer, a repressor will be bound to the inducer instead, forming an inducer-repressor complex. This complex cannot bind to an operator and thus gene expression is permitted.
2. A promoter which is a sequence of DNA where RNA polymerase attaches to begin transcription.
3. Operators which can block the action of RNA polymerase if there is a repressor present.
4. A regulator which codes for the synthesis of a repressor that can bind to the operator and block gene transcription.
5. Structural genes that code for several related enzymes that are responsible for production of a specific end product.

The *lac operon* controls the breakdown of lactose and is the simplest way of illustrating how gene regulation in bacteria works. In the lac operon system there is an active repressor that binds to the operator. In this scenario RNA polymerase is unable to transcribe the structural genes necessary to control the uptake and subsequent breakdown of lactose. When the repressor is inactivated (in the presence of lactose) the RNA polymerase is now able to transcribe the genes that code for the required enzymes. These enzymes are said to be *inducible* as it is the lactose that is required to turn on the operon.

Lac Operon

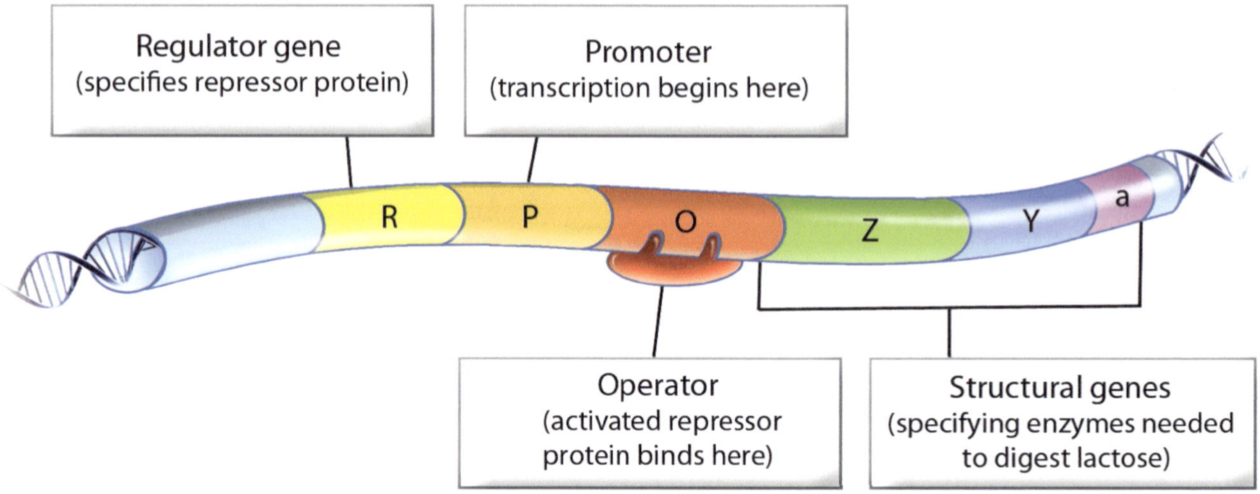

2.3 Fungi

Fungi are eukaryotic (= true nucleus) organisms which absorb their food through their chitinous cell walls. They may either be unicellular (i.e. yeast) or filamentous (i.e. mushrooms, molds) with individual filaments called hyphae which collectively form a mycelium. Fungal cell membranes contain ergosterol rather than cholesterol found in cell membranes of other eukaryotes.

Fungi often reproduce asexually. In molds, spores can be produced and then liberated from outside of a sporangium; or, as in yeast, a simple asexual budding process may be used. Sexual reproduction can involve the fusion of opposite mating types to produce asci (singular: ascus), basidia (singular: basidium), or zygotes. All of the three preceding diploid structures must undergo meiosis to produce haploid spores. If resources are unlimited, exponential growth would be expected.

Fungi are relatively important for humans as a source of disease and a decomposer of both food and dead organic matter. On the lighter side, they also serve as food (mushrooms, truffles), for alcohol and food production (cheese molds, bread yeast) and they have given us the breakthrough antibiotic, penicillin (from penicillium molds).

A vector can be a person, animal or microorganism that carries and transmits an infectious organism (i.e. bacteria, viruses, etc.) into another living organism. Examples: the mosquito is a vector for malaria; bats are vectors for rabies and a SARS-like virus.

2.5 The Scientific Method

The scientific method could be used in conjunction with any GAMSAT Biology experiment but microbiology is most common.

The point of the experiment is to test your ability to read scientific material, understand what is being tested, and determine if the hypothesis has been proved, refuted or neither. When a hypothesis survives rigorous testing, it graduates to a *theory*.

Observation, formulation of a theory, and testing of a theory by additional observation is called the scientific method. In biology, a key aspect to evaluate the validity of a trial or experiment is the presence of a *control group*. Generally, treatment is withheld from the control group but given to the *experimental group*.

First we will make an observation and then use deductive reasoning to create an appropriate hypothesis which will result in an experimental design. Consider the following: trees grow well in the sunlight. Hypothesis: exposure to light is directly related to tree growth. Experiment: two groups of trees are grown in similar conditions except one group (*experimental*) is exposed to light while the other group (*control*) is not exposed to light. Growth is carefully measured and the two groups are compared. Note that tree growth (*dependent variable*) is dependent on light (*independent variable*).

There are experiments where it is important to expose the control group to some factor different from the factor given to the experimental group (= *positive control*); as opposed to not giving the control group any exposure at all (= *negative control*). Exposure for a control group is used in medicine and dentistry because of the "Placebo Effect."

Experiments have shown that giving a person a pill that contains no biologically active material will cure many illnesses in up to 30% of individuals. Thus if Drug X is developed using a traditional control group, and the "efficacy" is estimated at 32%, it may be that the drug is no more effective than a sugar pill! In this case, the control group must be exposed to an unmedicated preparation to negate the Placebo Effect. To be believable the experiment must be well-grounded in evidence (= *valid,* based on the scientific method) and then one must be able to reproduce the results.

Medium-level Importance

2.5.1 The Experiment

A lab in Sydney reports 15% cell death when maximally stimulating the APO-1 receptor. In order to appropriately interpret the results, it must first be compared to:

A. data from other labs.
B. the attrition rate of other cell types.
C. the actual number of APO-1 cells dying in the tissue culture.
D. the rate of cell death without stimulation of APO-1.

- The experiment: stimulating a specific receptor on cells led to a 15% rate of cell death.
- Treatment is the stimulation of a receptor.
- The control (*group without treatment*): under the same conditions, do not stimulate the receptor (choice **D.**).

Choice **C.** does not answer the question. Choices **A.** and **B.** are most relevant if the initial data is shown to be significant. To prove that the data is significant or valid, one must first compare to a control group (choice **D.**).

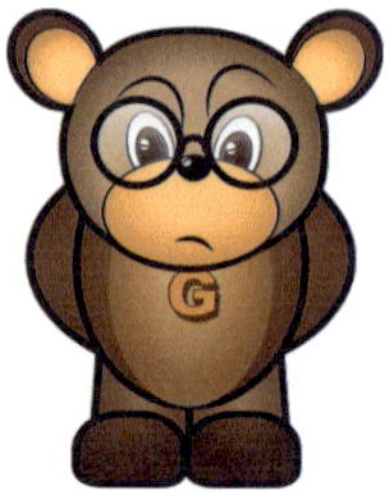

Excuse me for feeling superia
to all the lowly bacteria;
You should know very well,
there's no organelle
inside their tiny interia.

CHAPTER 2: Microbiology

GOLD STANDARD FOUNDATIONAL GAMSAT PRACTICE QUESTIONS

1) All viruses contain:

A. ribosomes.
B. antibodies.
C. nucleic acid.
D. lysosomes.

2) Both bacteria and eukaryotic cells may share all of the following features EXCEPT:

A. phospholipid bilayer.
B. cell wall.
C. ribosomes.
D. nuclear membrane.

3) Consider consulting Figure IV.A.2.5 and its caption (BIO 2.2). *Streptococcus mutans* and *Lactobacillus* are, respectively:

A. spherical and helical.
B. spherical and cylindrical.
C. cylindrical and helical.
D. helical and cylindrical.

4) Given that the time for one TS type *E. coli* to divide at 30 °C is approximately 15 minutes, if 10 bacteria should begin dividing in ample culture media, approximately how many would be present 2 hours later?

A. 500
B. 1000
C. 2500
D. 5000

5) Given unlimited resources, which of the following lines shows the population growth curve for the yeast *Candida albicans* once infection occurs?

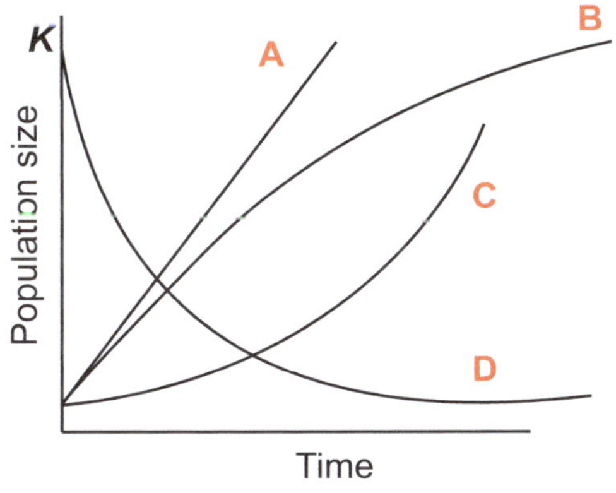

6) *Streptococcus mutans* is associated with the tooth surface and appears to be the major causative agent of dental caries, or tooth decay. *Streptococcus mutans* produces glucan, a sticky polymer of glucose that acts like a cement and binds the bacterial cells together and to the tooth surface. The enzyme which catalyses the formation of glucan is likely located:

A. in the cytosol of the cocci.
B. in lysosomes within the cytoplasm of the cocci.
C. in the nuclei of the cocci.
D. on the cell surface membrane of the cocci.

GOLD STANDARD GAMSAT-LEVEL PRACTICE QUESTIONS

Questions 7–9

In microbiology, a colony-forming unit (CFU) is a unit used to estimate the number of viable bacterial cells in a sample. Consider the following diagram.

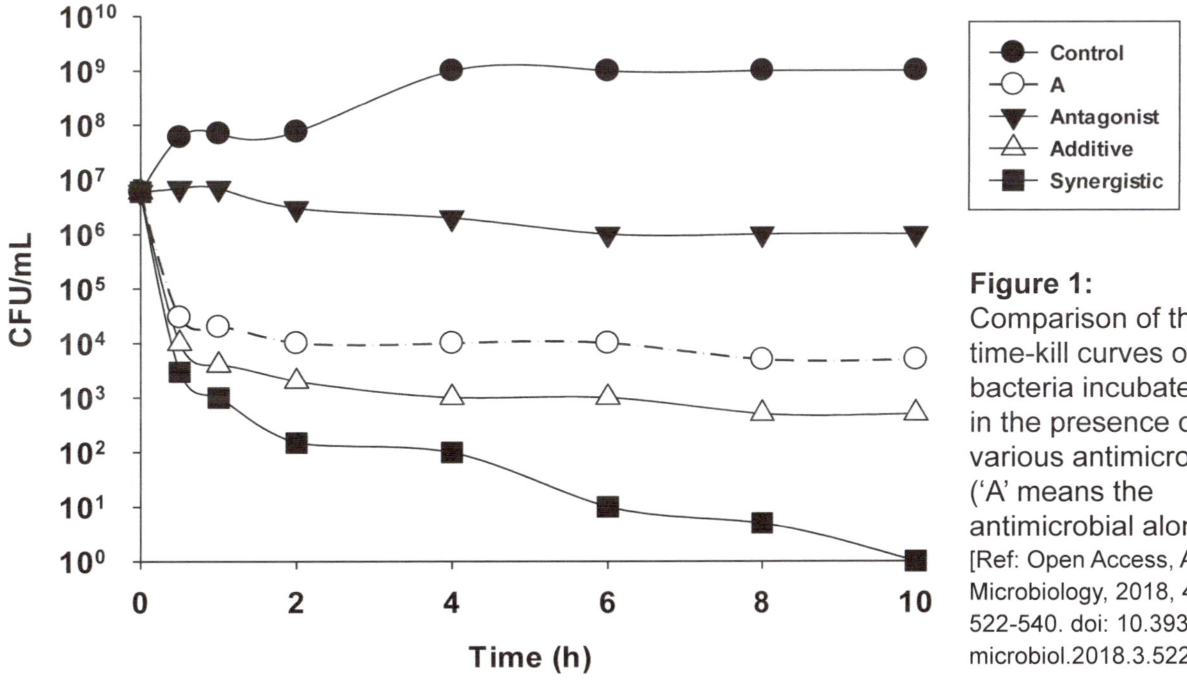

Figure 1: Comparison of the time-kill curves of bacteria incubated in the presence of various antimicrobials ('A' means the antimicrobial alone). [Ref: Open Access, AIMS Microbiology, 2018, 4(3): 522-540. doi: 10.3934/microbiol.2018.3.522]

High-level Importance

7) According to Figure 1, the largest drop in the number of viable bacterial cells per mL, between hour 1 and hour 10, occurs with which of the following trials?

A. Antimicrobial alone
B. Antagonist
C. Additive
D. Synergistic

8) At hour 6 in Figure 1, which of the following best approximates the difference in viable bacterial cell numbers per mL between the trial with the Control and the trial with Antimicrobial alone?

A. 1000
B. 100 000
C. 10 000 000
D. 1 000 000 000

9) Based on Figure 1, the fastest increase in the numbers of viable bacterial count per mL per hour occurs in the 'Control' group between which of the following time periods?

A. Hour 0 and 0.5
B. Hour 0 and 2
C. Hour 2 and 3
D. Hour 3 and 4

10) In a rich *medium* (i.e. solution with nutrients), one *E. coli* bacterium can divide in approximately 20 minutes. If ten *E. coli* begin to divide in a rich medium with no damaging radiation, approximately how many *E. coli* will be present 3 hours later?

A. Less than 700
B. 2500
C. 5000
D. 10 000

11) Cephalexin, at even a low dose, is excellent at killing gram-positive bacteria such as *Staphylococcus aureus* (*S. aureus*). In a normal population of *S. aureus*, approximately 1 in 10^8 cells are mutants that are resistant to cephalexin and thus can grow and divide. Consider a population of *S. aureus* in an exponential growth phase and then exposed to a low dose of cephalexin. After 20 generations of exposure to the antibiotic, what percentage of the cells would be resistant to cephalexin?

A. Approximately 100%
B. Between 10% and 50%
C. Approximately 0.000001%
D. None of the cells

12) The rate of growth of yeast cells decreases markedly when the inhibitor TX-22 is added to the medium.

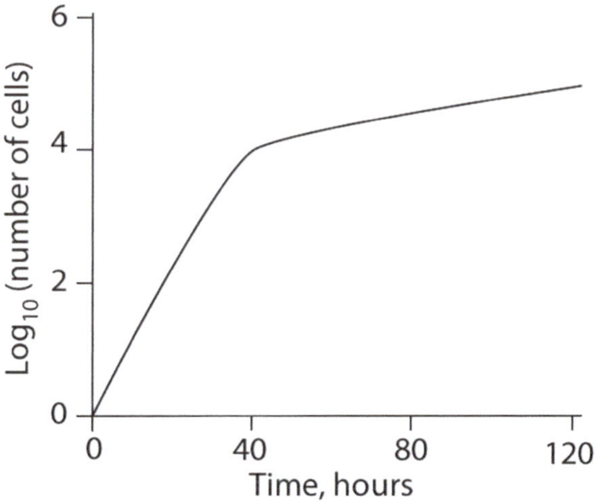

Figure 1: Yeast cell numbers as a function of time

According to Figure 1, when TX-22 is added, what is the approximate number of yeast cells in the medium?

A. 4
B. 40
C. 4000
D. 10 000

Questions 13–15

UV radiation can damage DNA by inhibiting proper replication and thus preventing cell division. Though exposure to intense and/or prolonged irradiation is fatal, most organisms, including the bacterium *Escherichia coli*, have mechanisms to repair DNA damaged by factors such as low levels of UV radiation.

A bacteriophage assay can be used to detect DNA repair activity because repair of bacterial DNA is not directly observable (note: a bacteriophage, or *phage*, is a virus that infects bacteria). When bacterial DNA has been mildly damaged, a generalised repair response is activated. In fact, the repair mechanisms of the bacteria will repair both bacterial and phage DNA. Therefore, the number of phages liberated at cell lysis is greater when damaged phages infect damaged *E. coli* than when they infect undamaged *E. coli*. The results obtained during an experiment testing the effect of UV radiation on phage repair are reported in Table 1.

Trial	Duration of bacterial irradiation (min)	Duration of phage irradiation (min)	Bacterial concentration (cells per mL)	Liberated phage concentration (phage per mL)
I	0	0	8×10^7	7×10^6
II	1	0	9×10^6	8×10^6
III	0	3	6×10^7	6×10^3
IV	1	3	5×10^6	8×10^4
V	2	3	4×10^4	4×10^4
VI	3	3	5×10^3	3×10^3
VII	45	3	0	0

Table 1

13) The liberated phage concentration in Trial VI is most likely lower than that in Trial V because in Trial VI there was/were:

A. fewer surviving infecting phages.
B. more damage to the phage DNA.
C. insufficient irradiation of the phage to activate the bacterial repair mechanism.
D. fewer surviving bacterial hosts.

14) If a scientist wishes to calculate the relative magnitude of bacteria-mediated phage repair, she must compare data from which of the following pairs of trials?

A. III and IV
B. I and VII
C. I and III
D. V and VI

15) An experiment is conducted to infect irradiated *E. coli* with irradiated phages and repaired-phage liberation is observed. In order to demonstrate that the repaired-phage liberation is due primarily to *E. coli's* DNA-repair mechanism, rather than a phage repair mechanism, an appropriate control in this experiment would be to infect:

A. nonirradiated bacteria with irradiated phages.
B. irradiated bacteria with irradiated phages.
C. nonirradiated bacteria with nonirradiated phages.
D. irradiated bacteria with nonirradiated phages.

High-level Importance

SPOILER ALERT

Gold Standard has cross-referenced the content in this chapter to examples from ACER's official GAMSAT practice materials. It is for you to decide when you want to explore these questions since you may want to preserve some of ACER's materials for timed mock-exam practice.

Examples – Easy question about the features of bacteria: Q47 of 1; graph-based exponential growth: Q104 and Q105 of 3; gene activation, promoters (BIO 2.2.1, 2.4): Q107 and Q108 of 5. Note that "Q" is followed by the question number, and, for example, "of 1" refers to booklet number 1 which is referenced in the Spoiler Alert table at the end of Chapter 1. The 15 full-length GAMSAT practice tests by Gold Standard, HEAPS-1 through HEAPS-15, contain specific cross-references to this chapter within the worked solutions. The graph-based colony-forming unit (CFU) questions in this chapter come from HEAPS-7.

Chapter Checklist

- ☐ Access your online account to view answers, worked solutions and discussion boards.
- ☐ Reassess your 'learning objectives' for this chapter: Go back to the first page of this chapter and re-evaluate the top 3 boxes and the Introduction.
- ☐ Complete a maximum of 1 page of notes using symbols/abbreviations to represent the entire chapter based on your learning objectives. These are your Gold Notes.
- ☐ Consider your multimedia options based on your optimal way of learning:
  - ☐ Download the free Gold Standard GAMSAT app for your Android device or iPhone.
  - ☐ Create your own, tangible study cards or try the free app: Anki.
  - ☐ Record your voice reading your Gold Notes onto your smartphone (audio files, e.g., *memo* or MP3s) and listen during exercise, transportation, etc.
  - ☐ Try out the Gold Standard GAMSAT online videos at gamsat-prep.com, or you can try other options on YouTube like Khan Academy or Crash Course Biology.
- ☐ Reassess your schedule for your full-length GAMSAT practice tests: ACER and/or HEAPS exams. Ensure that you have scheduled one full day to complete a practice test and 1-2 days for a thorough assessment of worked solutions while adding to your abbreviated Gold Notes.
- ☐ Reassess your progress in scheduling and/or evaluating stress reduction techniques such as regular exercise (sports), yoga, meditation and/or mindfulness exercises (*see* YouTube for suggestions).

References

α: Figure IV.A.2.1.1
Professor Graham Beards, Wikimedia Commons, 2022.

β: Figure IV.A.2.2.1
Alexey Solodovnikov; Wikimedia Commons; Protein Data Bank: 2mls, 6y3y, 5x29, 6yyt Charmmgui: 6vsb_1_1_1_S309; May 4, 2021.

δ: Figure IV.A.2.2.2
Funk CD, Laferrière C and Ardakani A (2020) A Snapshot of the Global Race for Vaccines Targeting SARS-CoV-2 and the COVID-19 Pandemic. Front. Pharmacol. 11:937.

PROTEIN SYNTHESIS

Chapter 3

Memorise

* The genetic code (triplet)
* Central Dogma: DNA ➡ RNA ➡ protein
* Definitions: mRNA, tRNA, rRNA
* Codon-anticodon relationship
* Initiation, elongation and termination

Understand

* Mechanism of transcription
* Mechanism of translation
* Roles of mRNA, tRNA, rRNA
* Role and structure of ribosomes
* One-gene–one-enzyme hypothesis
* The biosynthetic pathway

Importance

Medium level: 6% of GAMSAT Biology questions released by ACER are related to content in this chapter (in our estimation).
* Note that approximately 75% of the questions in GAMSAT Biology are related to just 7 chapters: 1, 2, 3, 4, 7, 12, and 15.

Introduction

Protein synthesis is the creation of proteins using DNA and RNA. Individual amino acids are connected to each other in peptide linkages in a specific order given by the sequence of nucleotides in DNA. Thus the process occurs through a precise interplay directed by the genetic code and involving mRNA, tRNA and amino acids - all in an environment provided by a ribosome. The “one-gene–one-enzyme hypothesis” and its relation to biosynthetic pathways comprise rather regular GAMSAT questions.

Multimedia Resources at GAMSAT-Prep.com

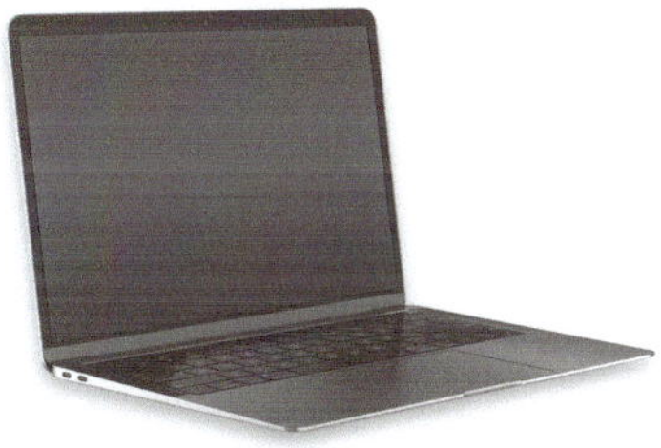

Open Discussion Boards
(*gamsat-prep.com/forum*)

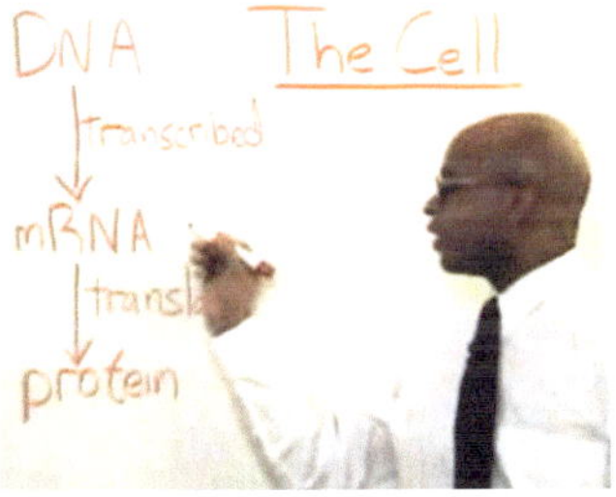

Foundational Videos

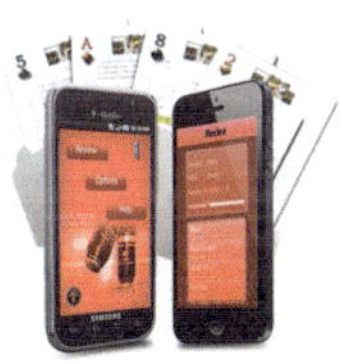

Flashcards

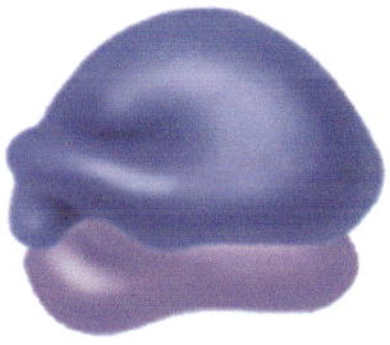

Special Guest

* The real GAMSAT may have advanced-level information presented (i.e. in a passage) but previous knowledge of said information is not required to answer the questions that would follow. Practice questions at the end of this chapter, as well as ACER and GS (HEAPS) practice GAMSATs can help you clarify this point.

3.1 Building Proteins

Proteins (which comprise many hormones, enzymes, antibodies, etc.) are long chains formed by peptide bonds between combinations of twenty amino acid subunits. Each amino acid is encoded in a sequence of three nucleotides (a triplet code = the *genetic code*). A gene is a conglomeration of such codes and thus is a section of DNA which encodes for a protein (or a polypeptide which is exactly like a protein but much smaller).

3.1.1 DNA Transcription

The information in DNA is rewritten (transcribed) into a messenger composed of RNA (= mRNA); the reaction is catalysed by the enzyme RNA polymerase. The newly synthesised mRNA is elongated in the 5′ to 3′ direction. It carries the complement of a DNA sequence.

Transcription can be summarised in 4 or 5 steps for prokaryotes or eukaryotes, respectively:

1. RNA polymerase moves the transcription bubble, a stretch of unpaired nucleotides, by breaking the hydrogen bonds between complementary nucleotides (*see* BIO 1.2.2 for nucleoside phosphates - nucleotides - and the binding of nitrogen bases).
2. RNA polymerase adds matching RNA nucleotides that are paired with complementary DNA bases.
3. The extension of the RNA sugar-phosphate

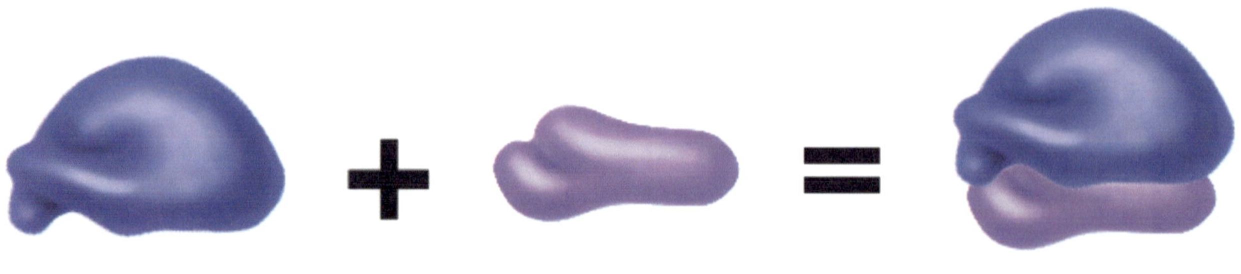

Figure IV.A.3.1: A ribosome provides the environment for protein synthesis. Ribosomes are composed of a large and a small subunit. The unit of measurement used is called the "Svedberg unit" (S) which is a measure of the rate of sedimentation in a centrifuge as opposed to a direct measurement of size. For this reason, fragment names do not add up (70S is made of 50S and 30S). Prokaryotes have 70S ribosomes, each comprised of a small (30S) and a large (50S) subunit. Eukaryotes have 80S ribosomes, each comprised of a small (40S) and large (60S) subunit. The ribosomes found in chloroplasts and mitochondria of eukaryotes also consist of large and small subunits bound together with proteins into one 70S ribosome. These organelles are believed to be descendants of bacteria ("Endosymbiotic theory") thus their ribosomes are similar to those of bacteria (*see* BIO 16.6.3).

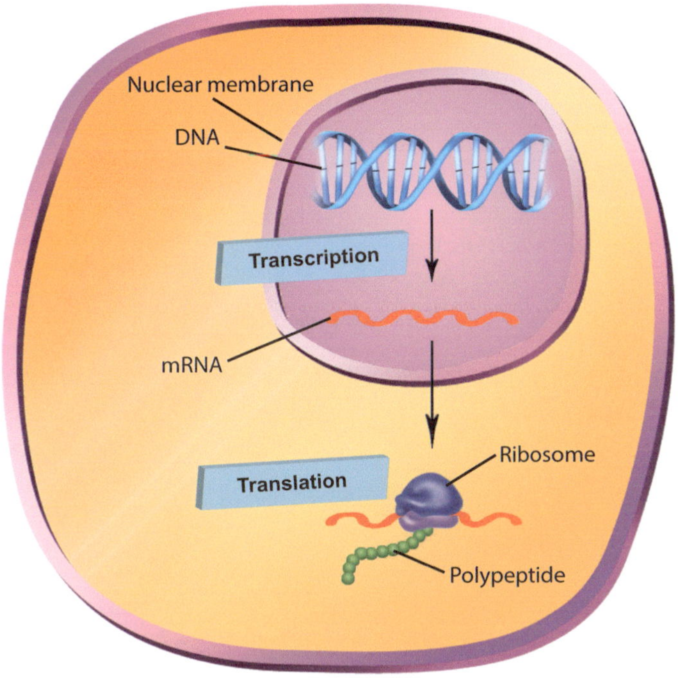

Figure IV.A.3.2: The central dogma of protein synthesis.

backbone is catalysed by RNA polymerase.

4. Hydrogen bonds of the untwisted RNA + DNA helix break, freeing the newly synthesised RNA strand.

5. If the cell has a nucleus, the RNA is further processed [addition of a 5′ cap and a 3′ poly(A) tail] and then exits through the nuclear pore to the cytoplasm.

The mRNA synthesis in eukaryotes begins with the binding of RNA polymerase at a specific DNA sequence known as promoters. Elongation continues until the RNA polymerase reaches a termination signal. The initially formed primary mRNA transcript, also called pre-mRNA, contains regions called introns that are not expressed in the synthesised protein. The introns are removed and the regions that are expressed (exons) are spliced together to form the final functional mRNA molecule. {EXons EXpressed; INtrons IN the garbage!}

Post-transcriptional processing of mRNA occurs in the nucleus. Even before transcription is completed, a 7-methylguanosine cap is added to the 5′ end of the growing mRNA serving as attachment site for protein synthesis and protection against degradation. The 3′ end is added with a poly(A) tail consisting of 20 to 250 adenylate residues as protection. Of course, "A" refers to adenine and the

Medium-level Importance

Note the following summary of protein synthesis[1]:

DNA —TRANSCRIBED in the nucleus—> mRNA —TRANSLATED in the cytosol—> protein

[1] for eukaryotes; in prokaryotes, some of the above-mentioned events occur simultaneously since they contain no nucleus. In fact, in bacterial cells it is common to have several ribosomes working in parallel on a single mRNA, forming what is called polyribosomes or polysome.

nucleotide is thus adenosine monophosphate or AMP (BIO 1.2.2, ORG 12.5) which *poly-merises* to create the tail of residues. The messenger then leaves the nucleus with the information necessary to make a protein.

Medium-level Importance

3.1.2 RNA Translation

The mRNA is constantly produced and degraded, which is the main method through which cells regulate the amount of a particular protein they synthesise. It attaches to a small subunit of a ribosome which will then attach to a larger ribosomal subunit thus creating a full ribosome. A ribosome is composed of a complex of protein and ribosomal RNA (= rRNA). The rRNA is the most abundant of all RNA types.

Floating in the cytoplasm is yet another form of RNA; this RNA specialises in taking amino acids and transfering them onto other amino acids when contained within the environment of the ribosome. More specifically, this transfer RNA (tRNA) molecule can be charged with a specific amino acid by aminoacyl-tRNA synthetase enzyme, bring the amino acid to the environment of ribosome, recognise the triplet code (= codon) on mRNA via its own triplet code anticodon, which is a three nucleotide sequence on tRNA that recognises the complementary codon in mRNA; and finally, tRNA can transfer its amino acid onto the preceding one thus elongating the polypeptide chain. In a way, tRNA translates the code that mRNA carries into a sequence of amino acids which can produce a protein.

Translation of mRNA into a protein involves three stages: initiation, elongation and termination. The direction of synthesis of the protein chain proceeds from the amino end/terminus to the carboxyl end/terminus. Synthesis begins when the ribosome scans the mRNA until it binds to a start codon (AUG), which specifies the amino acid methionine. During elongation, a peptide bond is formed between the existing amino acid in the protein

The 20 Amino Acids	The 64 DNA Codons
Alanine	GCT, GCC, GCA, GCG
Arginine	CGT, CGC, CGA, CGG, AGA, AGG
Asparagine	AAT, AAC
Aspartic acid	GAT, GAC
Cysteine	TGT, TGC
Glutamic acid	GAA, GAG
Glutamine	CAA, CAG
Glycine	GGT, GGC, GGA, GGG
Histidine	CAT, CAC
Isoleucine	ATT, ATC, ATA
Leucine	CTT, CTC, CTA, CTG, TTA, TTG
Lysine	AAA, AAG
Methionine	ATG
Phenylalanine	TTT, TTC
Proline	CCT, CCC, CCA, CCG
Serine	TCT, TCC, TCA, TCG, AGT, AGC
Threonine	ACT, ACC, ACA, ACG
Tyrosine	TAT, TAC
Tryptophan	TGG
Valine	GTT, GTC, GTA, GTG
Stop codons	TAA, TAG, TGA

Table IV.A.3.1: The 20 standard amino acids. Do not memorise.

chain and the incoming amino acid. Following peptide bond formation, the ribosome shifts by one codon in the 5′ to 3′ direction along mRNA and the uncharged tRNA is expelled and the peptidyl-tRNA grows by one amino acid. Protein synthesis terminates when the ribosome binds to one of the three mRNA termination codons (UAA, UAG or UGA; notice the similarity with the DNA stop codons in Table IV.A.3.1 except that U replaces T in this RNA molecule).

The 20 standard amino acids are encoded by the genetic code of 64 codons. Notice that since there are 4 bases (A, T, G, C), if there were only two bases per codon, then only 16 amino acids could be coded for ($4^2=16$). However, since at least 21 codes are required (20 amino acids plus a stop codon) and the next largest number of bases is three, then 4^3 gives 64 possible codons, meaning that some degeneracy exists.

Medium-level Importance

Degeneracy is the redundancy of the genetic code. Degeneracy occurs because there are more codons than encodable amino acids. This makes the genetic code more tolerant to point mutations (BIO 15.5). For example, in theory, fourfold degenerate codons can tolerate any point mutation at the third position (*see* valine, alanine, glycine, etc. in Table IV.A.3.1 and notice that any 3rd base codes for the same amino acid). The structure of amino acids is discussed in ORG 12.1.

A nonsense mutation is a point mutation (BIO 15.5) in a sequence of DNA that results in a premature stop codon (UAA, UAG, UGA), or a nonsense codon in the transcribed mRNA. Either way, an incomplete, and usually nonfunctional protein is the result. A missense mutation is a point mutation where a single nucleotide is changed to cause substitution of a different amino acid. Some genetic disorders (i.e. thalassemia) result from nonsense mutations.

Protein made on free ribosomes in the cytoplasm may be used for intracellular purposes (i.e. enzymes for glycolysis, etc.). Whereas proteins made on RER ribosomes are usually modified by both RER and the Golgi apparatus en route to the plasma membrane or exocytosis (i.e. antibodies, intestinal enzymes, etc.).

DNA	Coding Strand (codons)	5′→ →------ T T C ------→ → 3′
	Template Strand (anticodons)	3′← ←------ A A G ------← ← 5′
mRNA	The Message (codons)	5′ → →------ U U C ------→ → 3′
tRNA	The Transfer (anticodons)	3′ ← ← A A G ← ← 5′
Protein	Amino Acid	N-terminus → → Phenylalanine → → C-terminus

Table IV.A.3.2. DNA, RNA and protein strands with directions of synthesis. For both DNA and RNA, strands are synthesised from the **5′** ends → → to the **3′** ends. Protein chains are synthesised from the **N-terminus** → → to the **C-terminus**. Colour code: the **old** end is **cold blue**; the **new** end is **red hot** where new residues are added. As shown in the table, mRNA is synthesised complementary and antiparallel to the **template strand (anticodons)** of DNA, so the resulting mRNA consists of codons corresponding to those in the coding strand of DNA. The **anticodons of tRNA** read each three-base mRNA codon and thus transfers the corresponding **amino acid** to the growing **polypeptide chain** or **protein** according to the genetic code.

3.1.3 Key Points

Note the following: **i)** the various kinds of RNA are single stranded molecules which are produced using DNA as a template; **ii)** hormones can have a potent regulatory effect on protein synthesis (esp. enzymes); **iii)** allosteric enzymes (= proteins with two different configurations - each with different biological properties) are important regulators of transcription; **iv)** there are many protein factors which trigger specific events in the initiation (using a start codon, AUG), elongation and termination (using a stop codon) of the synthesis of a protein; **v)** one end of the protein has an amine group ($-NH_2$, which projects from the first amino acid), while the other end has a carboxylic acid group (-COOH, which projects from the last amino acid). {Amino acids and protein structure are explored in ORG 12.1 and 12.2}

Note that the free amine group end, the start of the protein, is also referred to as: N-terminus, amino-terminus, NH_2-terminus, N-terminal end or amine-terminus. The free carboxylic acid end, which is the end of the protein, is also referred to as: C-terminus, carboxyl-terminus, carboxy-terminus, C-terminal tail, C-terminal end, or COOH-terminus.

Differences in translation between prokaryotes and eukaryotes:

1) Ribosomes: in prokaryotes it is 70S, in eukaryotes it is 80S
2) Start codon: the start codon AUG specifies formyl-methionine [f-Met] in prokaryotes, in eukaryotes it is methionine
3) Location of translation: in prokaryotes translation occurs at the same compartment and same time as transcription, in eukaryotes transcription occurs in the nucleus while translation occurs in the cytosol.

Because of the incredible variety of organisms that use the genetic code, it was thought to be a *truly* 'universal' code but that is not quite accurate. Variant codes have evolved. For example, protein synthesis in human mitochondria relies on a genetic code that differs from the standard genetic code.

Furthermore, not all genetic information is stored using the genetic code. DNA also has regulatory sequences, chromosomal structural areas and other non-coding DNA that can contribute greatly to phenotype. Such elements operate under sets of rules that are different from the codon-to-amino acid standard underlying the genetic code.

Medium-level Importance

3.2 One Gene, One Enzyme, and the Biosynthetic Pathway

Duchenne muscular dystrophy (DMD) is a disease caused by a mutation in the DNA (X-linked recessive mutation; BIO 15.3). DMD patients have a mutation in the gene coding for the protein dystrophin. This protein connects the cytoskeleton to the extracellular matrix (thus through the plasma membrane) in muscle cells and appears to stabilise the muscle during contraction. Without dystrophin, the plasma membrane ruptures during muscle contraction and degeneration of the muscle tissue occurs (most DMD patients become wheelchair-dependent early in life). One gene, one protein and we can see how it is expressed in the organism (phenotype; BIO 15.1).

Experiments done in the 1940s, that would later give birth to Molecular Biology, used the bread mold *Neurospora* (a fungus; BIO 2.3) to conclude the following:

- Molecules are synthesised in a series of steps (= biosynthetic pathway, or, more generally: metabolic pathway)
- Each step is catalysed by a unique enzyme (of course, enzymes are proteins)
- Each enzyme is specified by a unique gene ("one gene, one enzyme").

As we will see in Chapter 4, in a metabolic pathway, a principal chemical is modified by a series of chemical reactions. Enzymes catalyse these reactions. Because of the many chemicals (= "metabolites") that may be involved, metabolic pathways can be complex. Consider the following straightforward synthetic pathway (Int = Intermediate):

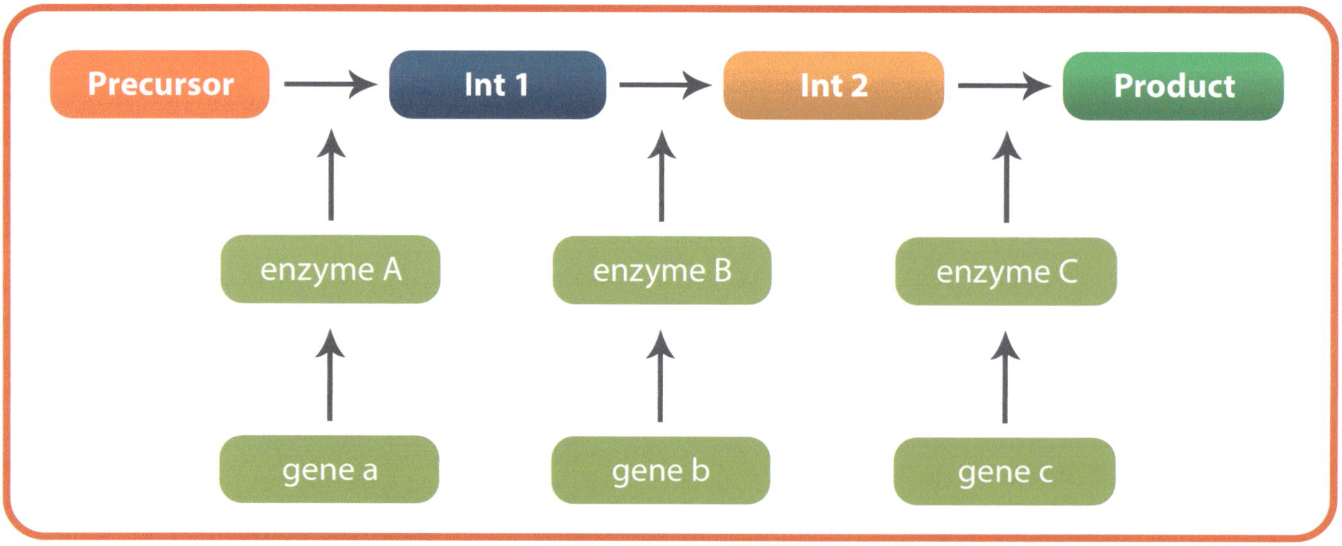

Consider the following questions:

1. Imagine that there was a mutation (or inactivation) in gene c, would any Product be produced? Would you expect the intermediates to be produced? Would their concentrations go up or down?
2. What would be the consequences of a mutation in gene b?
3. What happens if we add Intermediate 1 or Intermediate 2 to the media of a gene b mutation? Would either case result in Product? {Note: "media" is plural and

refers to a growth medium or culture medium which is a liquid or gel designed to support the growth of cells}

Consider your answers before continuing. You can expect questions like this on the real exam.

1. If there is a mutation at gene c then enzyme C is blocked (i.e. it is either not being produced or it is not functioning normally) which means the Product would not be produced and we would expect Intermediate 2 to increase in concentration (imagine a production line where one worker stops working but there continues to be items arriving at their desk, the result is accumulation at that point and non-production beyond that point).

2. A mutation at gene b stops the function of enzyme B thus the production of Intermediate 2 is blocked thus no Product is formed. Intermediate 1 begins to accumulate.

3. Adding Intermediate 1 just leads to its accumulation since we are presented with one way arrows so the reaction can only move forward but it is blocked because of the gene b mutation [had the arrows been double sided, which is quite normal in nature, then Le Chatelier's principle (CHM 9.9) would suggest that Precursor would be produced because of the stress of increasing Intermediate 1].

However, if Intermediate 2 is added to the media with the gene b mutation, since gene c is not mutated, the Product will be formed. Being beyond the 'blockage' caused by enzyme B dysfunction, the medium supplemented with Intermediate 2 bypasses the problem and is able to produce Product because there are no issues with gene c.

It should be noted that the one gene-one enzyme hypothesis predated the understanding of the genetic code and our modern understanding of enzymes – many of which are composed of multiple polypeptides (ORG 12.2), each of which is coded for by one gene. Thus "one gene-one polypeptide" would be more accurate but even so, remains incomplete because of more recent discoveries outside the scope of this exam.

Peptide: The result of the moon pulling on the Pepsi. ;)

At the time of publication, the preceding information would be helpful to solve ACER GAMSAT Red Booklet Unit 16, and Blue Booklet Unit 17, and somewhat helpful for Purple Booklet questions 87 and 88. In other words, the reasoning may be helpful during the real exam. Of course, your understanding will be tested in the GAMSAT-level practice questions in the next few pages.

CHAPTER 3: Protein Synthesis

GOLD STANDARD FOUNDATIONAL GAMSAT PRACTICE QUESTIONS

1) Which of the following enzymes is most important in RNA synthesis during transcription?

   A. DNA polymerase
   B. RNA replicase
   C. RNA polymerase
   D. Reverse transcriptase

2) The 3 base-pair sequence found on an mRNA strand is called which of the following?

   A. Codon
   B. Anticodon
   C. Genome
   D. Gene

3) Human mRNA with a length of 210 nucleotides likely codes for a protein of:

   A. approximately 210 amino acids.
   B. between 70 – 210 amino acids.
   C. exactly 70 amino acids.
   D. less than 70 amino acids.

4) A radioactive tracer can be used to track the distribution of a substance in the body or in a cell. If such a tracer is applied to amino acids which are then introduced into a cell, in which cellular structure would the radioactivity first become concentrated?

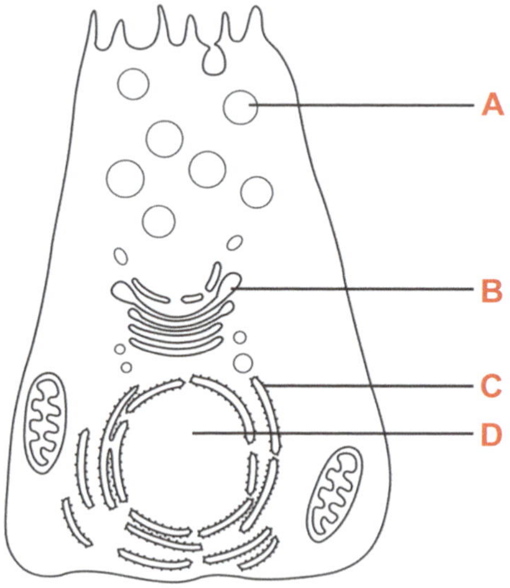

5) Given the nucleotide binding of A:T and G:C, and that in RNA U replaces T and binding is antiparallel, consider a segment of DNA that is 5′ AGT 3′. Which of the following represents the corresponding codon for the mRNA transcribed?

   A. 3′ ACU 5′
   B. 5′ TCA 3′
   C. 3′ UCA 5′
   D. 3′ UGA 5′

High-level Importance

GOLD STANDARD GAMSAT-LEVEL PRACTICE QUESTIONS

Questions 6–7

The red bread mold *Neurospora crassa* grows well on a cultural plate with "minimal" medium which is a fluid containing only a few simple sugars, inorganic salts, and vitamin. *Neurospora* that grows normally in nature (wild type) has enzymes that convert these simple substances into the amino acids necessary for growth. Mutating any one of the genes that makes an enzyme can produce a *Neurospora* strain that cannot grow on minimal medium. The mutant would only grow if the enzyme product were to be added as a supplement. On the other hand, if a "complete" medium is provided, containing all required amino acids, then *Neurospora* would grow, with or without mutation.

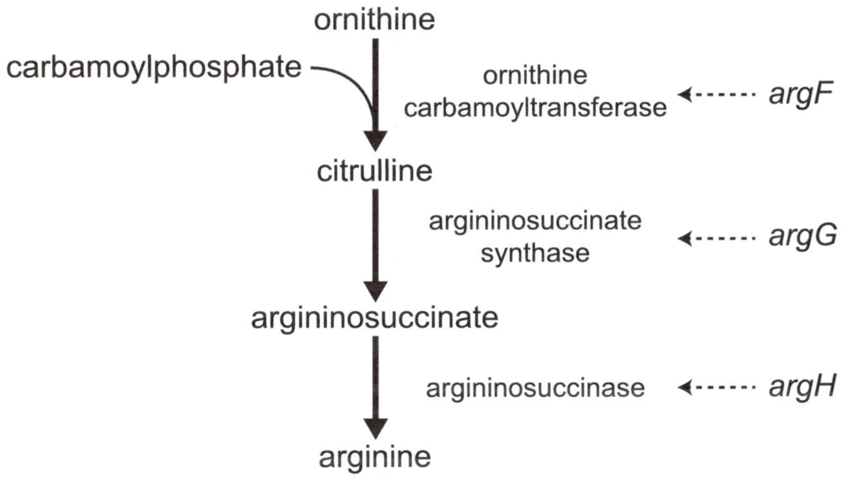

Figure 1: A synthesis pathway for the amino acid arginine. Each gene in italics in the diagram produces one enzyme necessary for the synthesis of this essential amino acid required for growth.

mutant strain	nothing	ornithine	citrulline	argininosuccinate	arginine
P	-	-	-	+	+
Q	-	-	-	+	+

Table 1: Growth response of mutant strains in "minimal" media with supplements as indicated. Growth is indicated by (+), and no growth is indicated by (-).

6) According to the information provided, a conclusion that can be made with certainty is that neither mutant strain P nor Q has the defective enzyme:

A. carbamoyltransferase.
B. argininosuccinate synthase.
C. argininosuccinase.
D. None of the above enzymes are defective in either mutant strain P nor Q.

7) Experiments using the two mutant strains P and Q, reveal that strain P accumulates citrulline, but strain Q does not. Which of the following statements is most consistent with the data provided?

A. Strain Q has only one mutation.
B. Strain P has a mutation in *argF* only.
C. Strain P has mutations in *argF*, *argG* and *argH*.
D. Strain P has a mutation in *argG* only.

Questions 8–12

A codon is a trinucleotide sequence of DNA or RNA that corresponds to a specific amino acid. The genetic code describes the relationship between the sequence of DNA bases (A, C, G, and T) in a gene and the corresponding protein/polypeptide (i.e. chain of amino acids) sequence that it encodes. Of the 64 three-letter codons, 1 is a start signal which begins the chain, and 3 are stop signals which end the chain but do not code for any amino acid. Consider Figure 1.

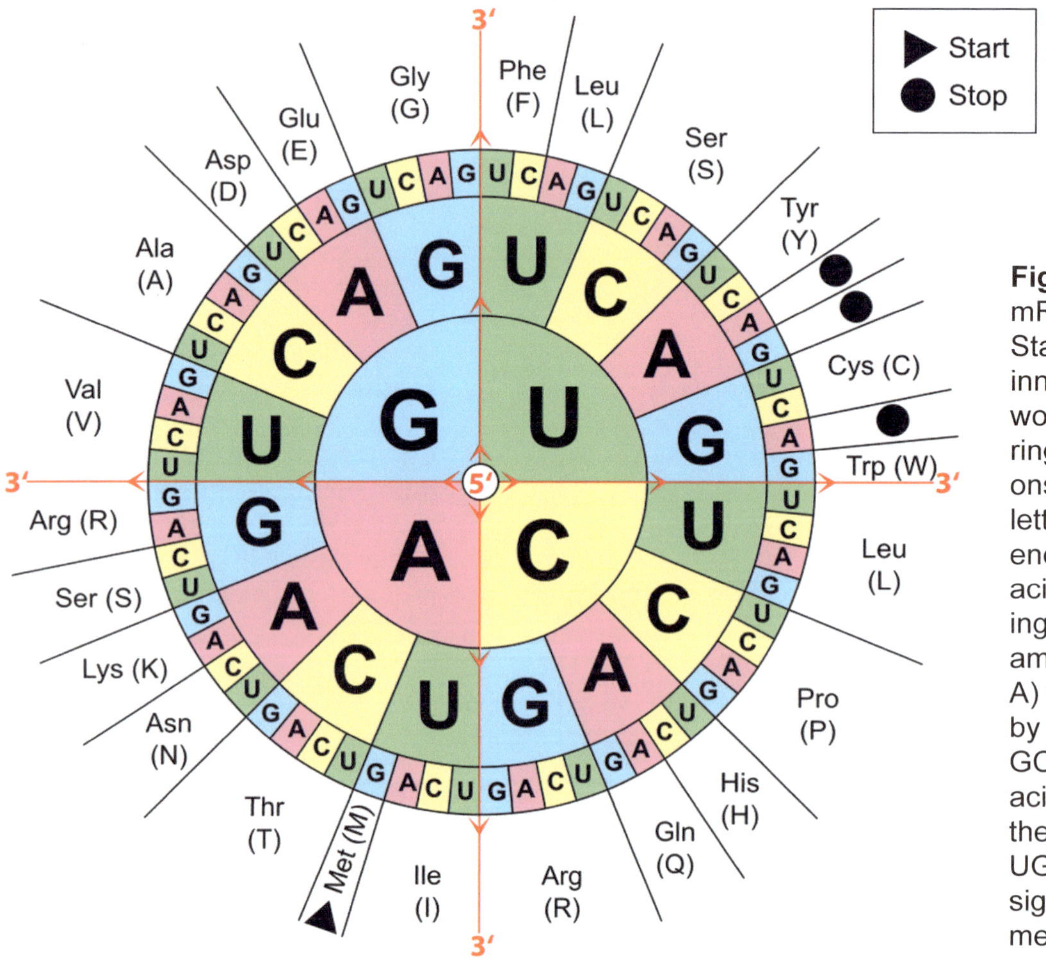

Figure 1: Amino acid mRNA codon wheel. Starting from the four innermost letters and working to the outermost ring, this chart demonstrates which three-letter base sequence encodes which amino acid. For example, reading from 5′ to 3′, the amino acid alanine (ala, A) can be represented by the three-letter codon GCU, and the amino acid cysteine (cys, C) by the three-letter codon UGU. Note the start signal AUG codes for methionine (met, M).

8) According to Figure 1, and reading from 5′ to 3′, which of the following represents a stop codon?

A. AUG
B. UAC
C. UGC
D. UGA

9) Consider the following mRNA codon sequence: 5′ AUGUCUUCGUUAUCC 3′. Based on Figure 1, which of the following represents the expected amino acid sequence?

A. met-leu-phe-arg-glu
B. met-ser-ser-leu-ser
C. met-glu-arg-arg-glu
D. met-ser-leu-ser-leu

10) Consider the following mRNA sequence:

5′-GCAUGCAAGUGAUGCAUAAAGAGUAGC-3′

If a polypeptide was encoded by the sequence above, how long (number of amino acids) would it be?

A. Less than 7
B. 7
C. 8
D. More than 8

11) Amino acids are sometimes identified by three-letter or one-letter abbreviations as can be seen in Figure 1 (i.e. Gly, G represents glycine). Considering the need for start and stop codons, how many different mRNA sequences can encode a polypeptide chain with the amino acid sequence M-L-R?

A. 12
B. 15
C. 36
D. 108

12) According to Figure 1, which of the following nucleotide sequences would code for the polypeptide sequence arg-gly-asp?

A. 5′-AGAGGAGAU-3′
B. 5′-GGGAAAUUU-3′
C. 5′-CGGGGUGAC-3′
D. More than one of the above is correct.

13) How many different tripeptides can be produced with the combination of one each of the amino acids Phe, Pro and Asp?

A. 2
B. 4
C. 6
D. 8

14) Consider tetrapeptides containing 2 equivalents each of the natural forms of arginine and proline. How many different linear tetrapeptides can be synthesised?

A. 2
B. 3
C. 6
D. 8

15) Minimum medium is a culture medium for microorganisms that contains inorganic salts, a carbon source, and water - which are the minimal necessities for growth of the wild-type (the organism that grows naturally in the wild). Consider the following branched biochemical pathway in the bacterium *P. syringae* which synthesises two related essential amino acids, alpha and beta in the presence of enzymes labelled 1 to 5:

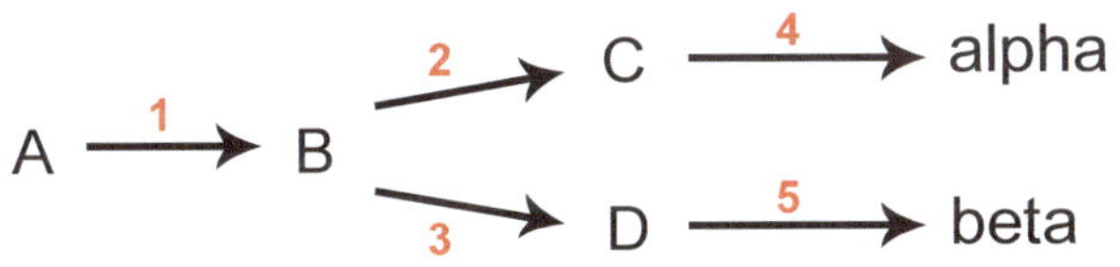

A mutant *P. syringae* defective for enzyme 1 will grow on minimal medium plus which of the following?

A. A only
B. B only
C. C or D
D. alpha or beta

High-level Importance

SPOILER ALERT

Gold Standard has cross-referenced the content in this chapter to examples from ACER's official GAMSAT practice materials. It is for you to decide when you want to explore these questions since you may want to preserve some of ACER's materials for timed mock-exam practice.

Examples – One gene, one enzyme pathway questions: 44-46 of 1; challenge: 48-50 of 2; central dogma of protein synthesis: Q77 of 4 (*see* Figure IV.A.3.2 in BIO 3.1); the antiparallel nature of DNA puzzle 90-93 of 5. Note that "Q" is followed by the question number, and, for example, "of 1" refers to booklet number 1 which is referenced in the Spoiler Alert table at the end of Chapter 1. The 15 full-length GAMSAT practice tests by Gold Standard, HEAPS-1 through HEAPS-15, contain specific cross-references to this chapter within the worked solutions. Note that the pathway unit ("The red bread mold") of the GAMSAT-level practice questions in this chapter come from HEAPS-6.

Chapter Checklist

- ☐ Access your online account to view answers, worked solutions and discussion boards.
- ☐ Reassess your 'learning objectives' for this chapter: Go back to the first page of this chapter and re-evaluate the top 3 boxes and the Introduction.
- ☐ Complete a maximum of 1 page of notes using symbols/abbreviations to represent the entire chapter based on your learning objectives. These are your Gold Notes.
- ☐ Consider your multimedia options based on your optimal way of learning:
    - ☐ Download the free Gold Standard GAMSAT app for your Android device or iPhone.
    - ☐ Create your own, tangible study cards or try the free app: Anki.
    - ☐ Record your voice reading your Gold Notes onto your smartphone (audio files, e.g., *memo* or MP3s) and listen during exercise, transportation, etc.
    - ☐ Try out the Gold Standard GAMSAT online videos at gamsat-prep.com, or you can try other options on YouTube like Khan Academy or Crash Course Biology.
- ☐ Reassess your schedule for your full-length GAMSAT practice tests: ACER and/or HEAPS exams. Ensure that you have scheduled one full day to complete a practice test and 1-2 days for a thorough assessment of worked solutions while adding to your abbreviated Gold Notes.
- ☐ Reassess your progress in scheduling and/or evaluating stress reduction techniques such as regular exercise (sports), yoga, meditation and/or mindfulness exercises (*see* YouTube for suggestions).

ENZYMES AND CELLULAR METABOLISM
Chapter 4

Memorise

* Define: catabolism, anabolism, activation energy
* Define: metabolism

Understand

* Enzyme basics, naming and classic graphs
* Feedback, competitive, non-competitive inhibition
* Krebs cycle, electron transport chain: basic features, follow the arrows
* Metabolism: carbohydrates (glucose), fats and proteins

Importance

Medium level: 7% of GAMSAT Biology questions released by ACER are related to content in this chapter (in our estimation).
* Note that approximately 75% of the questions in GAMSAT Biology are related to just 7 chapters: 1, 2, 3, 4, 7, 12, and 15.

GAMSAT-Prep.com

Introduction

Cells require energy to grow, reproduce, maintain structure, respond to the environment, etc. Biochemical reactions and other energy-producing processes that occur in cells, including cellular metabolism, are regulated in part by enzymes. GAMSAT tests almost always include multiple questions exploring your understanding of a cycle or biochemical mechanism with or without negative or positive feedback. The questions do not centre on your memorising details but rather having an understanding as to how the presented cycle functions or how it can be stimulated or inhibited. The end of Chapter 6 will focus on feedback loops with respect to hormones. Metabolism can be complex and it forms a story that you should be familiar with but that you should not spend time trying to memorise for the GAMSAT.

Multimedia Resources at GAMSAT-Prep.com

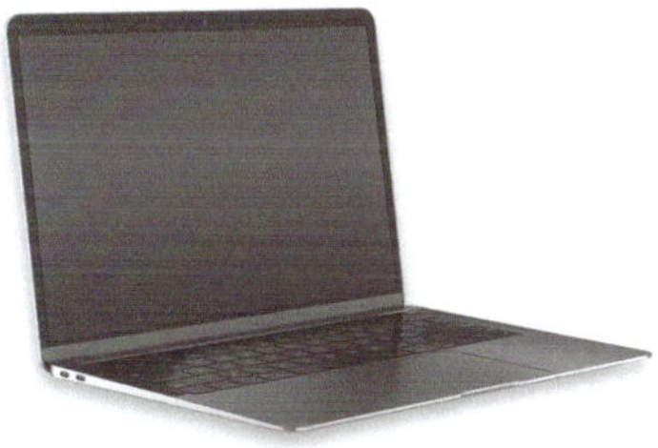

Open Discussion Boards
(*gamsat-prep.com/forum*)

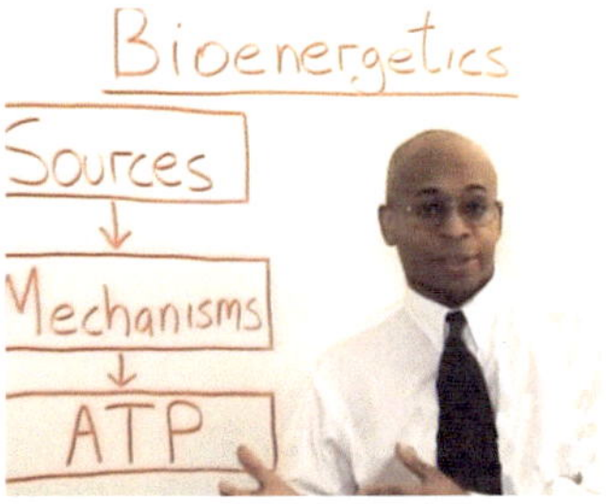

Foundational Videos

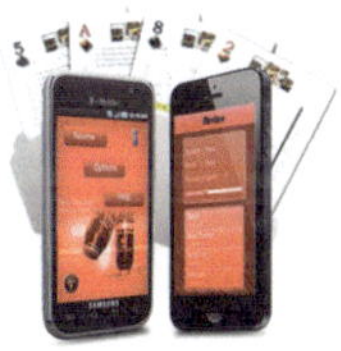

Flashcards

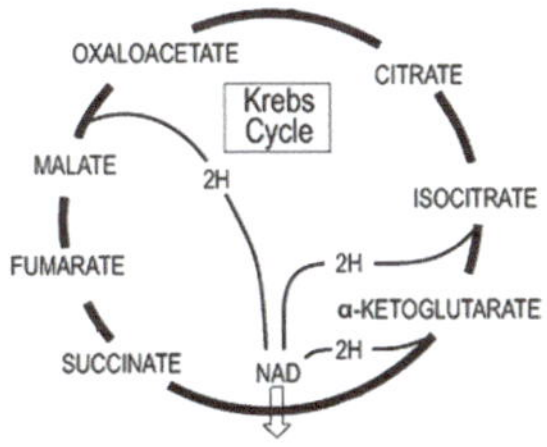

Special Guest

* The real GAMSAT may have advanced-level information presented (i.e. in a passage) but previous knowledge of said information is not required to answer the questions that would follow. Practice questions at the end of this chapter, as well as ACER and GS (HEAPS) practice GAMSATs can help you clarify this point.

4.1 Overview of Enzymes

Biochemical reactions are a necessary part of life, occuring in all organisms, and encompassing a wide variety of critical functions. All these biochemical reactions are collectively termed metabolism. In general, metabolism can be broadly divided into two main categories. They are:

(a) Catabolism which is the breakdown of macromolecules (larger molecules) such as glycogen to micromolecules (smaller molecules) such as glucose.

(b) Anabolism which is the building up of macromolecules such as protein using micromolecules such as amino acids. A good way to remember both is to break the terms down into their Greek roots - "cata" means "downward" (think catacombs), like the breaking *down* of macromolecules in catabolism, while "ana" means "upward." It's the same root words that give "cation" (a substance with fewer electrons than protons: +) and "anion" (a substance with more electrons than protons: -) their name.

As we all know, chemical reactions in general involve great energy exchanges when they occur. Similarly, most catabolic and anabolic reactions would involve massive amounts of energy if they were to occur *in vitro* (outside a living organism). However, all these reactions could be carried out *in vivo* (in a living organism) which is an environment of less free energy exchange, using molecules called enzymes.

What is an enzyme?

An enzyme is a protein catalyst. A protein is a large polypeptide made up of amino acid subunits. A catalyst is a substance that alters the rate of a chemical reaction without itself being permanently changed into another compound. A catalyst accelerates the rate of the reaction by decreasing the free energy of activation (E_a, the minimum energy the reactants need in order to form products; also discussed in CHM 9.5, 9.7). Note that although enzymes can reduce E_a, neither the overall energy of the reaction (ΔH) nor the equilibrium of the reaction is affected. The major observations are reflected in Fig. IV.A.4.0: The potential energy diagram for the complete oxidation (i.e. *combustion*) of glucose which produces carbon dioxide and water. This famous exothermic reaction (i.e. *releases heat/energy*) is a central component of bioenergetics (BIO 4.4).

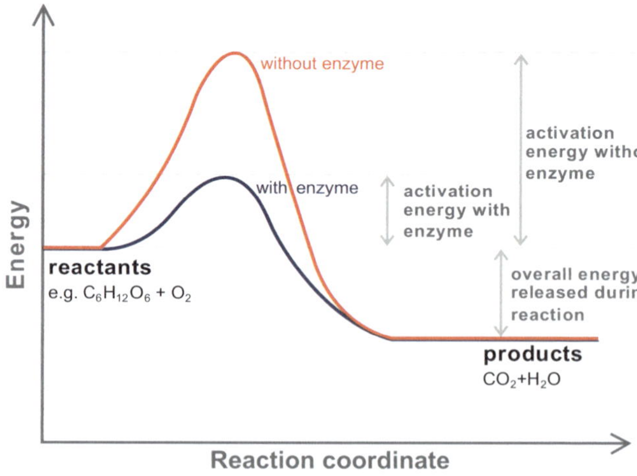

Figure IV.A.4.0: Potential energy diagram of the oxidation of glucose.

Enzymes fall into two general categories:

(a) Simple proteins, which contain only amino acids like the digestive enzymes ribonuclease, trypsin and chymotrypsin.

(b) Complex proteins, which contain amino acids and a non-amino acid cofactor.

Thus the complete enzyme is called a holoenzyme and is made up of a protein portion (apoenzyme) and a cofactor. Again, a helpful hint from Greek roots - "Apo" means "away from/separate," while "holo" means "whole."

Holoenzyme = Apoenzyme + Cofactor

A metal may serve as a cofactor. Zinc, for example, is a cofactor for the enzymes carbonic anhydrase and carboxypeptidase. An organic molecule such as pyridoxal phosphate or biotin may serve as a cofactor. Cofactors such as biotin, which are covalently linked to the enzyme, are called prosthetic groups or ligands.

The suffix "-ase" is a dead giveaway that the molecule in question is an enzyme. It also gives a hint as to the function of the enzyme. For instance, lactase is responsible for breaking down lactose into glucose and galactose; ligases ligate two molecules with covalent bonds; transferases transfer functional groups. Be careful, though - there are also many important enzymes that don't end with -ase, but as a general hint, it works.

Six Basic Types of Enzymes

Class of Enzymes	*What They Catalyse*
Oxidoreductases	Redox Reactions
Transferases	The transfer of groups of atoms
Hydrolases	Hydrolysis
Lyases	Additions to a double bond, or the formation of a double bond
Isomerases	The isomerisation of molecules
Ligases or synthetases	The joining of two molecules

In addition to their enormous catalytic power, which accelerates reaction rates, enzymes exhibit exquisite specificity in the types of reactions that each catalyses, as well as specificity for the substrates upon which they act. Their specificity is linked to the concept of an active site. An *active site* is a cluster of amino acids within the tertiary (i.e. 3-dimensional) configuration of the enzyme where the actual catalytic event occurs. The active site is often similar to a pocket or groove with properties (chemical or structural) that accommodate the intended substrate with high specificity.

Examples of such specificity are as follows: Phosphofructokinase catalyses a reaction between ATP and fructose-6-phosphate. The enzyme does not catalyse a reaction between other nucleoside triphosphates. It is worth mentioning the specificity of trypsin and chymotrypsin, though both of them are proteolytic (i.e. they degrade or hydrolyse proteins). Trypsin catalyses the hydrolysis of peptides

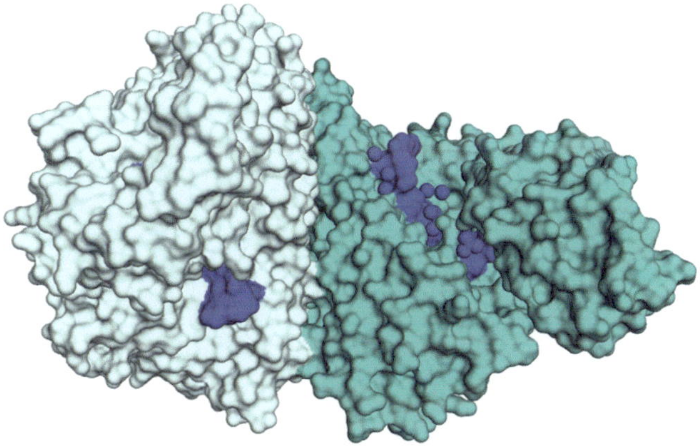

Figure IV.A.4.0a: Two molecules of human O-GlcNAc transferase, bound to their peptide substrates (dark blue), as determined my X-ray protein crystallography. The active site resembles a groove that selectively binds to its substrate with high specificity. (Protein Data Bank [pdb.org] code: 3PE4)

Medium-level Importance

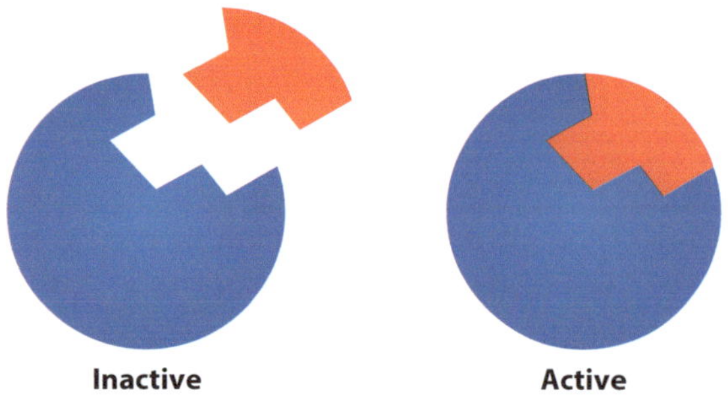

Figure IV.A.4.0b: Lock and Key model. On the left, the enzyme (blue) is rigid, with a pocket that is highly specific to a particular key, the substrate (red). On the right, when the key enters the lock, the enzyme becomes active.

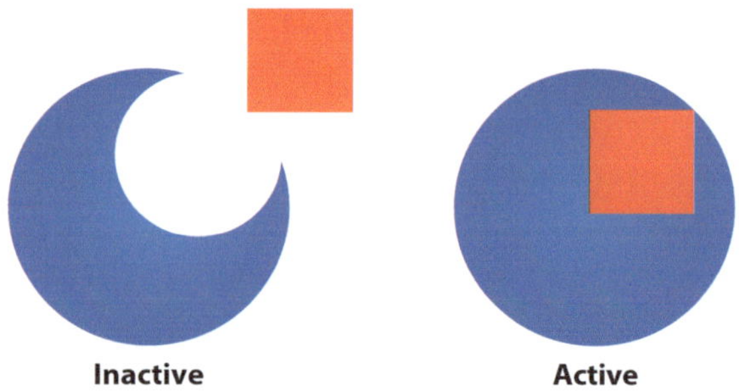

Figure IV.A.4.0c: Induced fit model. On the left, the active site of the enzyme (blue) is more flexible, but still specific to its substrate (red). On the right, upon binding, the substrate induces a conformational change, allowing the enzyme to change from an inactive form to an active form.

Medium-level Importance

and proteins only on the carboxyl side of the lysine and arginine. Chymotrypsin catalyses the hydrolysis of peptides and proteins on the carboxyl side of polypeptidic amino acids phenylalanine, tyrosine and tryptophan.

The degree of specificity described in the previous examples originally led to the **Lock and Key Model** which has been generally replaced by the **Induced Fit Hypothesis**. While the former suggests that the spatial structure of the active site of an enzyme fits exactly that of the substrate, the latter is more widely accepted and describes a greater flexibility at the active site and a conformational change in the enzyme to strengthen binding to the substrate.

4.2 Enzyme Kinetics and Inhibition

There is an increase in reaction velocity (= reaction rate) with an increase in the concentration of substrate. At increasingly higher substrate concentrations, the increase in activity is progressively smaller. From this, it could be inferred that enzymes exhibit saturation kinetics. The mechanism of the preceding lies largely with saturation of the enzyme's active sites. As substrate concentration increases, more and more enzymes are converted to the substrate bound enzyme complex until all the enzyme active sites are bound to substrate. After this point, further increase in substrate concentration will not increase reaction rate.

Enzyme inhibitors are classified as: competitive inhibitor, noncompetitive inhibitor and irreversible inhibitor. In competitive inhibition, the inhibitor and the substrate are analogues that compete for binding to the active site, forming an unreactive enzyme-inhibitor complex. However, at higher substrate concentration, the inhibition can be reversed. In noncompetitive inhibition, the inhibitor can bind to the enzyme at a site different from the active site where the substrate binds to, thus forming either an unreactive enzyme-inhibitor complex or enzyme-substrate-inhibitor complex. However, a higher substrate concentration does not reverse the inhibition. In irreversible inhibition, the inhibitor binds permanently to the enzyme and inactivates it (e.g. heavy metals, aspirin, organophosphates). The effects caused by irreversible inhibitors are only overcome by synthesis of new enzyme.

4.3 Regulation of Enzyme Activity

The activity of enzymes in the cell is subject to a variety of regulatory mechanisms. The amount of enzyme can be altered by increasing or decreasing its synthesis or degradation. Enzyme induction refers to an enhancement of its synthesis. Repression refers to a decrease in its biosynthesis.

Enzyme activity can also be altered by covalent modification. Phosphorylation of specific serine residues by protein kinases increases or decreases catalytic activity depending upon the enzyme. Proteolytic cleavage of proenzymes (e.g., chymotrypsinogen, trypsinogen, protease and clotting factors) converts an inactive form to an active form (e.g., chymotrypsin, trypsin, etc.).

Enzyme activity can be greatly influenced by its environment (esp. pH and temperature). For example, most enzymes exhibit optimal activity at a pH in the range 6.5 to 7.5. However, pepsin (an enzyme found in the stomach) has an optimum pH of ~ 2.0. Thus it cannot function adequately at a higher pH (i.e. in the small intestine). Likewise, enzymes function at an optimal temperature. When the temperature is lowered, kinetic energy decreases and thus the rate of reaction decreases. If the temperature is raised too much then the enzyme may become denatured and thus non-functional.

Enzyme activity can also be modified by an *allosteric* mechanism which involves binding to a site other than the active site. Isocitrate dehydrogenase is an enzyme in the Krebs Tricarboxylic Acid Cycle, which is activated by ADP. ADP is not a substrate or substrate analogue. It is postulated to bind a site *distinct* from the active site called the *allosteric site.* Positive effectors stabilise the more active form of enzyme and enhance enzyme activity while negative effectors stabilise the less active form of enzyme and inhibit enzyme activity.

Some enzymes fail to behave by simple saturation kinetics. In such cases a phenomenon called positive cooperativity is explained in which binding of one substrate or ligand shifts the enzyme from the less active form to the more active form and makes it easier for the second substrate to bind. Instead of a hyperbolic curve of velocity vs. substrate concentration [S] that many enzymes follow, a sigmoid-shaped curve of velocity vs. [S] characterises cooperativity (*see* the Enzyme Kinetic Curve Plot in this section, Figure IV.A.4.1, as well as myoglobin vs. hemoglobin, BIO 7.5.1).

Medium-level Importance

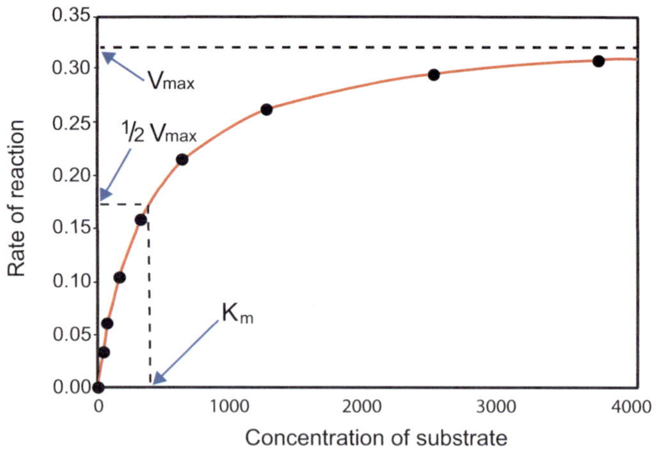

Michaelis-Menten Kinetics: Enzymes with single-substrate mechanisms usually follow the Michaelis-Menten model, in which the plot of velocity vs. substrate concentration [S] produces a rectangular hyperbola. Initially, the reaction rate [V] increases as substrate concentration [S] increases over a range of substrate concentration. However, as [S] gets higher, the enzyme becomes saturated with substrate and eventually the reaction rate [V] reaches maximum velocity V_{max} when the enzyme is fully saturated with substrate. Compare the diagram above with the curve of carrier-mediated transport (i.e. showing saturation kinetics) for solutes crossing the plasma membrane in BIO 1.1.2. The K_m is the substrate concentration at which an enzyme-catalysed reaction occurs at half its maximal velocity, $V_{max}/2$. K_m is called the Michaelis constant. Each enzyme has a unique K_m value. Famously, the hyperbolic curve traces the oxygen dissociation curve for myoglobin (BIO 7.5.1).

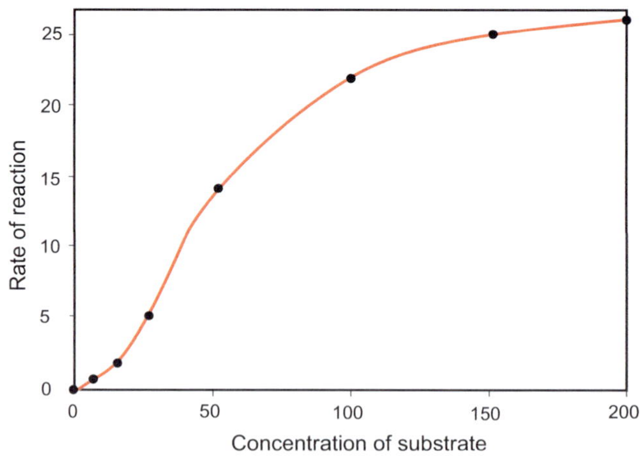

Non-Michaelis-Menten Kinetics: Some enzymes with multiple-substrate mechanisms exhibit the non-Michaelis-Menten model, in which the plot of velocity vs. substrate concentration [S] produces a sigmoid curve. This characterises cooperative binding of substrate to the active site, which means that the binding of one substrate to one subunit affects the binding of subsequent substrate molecules to other subunits. This behavior is most common in multimeric enzymes with several active sites. Positive cooperativity occurs when binding of the first substrate increases the affinity of the other active sites for the following substrates. Negative cooperativity occurs when binding of the first substrate decreases the affinity of the other active site for the following substrates. Famously, the sigmoidal curve traces the oxygen dissociation curve for hemoglobin (BIO 7.5.1).

Fig. IV. A. 4.1 Enzyme Kinetic Curve Plot.

Medium-level Importance

4.4 Bioenergetics

Biological species must transform energy into readily available sources in order to survive. ATP (adenosine triphosphate) is the body's most important short term energy storage molecule. It can be produced by the breakdown or oxidation of protein, lipids (i.e. fat) or carbohydrates (esp. glucose). If the body is no longer ingesting sources of energy it can access its own stores: glucose is stored in the liver as glycogen, lipids are stored throughout the body as fat, and ultimately, muscle can be catabolised to release protein (esp. amino acids).

We will be examining four key processes that can lead to the production of ATP: glycolysis, Krebs Citric Acid Cycle, the electron transport chain (ETC), and oxidative phosphorylation. Figure IV.A.4.2 is a schematic summary.

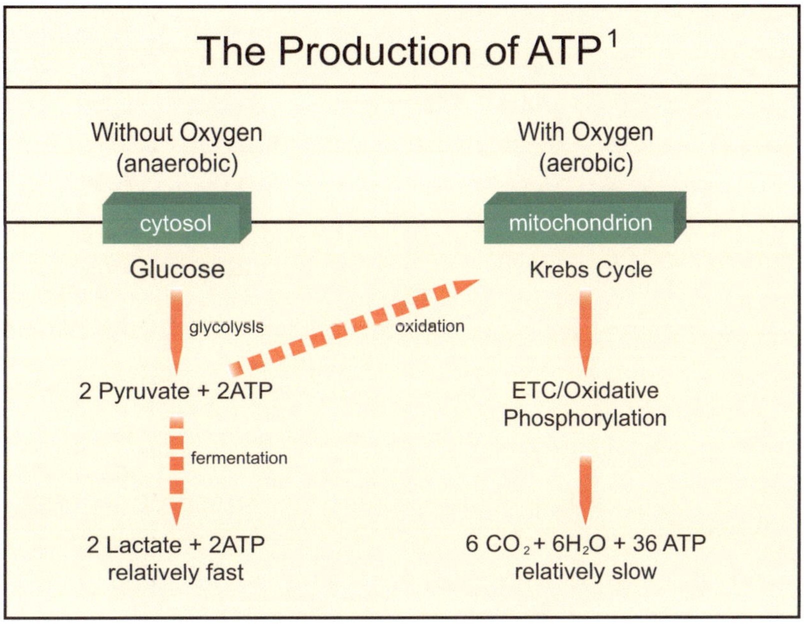

[1]from 1 molecule of glucose

Figure IV.A.4.2: Summary of ATP production.

4.5 Glycolysis

The initial steps in the catabolism or *lysis* of D-glucose constitute the Embden - Meyerhof glyco*lytic* pathway. This pathway can occur in the absence of oxygen (anaerobic). The enzymes for glycolysis are present in all human cells and are located in the cytosol. The overall reaction can be depicted as follows (ADP: adenosine diphosphate, NAD: nicotinamide adenine dinucleotide, P_i: inorganic phosphate):

$$\text{Glucose} + 2\text{ADP} + 2\ \text{NAD}^+ + 2\text{P}_i \longrightarrow 2\text{Pyruvate} + 2\text{ATP} + 2\text{NADH} + 2\text{H}^+$$

The first step in glycolysis involves the phosphorylation of glucose by ATP. The enzyme that catalyses this irreversible reaction is either hexokinase or glucokinase. Phosphohexose isomerase then catalyses the conversion of glucose-6-phosphate to fructose-6-phosphate. Phosphofructokinase (PFK) catalyses the second phosphorylation. It is an irreversible reaction. This reaction also utilises 1 ATP. This step, which produces fructose-1,6-diphosphate, is said to be the rate limiting or pacemaker step in glycolysis. Aldolase then catalyses the cleavage of fructose-1,6-diphosphate to glyceraldehyde-

Medium-level Importance

3-phosphate and dihydroxyacetone phosphate (= 2 triose phosphates). Triose phosphate isomerase catalyses the interconversion of the two preceding compounds. Glyceraldehyde-3-phosphate dehydrogenase mediates a reaction between the designated triose, NAD^+ and P_i to yield 1,3-diphosphoglycerate.

Next, phosphoglycerate kinase catalyses the reaction of the latter, an energy rich compound, with ADP to yield ATP and phosphoglycerate. This reaction generates 2 ATP per glucose molecule. Phosphoglycerate mutase catalyses the transfer of the phosphoryl group to carbon two to yield 2-phosphoglycerate. Enolase catalyses a dehydration reaction to yield phosphoenolpyruvate and water. The enzyme enolase is inhibited by fluoride at high, nonphysiological concentrations. This is why blood samples that are drawn for estimation of glucose are added to fluoride to inhibit glycolysis. Phosphoenolpyruvate is then acted upon by pyruvate kinase to yield pyruvate which is a three carbon compound and 2 ATP.

NADH produced in glycolysis must regenerate NAD^+ so that glycolysis can continue. Under **aerobic** conditions (i.e. in the presence of oxygen) pyruvate is converted to acetyl CoA which will enter the Krebs cycle followed by oxidative phosphorylation producing a total of 38 ATP per molecule of glucose (i.e. 2 pyruvate). Electrons from NADH are transferred to the electron transfer chain located on the inside of the inner mitochondrial membrane and thus NADH produced during glycolysis in the cytosol is converted back to NAD^+.

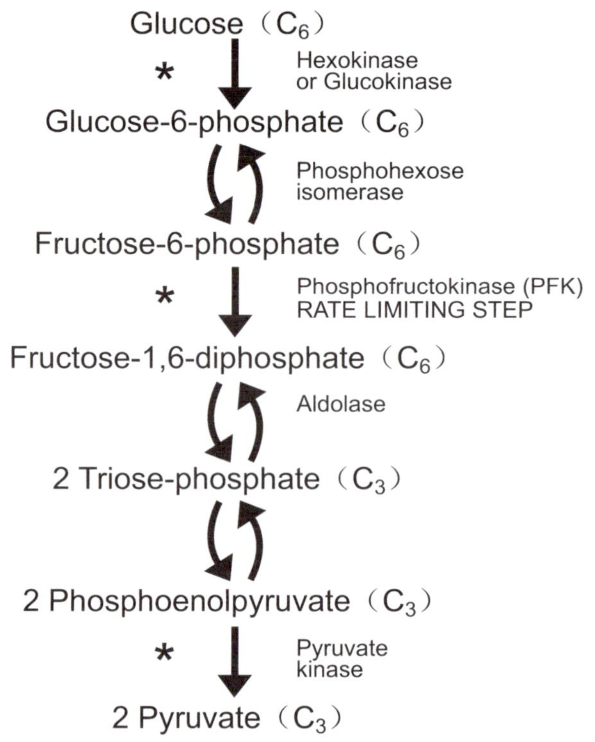

The symbol in brackets represents the number of carbons in each compound. The asterix represents steps which are functionally irreversible under physiologic conditions. PFK is involved in the rate limiting step which is activated by ADP and inhibited by ATP.

Figure IV.A.4.3: Summary of glycolysis.

Under **anaerobic conditions**, pyruvate is quickly reduced by NADH to lactic acid using the enzyme lactate dehydrogenase and NAD^+ is regenerated. A net of only 2 ATP is produced per molecule of glucose (this process is called *fermentation*).

Oxygen Debt: after running a 100m dash you may find yourself gasping for air even if you have completely ceased activity. This is because during the race you could not get an

Medium-level Importance

adequate amount of oxygen to your muscles and your muscles needed energy quickly; thus the anaerobic pathway was used. The lactic acid which built up during the race will require you to *pay back* a certain amount of oxygen in order to oxidise lactate to pyruvate and continue along the more energy efficient aerobic pathway.

4.6 Glycolysis: A Negative Perspective

Medium-level Importance

An interesting way to summarise the main events of glycolysis is to follow the fate of the phosphate group which contains a negative charge. Note that *kinases* and *phosphatases* are enzymes that can add or subtract phosphate groups, respectively.

The first event in glycolysis is the phosphorylation of glucose. Thus glucose becomes negatively charged which prevents it from leaking out of the cell. Then glucose-6-phosphate becomes its isomer (= *same* molecular formula, *different* structure) fructose-6-phosphate which is further phosphorylated to fructose-1,6-diphosphate. Imagine that this six carbon sugar (*fructose*) now contains two large negatively charged ligands which repel each other! The six carbon sugar (*hexose*) sensibly breaks into two three-carbon compounds (*triose phosphates*).

A triose phosphate is ultimately converted to 1,3-diphosphoglycerate which is clearly an unstable compound (i.e. *two negative phosphate groups*). Thus it transfers a high energy phosphate group onto ADP to produce ATP. When ATP is produced from a substrate (i.e. 1,3-diphosphoglycerate), the reaction is called *substrate level phosphorylation*.

A closer look at ATP and glycolysis: from one molecule of glucose, 2 molecules of pyruvate are obtained. During the glycolytic reaction, 2 ATP are used (one used in the phosphorylation of glucose to glucose 6-phosphate and one used in the phosphorylation of fructose 6-phosphate to fructose 1,6-bisphosphate) and 4 ATP are generated (two in the conversion of 1,3-bisphophoglycerate to 3-phosphoglycerate and two in the conversion of phosphoenolpyruvate to pyruvate).

4.7 Krebs Citric Acid Cycle

Aerobic conditions: for further breakdown of pyruvate it has to enter the mitochondria where a series of reactions will cleave the molecule to water and carbon dioxide. All these reactions (which were discovered by Hans. A. Krebs) are collectively known as the Tricarboxylic Acid Cycle (TCA) or Krebs Citric Acid Cycle. Not only carbohydrates but also lipids and proteins use the TCA for channelling their metabolic pathways. This is why

TCA is often called the final common pathway of metabolism.

The glycolysis of glucose (C_6) produces 2 pyruvate (C_3) which in turn produces 2 CO_2 and 2 acetyl CoA (C_2). Pyruvate is oxidised to acetyl CoA and CO_2 by the pyruvate dehydrogenase complex (PDC). The PDC is a complex of 3 enzymes located in the mitochondria of eukaryotic cells (and of course, in the cytosol of prokaryotes). This step is also known as the *link reaction* or *transition step* since it links glycolysis and the TCA cycle.

The catabolism of both glucose and fatty acids yields acetyl CoA. Metabolism of amino acids yields acetyl CoA or actual intermediates of the TCA Cycle. The Citric Acid Cycle provides a pathway for the oxidation of acetyl CoA. The pathway includes eight discrete steps. Seven of the enzyme activities are found in the mitochondrial matrix; the eighth (succinate dehydrogenase) is associated with the Electron Transport Chain (ETC) within the inner mitochondrial membrane.

The following includes key points to remember about the TCA Cycle: **i)** glucose → 2 acetyl CoA → 2 turns around the TCA Cycle; **ii)** 2 CO_2 per turn is generated as a waste product which will eventually be blown off in the lungs; **iii)** one GTP (guanosine triphosphate) per turn is produced by substrate level phosphorylation; one GTP is equivalent to one ATP (*GTP + ADP → GDP + ATP*); **iv)** *reducing equivalents* are hydrogens which are carried by NAD^+ (→ NADH + H^+) three times per turn and FAD (→ $FADH_2$) once per turn; **v)** for each molecule of glucose, 2 pyruvates are produced and oxidised to acetyl CoA in the "fed" state (as opposed to the "fasting" state). The acetyl CoA then enters the TCA cycle, yielding 3 NADH, 1 $FADH_2$, and 1 GTP per acetyl CoA. These reducing equivalents will eventually be oxidised to produce ATP (*oxidative phosphorylation*) and eventually produce H_2O as a waste product (the last step in the ETC); **vi)** the hydrogens (*H*) which are reducing equivalents are not protons (*H^+*) - quite the contrary! Often the reducing equivalents are simply called electrons.

4.8 Oxidative Phosphorylation

The term oxidative phosphorylation refers to reactions associated with oxygen consumption and the phosphorylation of ADP to yield ATP. The synthesis of ATP is coupled to the flow of electrons from NADH and $FADH_2$ to O_2 in the electron transport chain. Oxidative phosphorylation is associated with an Electron Transport Chain or Respiratory Chain which is found in the inner mitochondrial membrane of eukaryotes. A similar process occurs within the plasma membrane of prokaryotes such as *E.coli*.

The importance of oxidative phosphorylation is that it accounts for the reoxidation of reducing equivalents generated in the reac-

Medium-level Importance

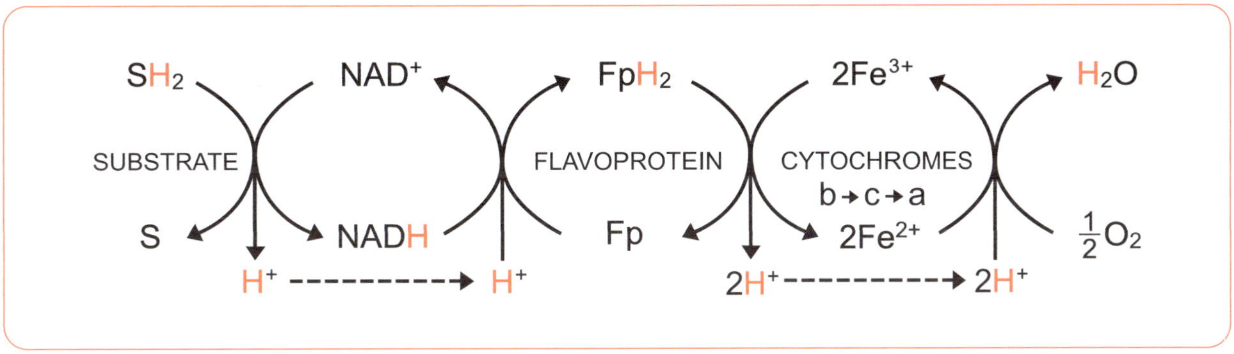

Figure IV.A.4.4: Transport of reducing equivalents through the respiratory chain. Examples of substrates (S) which provide reductants are isocitrate, malate, etc. Cytochromes contain iron (Fe).

tions of the Krebs Cycle as well as in glycolysis. This process accounts for the preponderance of ATP production in humans. The electron flow from NADH and $FADH_2$ to oxygen by a series of carrier molecules located in the inner mitochondrial membrane (IMM) provides energy to pump hydrogens from the mitochondrial matrix to the intermembrane space against the proton electrochemical gradient. The proton motive force then drives the movement of hydrogen back into the matrix thus providing the energy for ATP synthesis by ATP synthase. A schematic summary is in Figure IV.A.4.4.

The term *chemiosmosis* refers to the movement of protons across the IMM (a selectively permeable membrane) down their electrochemical gradient using the kinetic energy to phosphorylate ADP making ATP. The generation of ATP by chemiosmosis occurs in chloroplasts and mitochondria as well as in some bacteria.

Medium-level Importance

4.9 Electron Transport Chain (ETC)

The following are the components of the ETC: iron - sulphur proteins, cytochromes c, b, a and coenzyme Q or *ubiquinone*. The respiratory chain proceeds from NAD specific dehydrogenases through flavoprotein, ubiquinone, then cytochromes and ultimately molecular oxygen. Reducing equivalents can enter the chain at two locations. Electrons from NADH are transferred to NADH dehydrogenase. In reactions involving iron - sulphur proteins electrons are transferred to coenzyme Q; protons are translocated from the mitochondrial matrix to the exterior of the inner membrane during this process. This creates a proton gradient, which is coupled to the production of ATP by ATP synthase.

Electrons entering from succinate dehydrogenase ($FADH_2$) are donated directly to coenzyme Q. Electrons are transported from reduced coenzyme Q to cytochrome b and then cytochrome c. Electrons are then carried by cytochrome c to cytochrome a. Cytochrome a is also known as *cytochrome oxidase*. It catalyses the reaction of electrons and protons with molecular oxygen to produce water. Cyanide and carbon monoxide are powerful inhibitors of cytochrome oxidase.

4.10 Summary of Energy Production

Note the following: **i)** 1 NADH produces 3 ATP molecules while 1 $FADH_2$ produces only 2 ATP; **ii)** there is a cost of 2 ATP to get the two molecules of NADH generated in the cytoplasm (*see* the preceding point # 2.) to enter the mitochondrion, thus the *net yield for eukaryotes is 36 ATP.*

The efficiency of ATP production is far from 100%. Energy is lost from the system primarily in the form of heat. Under standard conditions, less than 40% of the energy generated from the complete oxidation of glucose is converted to the production of ATP. As a comparison, a gasoline engine fairs much worse with an efficiency rating generally less than 30%. Further inefficiencies reduce the net theoretical yield in the (non-GAMSAT!) real world.

Process of reaction	ATP yield
1. Glycolysis (Glucose → 2 Pyruvate)	2
2. Glycolysis (2NADH from glyceraldehyde-3-phosphate dehydrogenase)	6
3. Pyruvate dehydrogenase (2NADH)	6
4. Isocitrate dehydrogenase (2NADH)	6
5. Alpha-ketoglutarate dehydrogenase (2NADH)	6
6. Succinate thiokinase (2GTP)	2
7. Succinate dehydrogenase ($2FADH_2$)	4
8. Malate dehydrogenase (2NADH)	6
TOTAL	38 ATP yield per hexose.

Medium-level Importance

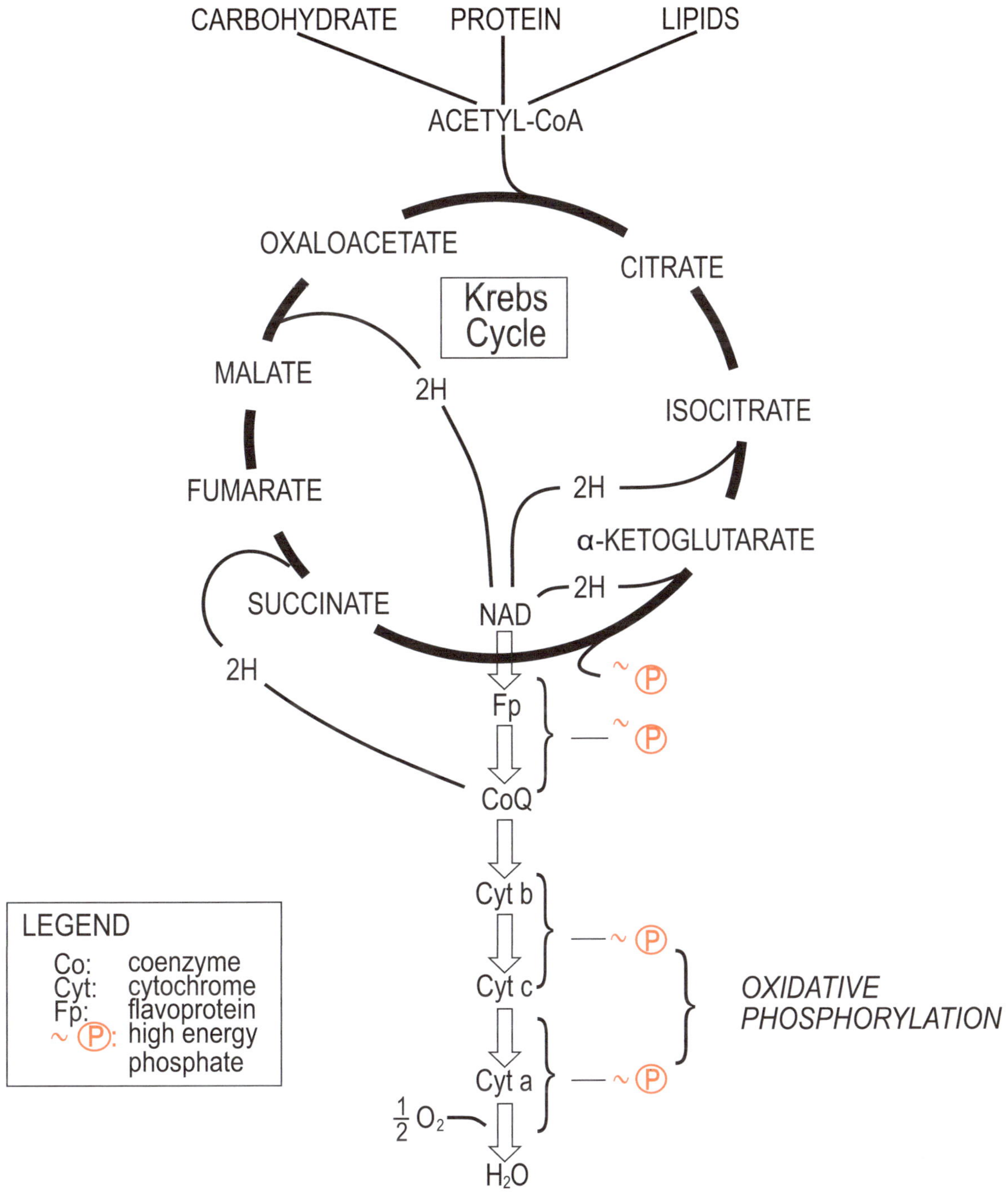

Figure IV.A.4.5: Summary of the Krebs Cycle and the Electron Transport Chain.

Note: Acetyl CoA can be the product of carbohydrate, protein, or lipid metabolism. Thick black arrows represent the Krebs Cycle while white arrows represent the Electron Transport Chain. High energy phosphate groups are transferred from ADP to produce ATP. Ultimately, oxygen accepts electrons and hydrogen from Cyt a to produce water.

High-level Importance

CHAPTER 4: Enzymes and Cellular Metabolism

GOLD STANDARD FOUNDATIONAL GAMSAT PRACTICE QUESTIONS

1) All of the following are characteristics of most enzymes, EXCEPT:
   - A. they affect the equilibrium of reaction.
   - B. they affect the rate of reaction.
   - C. they are specific to particular substrates.
   - D. they lower the energy of activation of a chemical reaction.

2) Phenylalanine hydroxylase most likely:
   - A. cleaves a $-OCH_3$ group from phenylalanine.
   - B. adds a $-OCH_3$ group to phenylalanine.
   - C. cleaves a $-OH_2$ group from phenylalanine.
   - D. adds a -OH group to phenylalanine.

3) Most body heat, under normal conditions, is produced by:
   - A. the reduction of foods.
   - B. the oxidation of foods.
   - C. the breakdown of skeletal muscle.
   - D. the blocking of thyroid stimulating hormone.

4) In eukaryotic cells, cellular respiration in the presence of oxygen occurs in the:
   - A. cytosol.
   - B. ATP.
   - C. ribosomes.
   - D. mitochondria.

GOLD STANDARD GAMSAT-LEVEL PRACTICE QUESTIONS

5) Consider Figure 1, where the black dots represent the active form of enzyme M and the white dots represent the active form of enzyme N at varying pH values and temperatures.

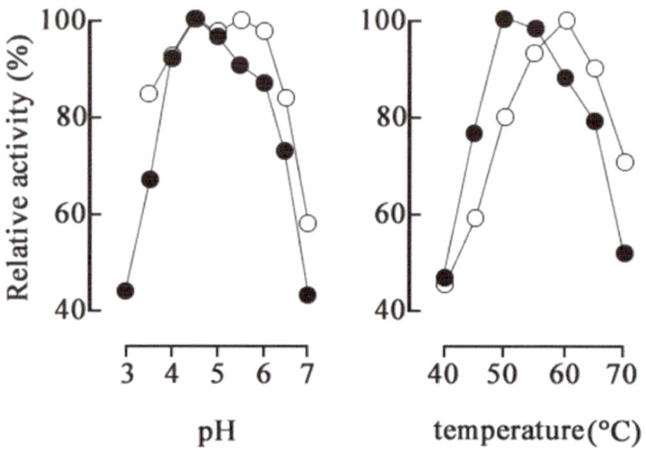

Figure 1

Which of the following can be correctly determined from Figure 1?

   - A. In reaching its peak, enzyme N exhibits the greater increase in activity per degree Celsius.
   - B. Enzyme M can sustain a percentage activity of more than 80% over a wider pH range.
   - C. Based on the data below 50 °C, extrapolating a linear regression line predicts that enzyme M would have less than 20% activity at 30 °C.
   - D. Given either a particular pH or temperature, there are instances of more than 30% difference in activity between the two enzymes under study.

6) Consider Figure 1.

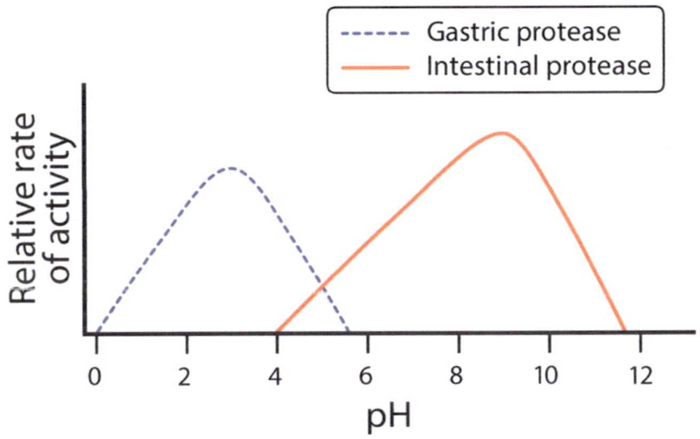

Figure 1

The optimal activity for the intestinal protease occurs in an environment that contains what factor of hydrogen ion concentration as compared to the optimal activity for the gastric protease?

A. 0.000001x
B. 2x
C. 3x
D. 1 000 000x

7) Consider Figure 1.

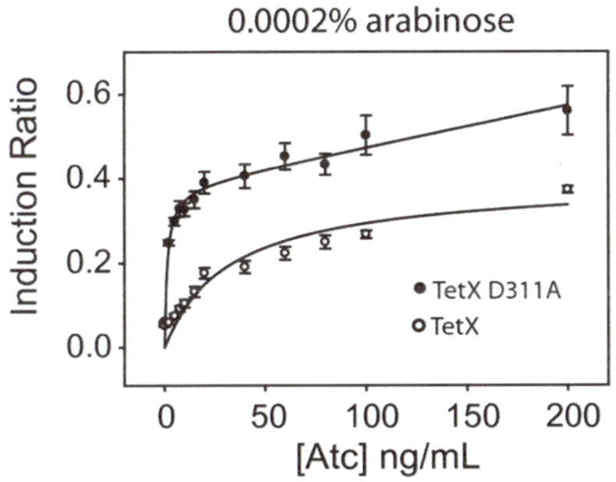

Figure 1: Induction ratios in the presence of inactive (•) and active (○) enzymes in the presence of increasing concentrations of anhydrotetracycline (Atc). Yu Z. et al, BMC Biochem, 2010.

The data in Figure 1 suggests that adding 500 ng/mL of anhydrotetracycline in the presence of active TetX will likely have an induction ratio within the range of which of the following?

A. Below 0.2
B. Between 0.3 and 0.4
C. Between 0.5 and 0.6
D. Above 0.6

8) Consider Figure 1 and the Michaelis-Menten equation.

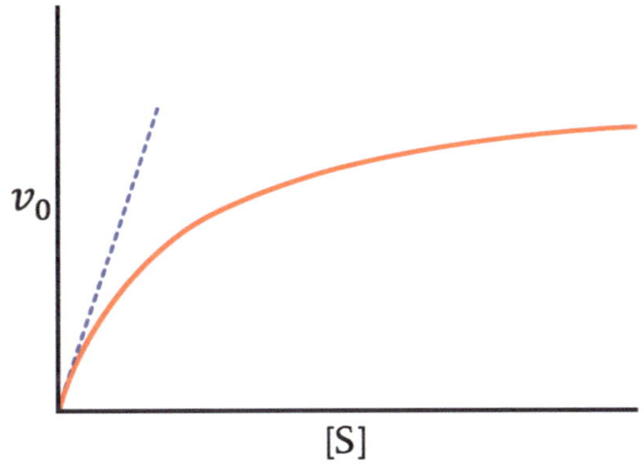

Figure 1: Initial velocity v_0 versus substrate concentration [S] in an enzyme-catalysed reaction demonstrating Michaelis-Menten kinetics. The dashed line indicates the slope of the curve when [S] << K_m.

The Michaelis-Menten equation:

$$v_0 = \frac{k_{cat}[E_t][S]}{[S] + K_m} = \frac{V_{max}[S]}{[S] + K_m}$$

Which of the following corresponds to the slope of the dashed line in Figure 1?

A. (1/2)[S]
B. V_{max}/K_m
C. k_{cat}/K_m
D. $1/V_{max}$

High-level Importance

Questions 9–14

Figure 1 is a diagram containing a summary of cellular respiration including glycolysis, the Krebs cycle (i.e. the citric acid cycle), and the electron transport chain. Note that the number of carbons in many of the molecules are designated, for example, "glucose C_6" indicates that glucose has 6 carbons.

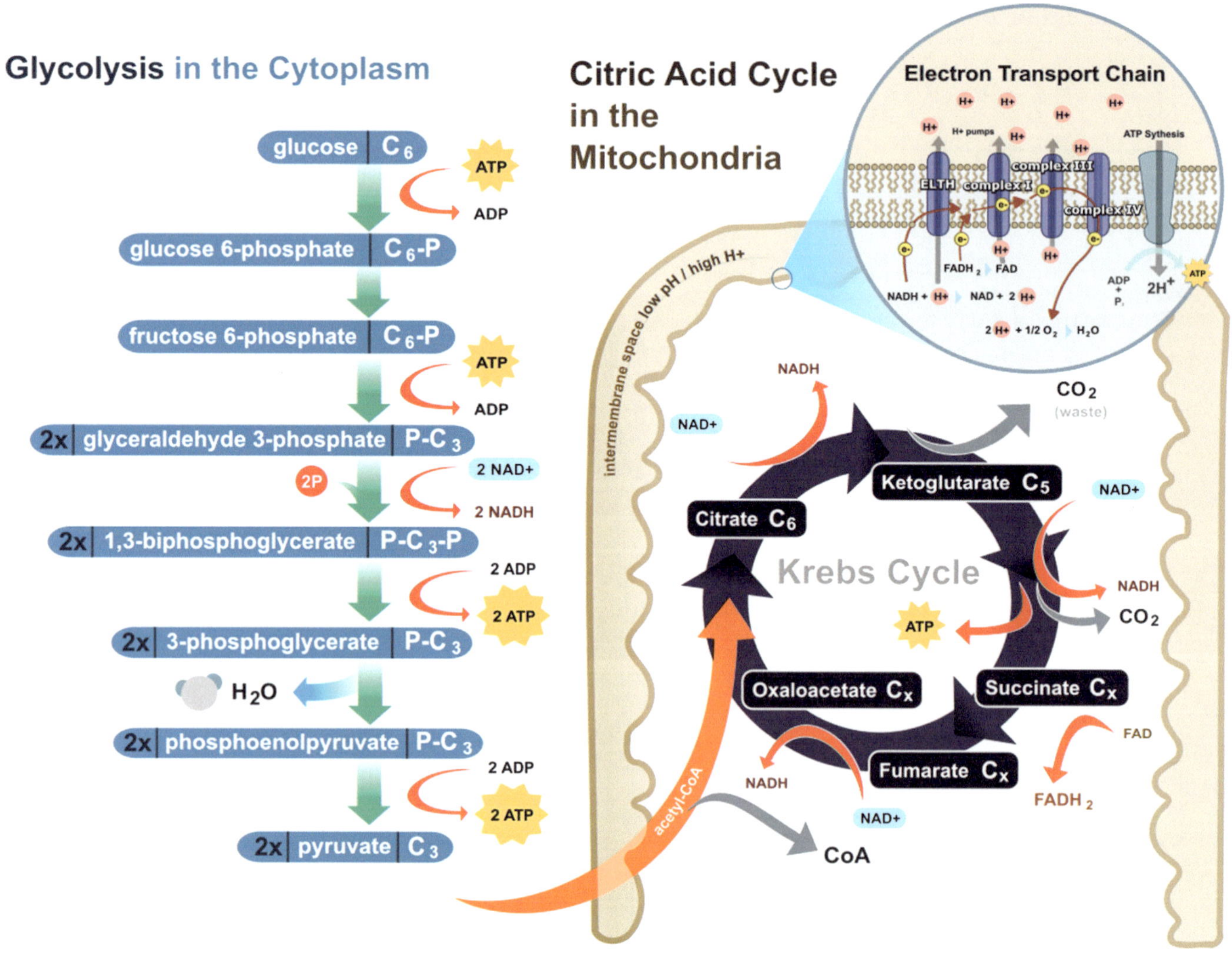

Figure 1 (ref: RegisFrey)

9) The cell in Figure 1 is likely:

A. a prokaryote.
B. a virus.
C. in metaphase.
D. in interphase.

10) In Figure 1, there are 3 intermediates in the Krebs cycle with the designation C_x. How many carbons would the intermediate fumarate be expected to have?

A. 3
B. 4
C. 5
D. 6

11) Based on Figure 1, per molecule of glucose, which of the following is true regarding the reactions that comprise glycolysis?

A. No ATP molecule is used and six ATP molecules are generated.
B. Two ATP molecules are used and four ATP molecules are generated.
C. Six ATP molecules are used and two ATP molecules are generated.
D. Six ATP molecules are used and four ATP molecules are generated.

12) What type of chemical reaction is responsible for the following step in glycolysis?

glyceraldehyde 3-phosphate → 1,3-biphosphoglycerate

A. Decarboxylation
B. Dehydration
C. Oxidation
D. Hydration

13) Consider that all glucose consumed by a particular yeast undergoes glycolysis to pyruvate and then produces ethanol and carbon dioxide. Based on Figure 1, how many molecules of each would be expected per molecule of glucose?

A. Two of carbon dioxide and two of ethanol
B. Two of carbon dioxide and one of ethanol
C. Three of carbon dioxide and one of ethanol
D. One of carbon dioxide and two of ethanol

14) Pyruvate kinase deficiency is an inherited, sometimes fatal metabolic disorder. Pyruvate kinase is the last enzyme involved in the glycolytic process, transferring the phosphate group from phosphoenolpyruvate to a waiting ADP. Based on Figure 1, all of the following would be expected to have a decrease in concentration with pyruvate kinase deficiency EXCEPT:

A. glucose.
B. pyruvate.
C. ATP.
D. succinate.

15) Consider the potential energy diagram in Figure 1 representing a biochemical reaction.

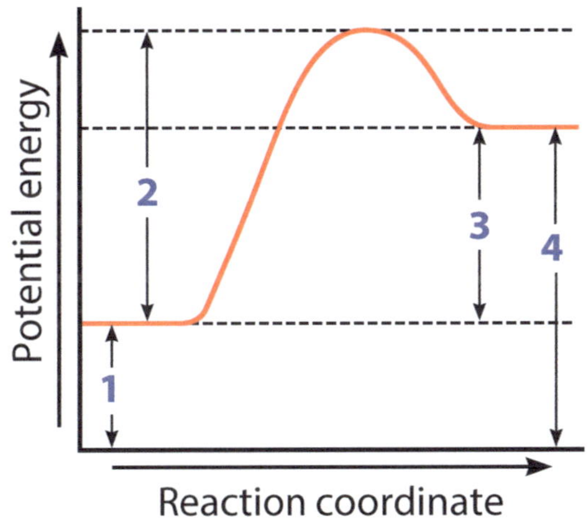

Figure 1

Which numbered interval in Figure 1 would change when an enzyme is added?

A. 1
B. 2
C. 3
D. 4

High-level Importance

High-level Importance

SPOILER ALERT ⚠

Gold Standard has cross-referenced the content in this chapter to examples from ACER's official GAMSAT practice materials. It is for you to decide when you want to explore these questions since you may want to preserve some of ACER's materials for timed mock-exam practice.

Examples – Potential energy diagram – activation energy: Q49-51 of 3; gastric enzyme pathway: Q1-5 of 4; type of cell with organelles: Q12-13 of 4; identify the name of an enzyme: Q78 of 4; following carbons and moles in a metabolic pathway: Q35-36 of 5. Note that "Q" is followed by the question number, and, for example, "of 1" refers to booklet number 1 which is referenced in the Spoiler Alert table at the end of Chapter 1. The 15 full-length GAMSAT practice tests by Gold Standard, HEAPS-1 through HEAPS-15, contain specific cross-references to this chapter within the worked solutions. The graph-based pH and temperature question in this chapter comes from HEAPS-5.

Chapter Checklist

- ☐ Access your online account to view answers, worked solutions and discussion boards.
- ☐ Reassess your 'learning objectives' for this chapter: Go back to the first page of this chapter and re-evaluate the top 3 boxes and the Introduction.
- ☐ Complete a maximum of 1 page of notes using symbols/abbreviations to represent the entire chapter based on your learning objectives. These are your Gold Notes.
- ☐ Consider your multimedia options based on your optimal way of learning:
  - ☐ Download the free Gold Standard GAMSAT app for your Android device or iPhone.
  - ☐ Create your own, tangible study cards or try the free app: Anki.
  - ☐ Record your voice reading your Gold Notes onto your smartphone (audio files, e.g., *memo* or MP3s) and listen during exercise, transportation, etc.
  - ☐ Try out the Gold Standard GAMSAT online videos at gamsat-prep.com, or you can try other options on YouTube like Khan Academy or Crash Course Biology.
- ☐ Reassess your schedule for your full-length GAMSAT practice tests: ACER and/or HEAPS exams. Ensure that you have scheduled one full day to complete a practice test and 1-2 days for a thorough assessment of worked solutions while adding to your abbreviated Gold Notes.
- ☐ Reassess your progress in scheduling and/or evaluating stress reduction techniques such as regular exercise (sports), yoga, meditation and/or mindfulness exercises (*see* YouTube for suggestions).

SPECIALISED EUKARYOTIC CELLS AND TISSUES
Chapter 5

Memorise	Understand	Importance
* Neuron: basic structure and function * Reasons for the membrane potential	* Resting potential: electrochemical gradient/action potential, graph * Excitatory and inhibitory nerve fibers: summation, frequency of firing * Organisation of contractile elements: actin and myosin filaments * Cross bridges, sliding filament model; calcium regulation of contraction	**Low level: 1% of GAMSAT Biology** questions released by ACER are related to content in this chapter (in our estimation). * Note that approximately 75% of the questions in GAMSAT Biology are related to just 7 chapters: 1, 2, 3, 4, 7, 12, and 15.

GAMSAT-Prep.com

Introduction

To build a living organism, with all the various tissues and organs, cells must specialise. Communication among cells and organs, movement, protection and support are achieved to a great degree by neurons, muscle cells, epithelial cells and the cells of connective tissue, respectively.

This chapter contains a lot of content with a small GAMSAT assumed-knowledge footprint. Read the chapter like a story that might be helpful to be familiar with, but avoid rote learning, and be guided by the learning objectives above. The GAMSAT-level practice questions at the end of this chapter offer significant graph and table analysis, including logs, that will help you for most Section 3 topics.

Multimedia Resources at GAMSAT-Prep.com

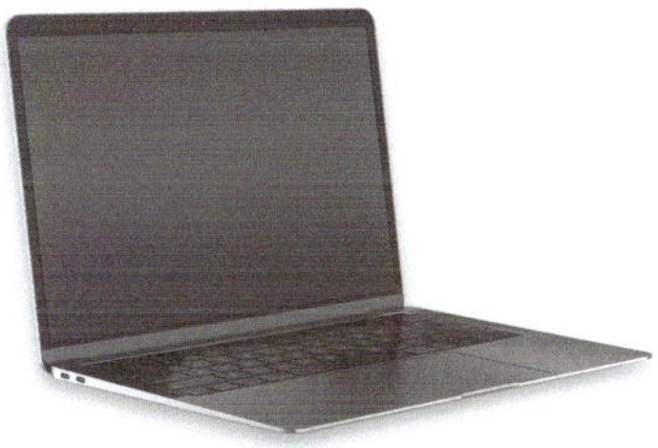

Open Discussion Boards
(*gamsat-prep.com/forum*)

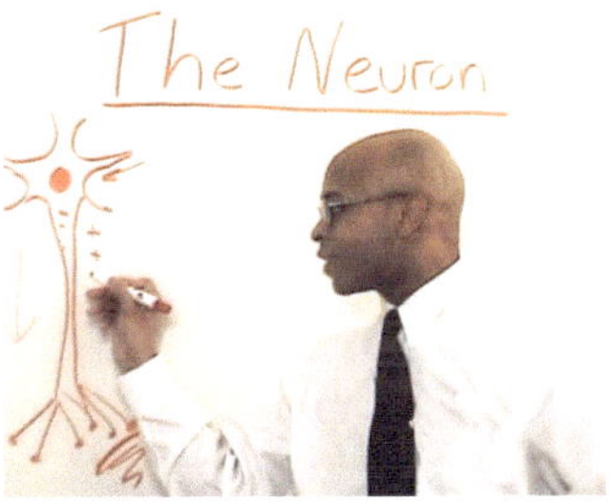

Foundational Videos

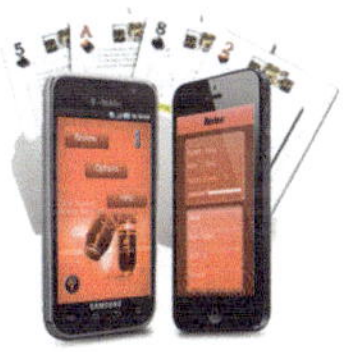

Flashcards

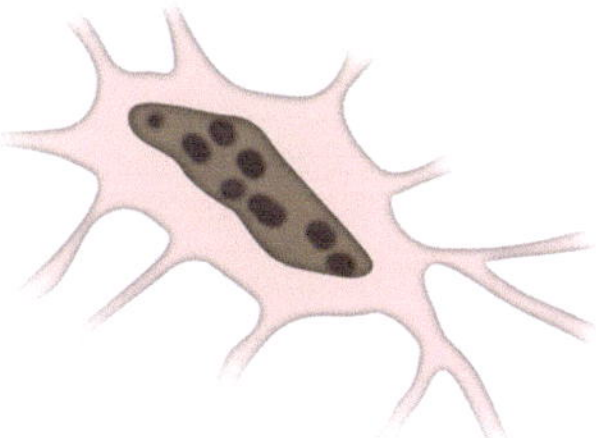

Special Guest

* The real GAMSAT may have advanced-level information presented (i.e. in a passage) but previous knowledge of said information is not required to answer the questions that would follow. Practice questions at the end of this chapter, as well as ACER and GS (HEAPS) practice GAMSATs can help you clarify this point.

5.1 Neural Cells and Tissues

The brain, spinal cord and peripheral nervous system are composed of nerve tissue. The basic cell types of nerve tissue is the *neuron* and the *glial cell*. Glial cells support and protect neurons and participate in neural activity, nutrition and defense processes. Neurons (= nerve cells) represent the functional unit of the nervous system. They conduct and transmit nerve impulses.

Neurons can be classified based on the shape or *morphology*. Unipolar neurons possess a single process. Bipolar neurons possess a single axon and a single dendrite. Multipolar neurons possess a single axon and more than one dendrite and are the most common type. Pseudounipolar neurons possess a single process that subsequently branches out into an axon and dendrite (note that in biology "pseudo" means "false"). Neurons can also be classified based on function. Sensory neurons receive stimuli from the environment and conduct impulses to the CNS. Motor neurons conduct impulses from the CNS to other neurons, muscles or glands. Interneurons connect other neurons and regulate transmitting signal between neurons.

Each neuron consists of a nerve cell body (*perikaryon or soma*), and its processes, which usually include multiple *dendrites* and a single *axon*. The cell body of a typical neuron contains a nucleus, *Nissl* material which is rough endoplasmic reticulum, free ribosomes, Golgi apparatus, mitochondria, many neurotubules, neurofilaments and pigment inclusions. The cell processes of neurons occur as axons and dendrites.

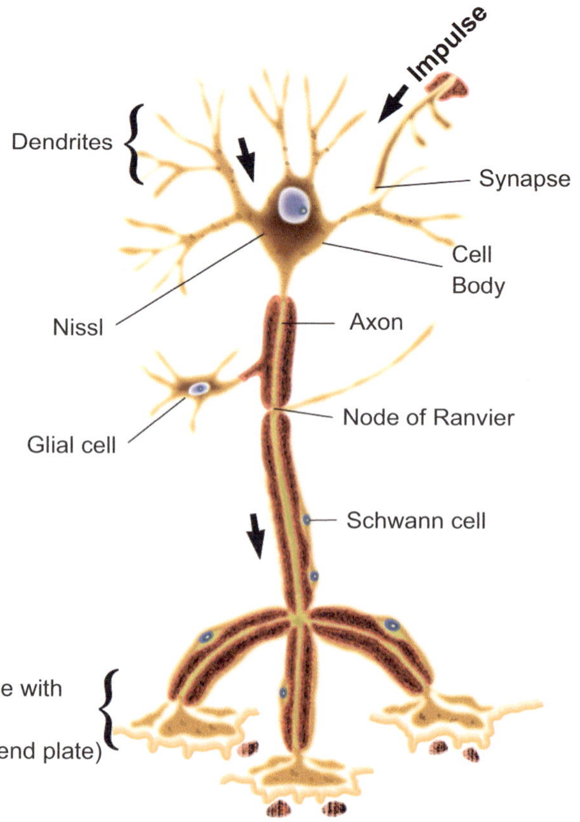

Figure IV.A.5.1: A neuron and other cells of nerve tissue, showing the neuromuscular junction, or motor end plate.

Dendrites contain most of the components of the cell, whereas axons contain major structures found in dendrites except for the Nissl material and Golgi apparatus. As a rule, dendrites receive stimuli from sensory cells, axons, or other neurons and conduct these impulses to the cell body of neurons and ultimately through to the axon. Axons are long cellular processes that conduct impulses away from the cell body of neurons. These originate from the axon hillock, a specialised region that contains many microtubules and neurofilaments. At the synaptic (terminal)

Low-level Importance

ends of axons, the presynaptic process contains vesicles from which are elaborated excitatory or inhibitory substances.

Unmyelinated fibers in peripheral nerves lie in grooves on the surface of the neurolemma (= plasma membrane) of a type of glial cell (*Schwann cell*). **Myelinated** peripheral neurons are invested by numerous layers of plasma membrane of Schwann cells or oligodendrocytes that constitute a *myelin sheath*, which allows axons to conduct impulses faster. The myelin sheath is produced by oligodendrocytes in the CNS and by Schwann cells in the PNS. In junctional areas between adjacent Schwann cells or oligodendrocytes, there is a lack of myelin. These junctional areas along the myelinated process constitute the nodes of Ranvier.

The neurons of the nervous system are arranged so that each neuron stimulates or inhibits other neurons and these in turn may stimulate or inhibit others until the functions of the nervous system are performed. The area between a neuron and the successive cell (i.e. another neuron, muscle fiber or gland) is called a *synapse*. Synapses can be classified as either a chemical synapse or an electrical synapse. A chemical synapse involves the release of a neurotransmitter by the presynaptic cell which then diffuses across the synapse and can act on the postsynaptic cell to generate an action potential. Signal transmission is delayed due to the time required for diffusion of the neurotransmitter across the synapse onto the membrane of the postsynaptic cell. An electrical synapse involves the movement of ions from one neuron to another via gap junctions (BIO 1.4.1). Signal transmission is immediate. Electrical synapses are often found in neural systems that require the fastest possible response, such as defensive reflexes.

When a neuron makes a synapse with muscle, it is called a *motor end plate* (*see* Fig. IV.A.5.1). The terminal endings of the nerve filament that synapse with the next cell are called presynaptic terminals, synaptic knobs, or more commonly - synaptic boutons. The postsynaptic terminal is the membrane part of another neuron or muscle or gland that is receiving the impulse. The synaptic cleft is the narrow space between the presynaptic and postsynaptic membrane.

At the synapse there is no physical contact between the two cells. The space between the dendrite of one neuron and the axon of another neuron is called the synaptic cleft and it measures about 200 - 300 angstroms (1 angstrom = 10^{-10} m) in a chemical synapse and about a tenth of that distance in an electrical synapse. The mediators in a chemical synapse, known as neurotransmitters, are housed in the presynaptic terminal and are exocytosed in response to an increase in intracellular Ca^{2+} concentration. The mediators or transmitters diffuse through the synaptic cleft when an impulse reaches the terminal and binds to receptors in the postsynaptic membrane. This transmitter substance may either excite the *postsynaptic* neuron or inhibit it. They are therefore called either excitatory or inhibitory transmitters (examples include *acetylcholine* and *GABA*, respectively).

Low-level Importance

5.1.1 The Membrane Potential

A membrane or resting potential (V_m) occurs across the plasma membranes of all cells. In large nerve and muscle cells, this potential amounts to about 70 millivolts with positivity outside the cell membrane and negativity inside (V_m = -70 mV). The development of this potential occurs as follows: every cell membrane contains a Na^+ - K^+ ATPase that pumps each ion to where its concentration is highest. The concentration of K^+ is higher inside the neuron and the concentration of Na^+ is higher outside; therefore, Na^+ is pumped to the outside of the cell and K^+ to the inside. However, more Na^+ is pumped outward than K^+ inward (3 Na^+ per 2 K^+). Also, the membrane is relatively permeable to K^+ so that it can leak out of the cell with relative ease. Therefore, the net effect is a loss of positive charges from inside the membrane and a gain of positive charges on the outside. The resulting membrane potential is the basis of all conduction of impulses by nerve and muscle fibers.

5.1.2 Action Potential

The action potential is a sequence of changes in the electric potential that occurs within a small fraction of a second when a nerve or muscle membrane impulse spreads over the surface of the cell. An excitatory stimulus on a postsynaptic neuron depolarises the membrane and makes the membrane potential less negative. Once the membrane potential reaches a critical threshold, the voltage-gated Na^+ channels become fully open, permitting the inward flow of Na^+ into the cell. The membrane potential is at the critical threshold when it is in a state where an action potential is inevitable. As a result, the positive sodium ions on the outside of the membrane now flow rapidly to the more negative interior. Therefore, the membrane potential suddenly becomes reversed with positivity on the inside and negativity on the outside. This state is called *depolarisation* and is caused by an inward Na^+ current.

Depolarisation also leads to the inactivation of the Na^+ channel and slowly opens the K^+ channel. The combined effect of the two preceding events repolarises the membrane back to its resting potential. This is called *repolarisation*. In fact, the neuron may shoot past the resting membrane potential and become even more negative, and this is called hyperpolarisation. The depolarised nerve goes on depolarising the adjacent nerve membrane in a wavy manner which is called an impulse. In other words, an impulse is a wave of depolarisation. Different axons can propagate impulses at different speeds. The increasing diameter of a nerve fiber or degree of myelination results in a faster impulse. The impulse is fastest in myelinated fibers since the wave of depolarisation "jumps" from node to node of Ranvier: this is called *saltatory* conduction because an action potential can be generated only at nodes of Ranvier.

Immediately following an action potential, the neuron will pass through three stages in the following order: a) it can no longer elicit

Low-level Importance

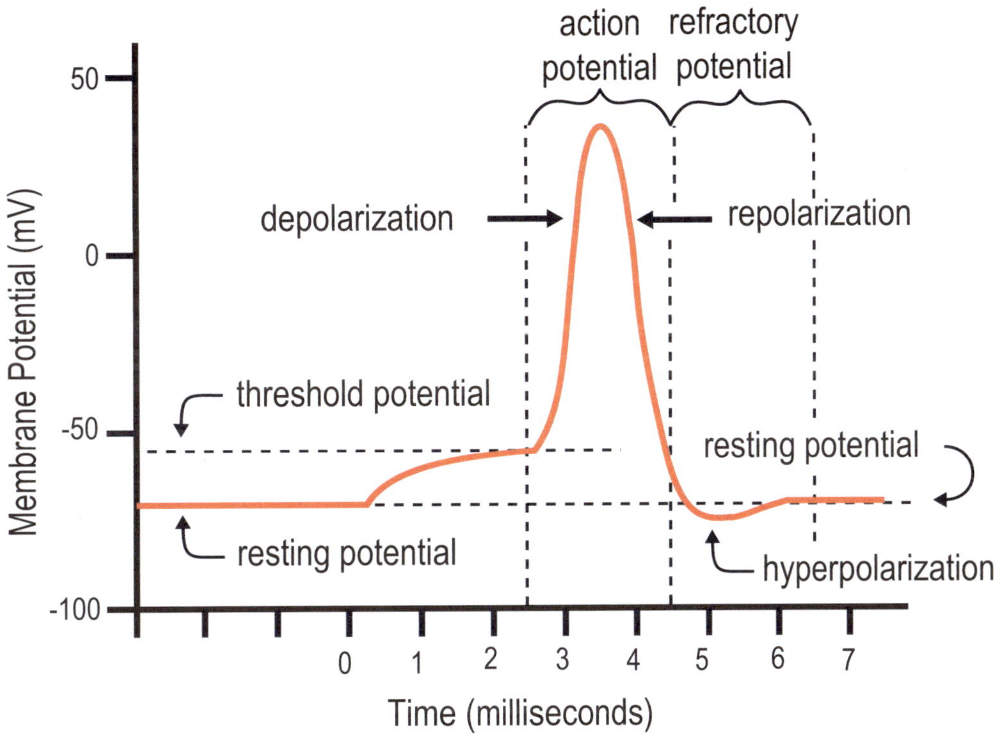

Figure IV.A.5.2: Action potential.

another action potential no matter how large the stimulus is = *absolute refractory period*; b) it can elicit another action potential only if a larger than usual stimulus is provided = *relative refractory period*; c) it returns to its original resting potential and thus can depolarise as easily as it originally did.

The action potential is an all-or-none event. The magnitude or strength of the action potential is not graded according to the strength of the stimulus. It occurs with the same magnitude each time it occurs, or it does not occur at all.

5.1.3 Action Potential: A Positive Perspective

To better understand the action potential, it is useful to take a closer look at what occurs to the positive ions Na^+ and K^+. To begin with, there are protein channels in the plasma membrane that act like gates which guard the passage of specific ions. Some gates open or close in response to V_m and are thus called *voltage gated channels.*

Low-level Importance

Once a threshold potential is reached, the voltage gated Na^+ channels open allowing the permeability or *conductance* of Na^+ to increase. The Na^+ ions can now diffuse across their chemical gradient: from an area of high concentration (*outside the membrane*) to an area of low concentration (*inside the membrane*). The Na^+ ions will also diffuse across their electrical gradient: from an area of relative positivity (*outside the membrane*) to an area of relative negativity (*inside the membrane*). Thus the inside becomes positive and the membrane is depolarised. Repolarisation occurs as the Na^+ channels close and the voltage gated K^+ channels open. As K^+ conductance increases to the outside (where K^+ concentration is lowest), the membrane repolarises to once again become relatively negative on the inside.

5.2 Contractile Cells and Tissues

There are three types of muscle tissue: smooth, skeletal and cardiac. All three types are composed of muscle cells (fibers) that contain myofibrils possessing contractile filaments of actin and myosin.

Smooth muscle: Smooth muscle cells are spindle shaped and are organised chiefly into sheets or bands of smooth muscle tissue. They contain a single nucleus and actively divide and regenerate. This tissue is found in blood vessels and other tubular visceral structures (i.e. intestines). Smooth muscles contain both actin and myosin filaments but actin predominates. The filaments are not organised into patterns that give cross striations as in cardiac and skeletal muscle. Filaments course obliquely in the cells and attach to the plasma membrane. Contraction of smooth muscle is involuntary and is innervated by the autonomic nervous system.

Skeletal muscle: Skeletal muscle fibers are characterised by their peripherally located multiple nuclei and striated myofibrils. Myofibrils are longitudinally arranged bundles of thick and thin myofilaments. Myofilaments are composed of thick and thin filaments present in an alternating arrangement responsible for the cross-striation pattern. The striations in a sarcomere consists of an A-band (dark), which contains both thin and thick filaments. These are bordered toward the Z-lines by I-bands (light), which contain thin filaments only. The mid-region of the A-band contains an H-band (light), which contains thick filaments only and is bisected by an M-line. The Z lines are dense regions bisecting each I-band and anchor the thin filaments. The filaments interdigitate and are cross-bridged in the A-band with myosin filaments forming a hexagonal pattern of one myosin filament surrounded by six actin filaments. In the contraction of a muscle fiber,

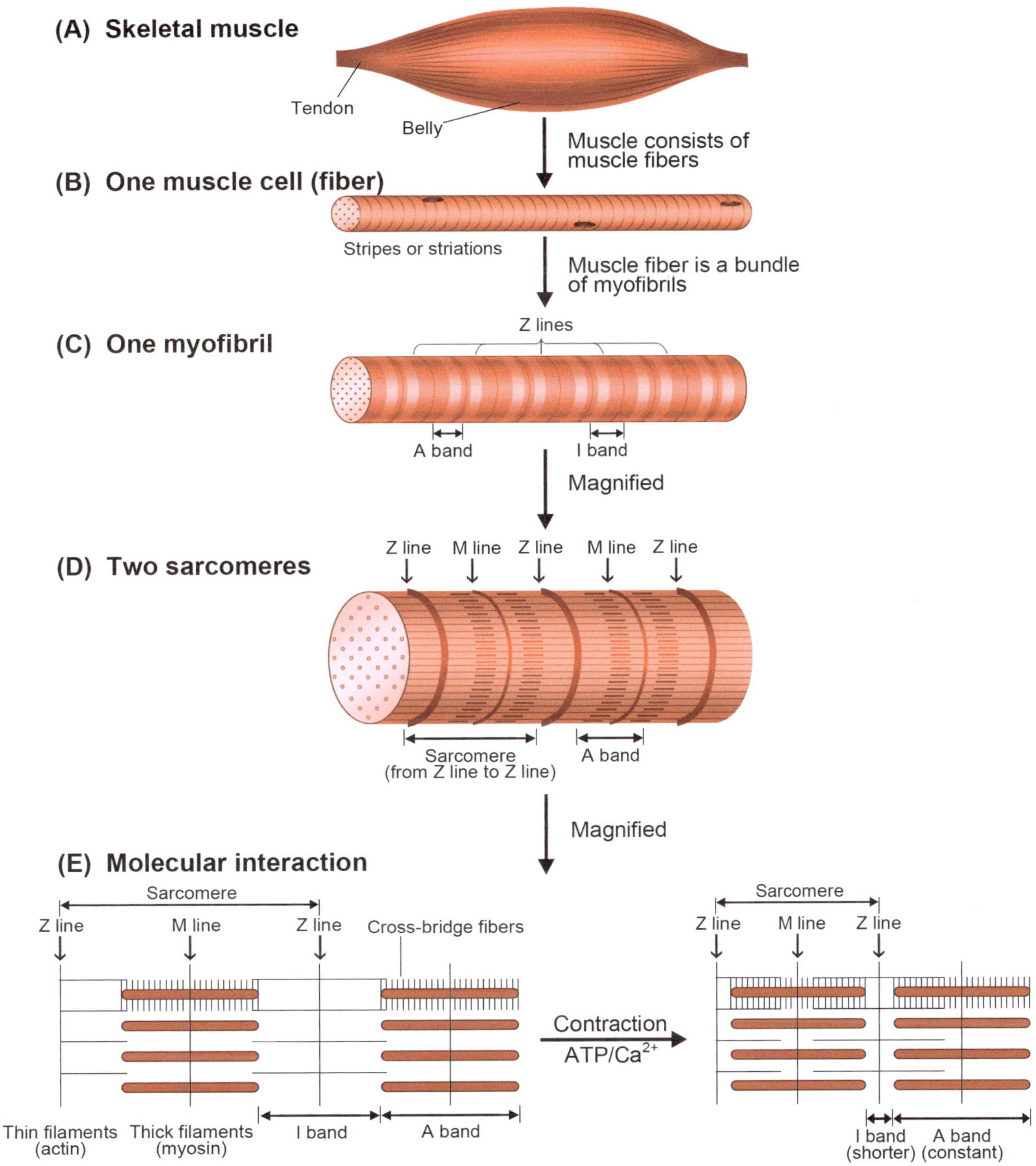

Figure IV.A.5.3: A schematic view of the molecular basis for muscle contraction. Note: the "H zone" is the central portion of an A band and is characterised by the presence of myosin filaments.

Low-level Importance

thick and thin filaments do not shorten but increase their overlap. The actin filaments of the I-bands move more deeply into the A-band, resulting in a shortening of the H-band and the I-bands as Z disks are brought closer. However, the A-band remains constant in length. {Mnemonic: "HI" bands shorten}

Each skeletal muscle fiber is invested with a sarcolemma (= plasmalemma = plasma membrane) that extends into the fiber as numerous small transverse tubes called T-tubules. These tubules ring the myofibrils at the A-I junction and are bounded on each side by terminal cisternae of the endoplasmic (sarcoplasmic) reticulum. The T-tubules, together with a pair of terminal cisternae form a triad. The triad helps to provide a uniform contraction throughout the muscle cell as it provides channels for ions to flow freely and helps to propagate action potentials. There are thousands of triads per skeletal muscle fiber.

The sarcoplasmic reticulum is a modified endoplasmic reticulum that regulates muscle contraction by either transporting Ca^{2+} into storage (muscle relaxation) or releasing Ca^{2+} during excitation-contraction coupling (muscle contraction).

The thick filaments within a myofibril are composed of about 250 myosin molecules arranged in an antiparallel fashion and some associated proteins. The myosin molecule is composed of two identical heavy chains and two pairs of light chains. The heavy chain consists of two "heads" and one "tail". The head contains an actin binding site which is involved in muscle contraction. The thin filaments within a myofibril are composed of actin and to a lesser degree two smaller proteins: *troponin and tropomyosin*. An action potential in the muscle cell membrane initiates depolarisation of the T tubules, which causes the nearby sarcoplasmic reticulum to release its Ca^{2+} ions and thus an increase in intracellular $[Ca^{2+}]$. Calcium then attaches to a subunit of troponin resulting in the movement of tropomyosin and the uncovering of the active sites for the attachment of actin to the cross bridging heads of myosin. Due to this attachment, ATP in the myosin head hydrolyses, producing energy, Pi and ADP which results in a bending of the myosin head and a pulling of the actin filament into the A-band. These actin-myosin bridges detach again when myosin binds a new ATP molecule and attaches to a new site on actin toward the plus end as long as Ca^{2+} is bound to troponin. Finally, relaxation of muscle occurs when Ca^{2+} is sequestered by the sarcoplasmic reticulum. Thus calcium is pumped out of the cytoplasm and calcium levels return to normal, tropomyosin again binds to actin, preventing myosin from binding.

There are three interesting consequences to the preceding:

i) neither actin nor myosin change length during muscle contraction; rather, shortening of the muscle fiber occurs as the filaments slide over each other increasing the area of overlap.

ii) initially a dead person is very stiff (*rigor mortis*) since they can no longer produce the ATP necessary to detach the actin-

Low-level Importance

myosin bridges thus their muscles remain locked in position.

iii) Ca^{2+} is a critical ion both for muscle contraction and for transmitter release from presynaptic neurons.

Cardiac muscle: Cardiac muscle contains striations and myofibrils that are similar to those of skeletal muscle. Contraction of cardiac muscle is involuntary and is innervated by the autonomic nervous system. It differs from skeletal muscle in several major ways. Cardiac muscle fibers branch and contain centrally located nuclei (characteristically, one nucleus per cell) and large numbers of mitochondria. Individual cardiac muscle cells are attached to each other at their ends by *intercalated* disks. These disks contain several types of membrane junctional complexes, the most important of which is the *gap junction* (BIO 1.4.1). Cardiac muscle cells do not regenerate: injury to cardiac muscle is repaired by fibrous connective tissue.

The gap junction electrically couples one cell to its neighbor (= *syncytium*) so that electric depolarisation is propagated throughout the heart by cell-to-cell contact rather than by nerve innervation to each cell. The sarcoplasmic reticulum - T-tubule system is arranged differently in cardiac muscle than in skeletal muscle. In cardiac muscle each T-tubule enters at the Z-line and forms a diad with only one terminal cisterna of sarcoplasmic reticulum.

5.3 Epithelial Cells and Tissues

Epithelia have the following characteristics:

1. they cover all body surfaces (i.e. skin, organs, etc.)
2. they are the principal tissues of glands
3. their cells are anchored by a nonliving layer (= the basement membrane)
4. they lack blood vessels and are thus nourished by diffusion.

Epithelial tissues are classified according to the characteristics of their cells. Tissues with elongated cells are called *columnar*, those with thin flattened cells are *squamous*, and those with cube-like cells are *cuboidal*. They are further classified as **simple** if they have a single layer of cells and **stratified** if they have multiple layers of cells. As examples of the classification, skin is composed of a stratified squamous epithelium while various glands (i.e. thyroid, salivary, etc.) contain a simple cuboidal epithelium. The former epithelium serves to protect against microorganisms, loss of water or heat, while the latter epithelium functions to secrete glandular products.

Low-level Importance

5.4 Connective Cells and Tissues

Connective tissue connects and joins other body tissue and parts. It also carries substances for processing, nutrition, and waste release. Connective tissue is characterised by the presence of relatively few cells surrounded by an extensive network of extracellular matrix, consisting of ground substance, extracellular fluid, and fibers.

The adult connective tissues are: connective tissue proper, cartilage, bone and blood (*see The Circulatory System*, section 7.5). Connective tissue proper is further classified into loose connective tissue, dense connective tissue, elastic tissue, reticular tissue and adipose tissue.

5.4.1 Loose Connective Tissue

Loose connective tissue is found in the superficial fascia. It is generally considered as the *packaging material* of the body, in part, because it frequently envelopes muscles. Fascia - usually a clear or white sheet (or band) of fibrous connective tissue - helps to bind skin to underlying organs, to fill spaces between muscles, etc. Loose connective tissue contains most of the cell types and all the fiber types found in the other connective tissues. The most common cell types are the fibroblast, macrophage, adipose cell, mast cell, plasma cell and wandering cells from the blood (which include several types of white blood cells).

Fibroblasts are the predominant cell type in connective tissue proper and have the capability to differentiate into other types of cells under certain conditions.

Macrophages are part of the *reticulo-endothelial system* (tissue which predominately destroys foreign particles). They are responsible for phagocytosing foreign bodies and assisting the immune response. They possess large lysosomes containing digestive enzymes which are necessary for the digestion of phagocytosed materials. Mast cells reside mostly along blood vessels and contain granules which include *heparin* and *histamine*. Heparin is a compound which prevents blood clotting and histamine is associated with allergic reactions. Mast cells mediate type I hypersensitivity.

Plasma cells are part of the immune system in that they produce circulatory antibodies (BIO 7.5, 8.2). They contain extensive amounts of rough endoplasmic reticulum (RER).

Adipose cells are found in varying quantities, when they predominate, the tissue is called adipose (fat) tissue.

Fibers are long protein polymers present in different types of connective tissue. Common types of fibers include collagen fiber, reticular fiber and elastic fiber.

Low-level Importance

Collagen fibers are usually found in bundles and provide **strength** to the tissue. Many different types of collagen fibers are identified on the basis of their molecular structure. Of the five most common types, collagen type I is the most abundant, being found in dermis, bone, dentine, tendons, organ capsules, fascia and sclera. Type II is located in hyaline and elastic cartilage. Type III is probably the collagenous component of reticular fibers. Type IV is found in a specific part (*the basal lamina*) of basement membranes. Type V is a component of placental basement membranes. **Reticular fibers** are smaller, more delicate fibers that form the basic framework of reticular connective tissue. **Elastic fibers** branch and provide elasticity and support to connective tissue.

Ground substance is the gelatinous material that fills most of the space between the cells and the fibers. It is composed of acid mucopolysaccharides and structural glycoproteins and its properties are important in determining the permeability and consistency of the connective tissue.

5.4.2 Dense Connective Tissue

Dense irregular connective tissue is found in the dermis, periosteum, perichondrium and capsules of some organs. All of the fiber types are present, but collagenous fibers predominate. Dense regular connective tissue occurs as aponeuroses, ligaments and tendons. In most ligaments and tendons collagenous fibers are most prevalent and are oriented parallel to each other. Fibroblasts are practically the only cell type present.

5.4.3 Cartilage

Cartilage is composed of chondrocytes (= cartilage cells) embedded in an intercellular (= extracellular) matrix, consisting of fibers and an amorphous firm ground substance. In cases of injury, cartilage repairs slowly since it has no direct blood supply. Three types of cartilage are distinguished on the basis of the amount of ground substance and the relative abundance of collagenous and elastic fibers. They are hyaline, elastic and fibrous cartilage.

Hyaline Cartilage is found as costal (rib) cartilage, articular cartilage and cartilage of the nose, larynx, trachea and bronchi. The extracellular matrix consists primarily of collagenous fibers and a ground substance rich in chondromucoprotein, a copolymer of a protein and chondroitin sulphates.

Elastic Cartilage is found in the pinna of the ear, auditory tube and epiglottis, and some laryngeal cartilage. Elastic fibers predominate and thus provide greater flexibility. Calcification of this type of cartilage is rare.

Fibrous Cartilage occurs in the anchorage of tendons and ligaments, in intervertebral disks, in the symphysis pubis, and in some interarticular disks and in some ligaments. Chondrocytes occur singly or in rows between large bundles of collagenous fibers. Compared with hyaline cartilage, only small amounts of hyaline matrix surround the chondrocytes of fibrous cartilage.

5.4.4 Bone

Bone tissue consists of three **cell types** and a calcified **extracellular matrix** that contains organic and inorganic components. The three cell types are: *osteoblasts* which synthesise the organic components of the matrix (osteoid) and become embedded in lacunae; *osteocytes* which are mature bone cells entrapped in their own lacunae within the matrix and maintain communication with each other via gap junctions; and *osteoclasts* which are large multinucleated cells functioning in resorption and remodeling of bone.

The organic matrix consists of dense collagenous fibers (primarily type I collagen) which is important in providing flexibility and tensile strength to bone. The inorganic component is responsible for the *rigidity* of the bone and is composed chiefly of calcium phosphate and calcium carbonate with small amounts of magnesium, fluoride, hydroxide, sulphate and hydroxyapatite.

Compact bone contains haversian systems (osteons), interstitial lamellae and circumferential lamellae. The Haversian system is the structural unit for bone and each osteon consists of a central haversian canal surrounded by a number of concentric deposits of bony matrix called lamellae. Haversian systems consist of extensively branching haversian canals that are oriented chiefly longitudinally in long bones. Each canal contains blood vessels and is surrounded by 8 to 15 concentric lamellae and osteocytes.

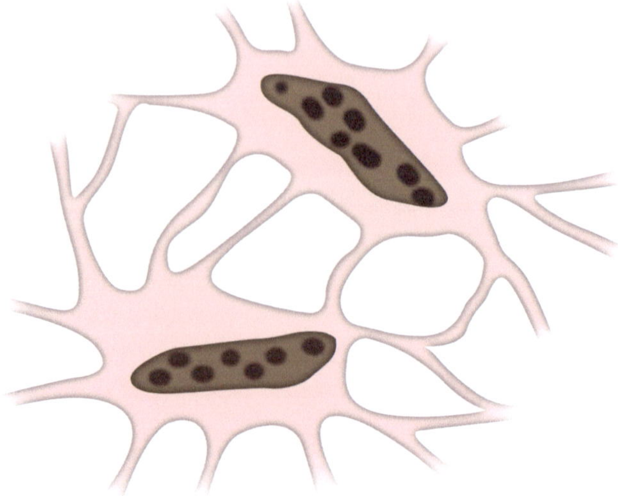

Figure IV.A.5.4: Osteocytes.

Low-level Importance

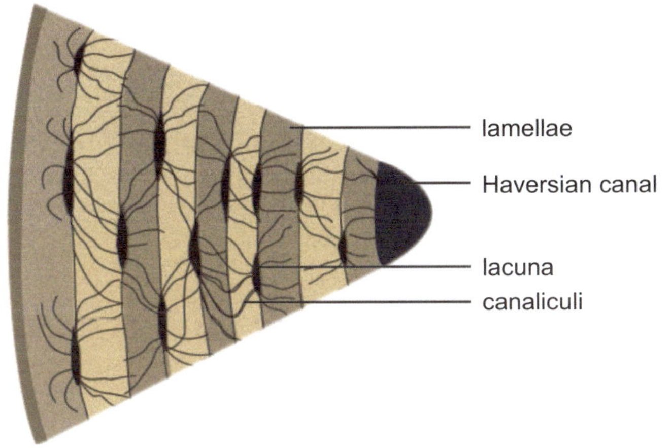

Figure IV.A.5.5: Schematic drawing of part of a haversian system.

Nutrients from blood vessels in the haversian canals pass through canaliculi and lacunae to reach all osteocytes in the system. Volkmann's canals traverse the bone transversely and interconnect the haversian systems. They enter through the outer circumferential lamellae and carry blood vessels and nerves which are continuous with those of the haversian canals and the periosteum. The periosteum is the connective tissue layer which envelopes bone. The endosteum is the connective tissue layer which lines the marrow cavities and supplies osteoprogenitor cells and osteoblasts for bone formation.

Bones are supplied by a loop of blood vessels that enter from the periosteal region, penetrate the cortical bone, and enter the medulla before returning to the periphery

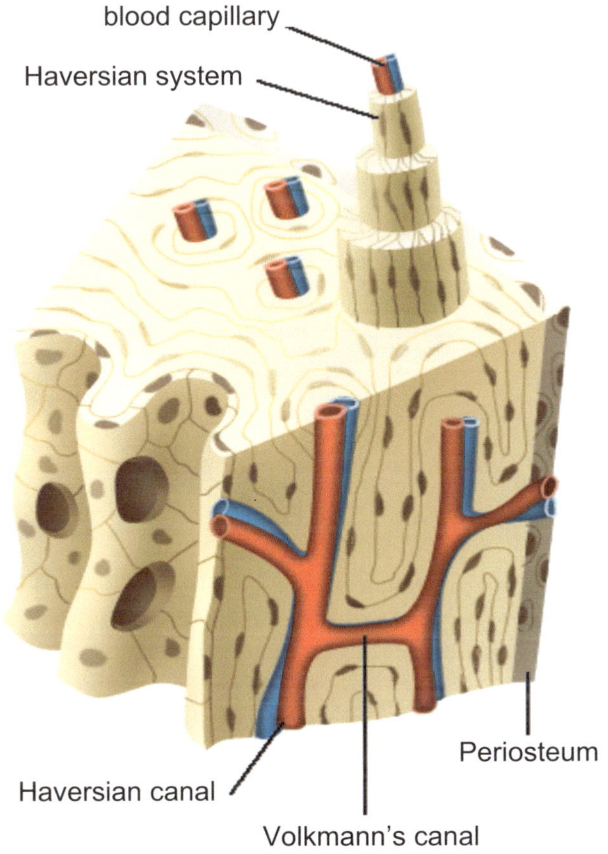

Figure IV.A.5.6
Schematic drawing of the wall of a long bone.

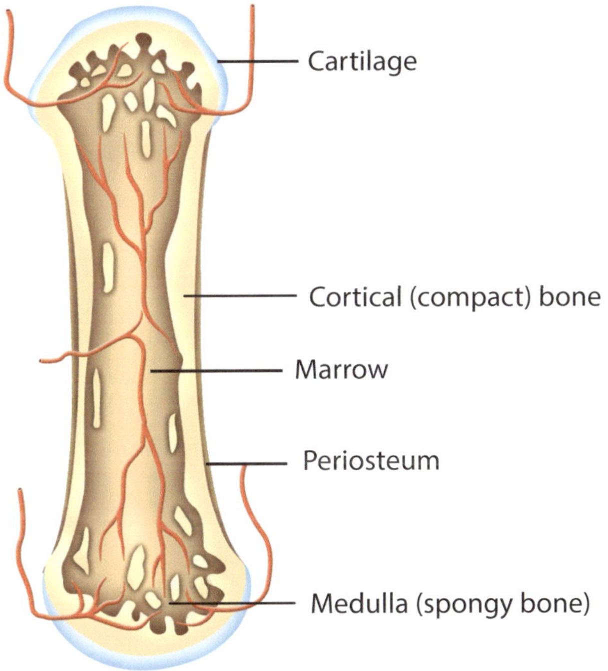

Figure IV.A.5.7
Schematic drawing of adult bone structure.

Low-level Importance

of the bone. Long bones are specifically supplied by arteries which pass to the marrow through diaphyseal, metaphyseal and epiphyseal arteries (for bone structure, *see* BIO 11.3.1).

Bone undergoes extensive remodelling, and harvesian systems may break down or be resorbed in order that calcium can be made available to other parts of the body. Bone resorption occurs by osteocytes engaging in osteolysis or by osteoclastic activity.

CHAPTER 5: Specialised Eukaryotic Cells and Tissues

GOLD STANDARD FOUNDATIONAL GAMSAT PRACTICE QUESTIONS

1) Most neurons are specialised to receive, conduct and transmit:

A. electrochemical signals.
B. action potentials.
C. chemical signals.
D. electrical signals.

2) Identify the ion released from the sarcoplasmic reticulum that combines with troponin and removes the blocking action of tropomyosin, resulting in the formation of cross bridges.

A. Acetylcholine
B. Ca^{2+}
C. Myosin
D. Troponin

3) A membrane potential is the difference in electrical charge between:

A. resting and action potentials.
B. sodium and potassium ions.
C. the inside and outside of the cell.
D. phospholipid and glycolipid layers.

4) Bone is occasionally compared to steel-reinforced concrete. The steel-reinforcing rods are analogous to collagen fibers and the concrete is analogous to which of the following?

A. Cartilage
B. Bone marrow
C. Haversian canals
D. Hydroxyapatite (calcium salts)

GOLD STANDARD GAMSAT-LEVEL PRACTICE QUESTIONS

Questions 5–9

Active transport is the energy-consuming transport of molecules against a concentration gradient. Energy is required because the substance must be moved in the opposite direction of its natural tendency to diffuse. Movement is usually unidirectional, unlike diffusion which is reversible.

When movement of ions is considered, two factors will influence the direction in which they diffuse: one is concentration, the other is electrical charge. An ion will usually diffuse from a region of its high concentration to a region of its low concentration. It will also generally be attracted towards a region of opposite charge, and move away from a region of similar charge. Thus ions are said to move down *electrochemical gradients*, which are the combined effects of both electrical and concentration gradients. Strictly speaking, active transport of ions is their movement against an electrochemical gradient powered by an energy source.

Research has shown that the cell surface membranes of most cells possess sodium pumps. Usually, though not always, the sodium pump is coupled with a potassium pump. The combined pump is called the sodium-potassium pump. This pump is an excellent example of active transport.

Ion	Concentration (mmol/L H_2O)		Equilibrium potential (mV)
	Inside cell	Outside cell	
Na^+	15.0	150.0	+60
K^+	150.0	5.5	-90
Cl^-	9.0	125.0	-75
Resting membrane potential (Vm) = -70 mV			

Table 1: Concentration of Na^+, K^+, and Cl^- inside and outside mammalian motor neurons. The sign of the potential (mV) is inside relative to the outside of the cell.

The value of the equilibrium potential for any ion depends upon the concentration gradient for that ion across the membrane. The equilibrium potential for any ion can be calculated using the Nernst equation.The following is an approximation of the equation for the equilibrium potential for potassium (E_k in mV) at room temperature:

$$E_k = 60 \log_{10} \frac{[K^+]_O}{[K^+]_i}$$

$[K^+]_o$ = extracellular K^+ concentration in mM

$[K^+]_i$ = intracellular K^+ concentration in mM

5) All of the following explain the ionic concentrations in Table 1 EXCEPT:

A. Na^+ and Cl^- ions passively diffuse more quickly into the extracellular fluid than K^+ ions.

B. Na^+ ions are actively pumped out of the intracellular fluid.

C. the negative charge of the cell contents repels Cl^- ions from the cell.

D. the cell membrane is more freely permeable to K^+ ions than to Na^+ and Cl^- ions.

6) If the concentration of potassium outside a mammalian motor neuron were changed to 0.55 mol/L, what would be the predicted change in the equilibrium potential?

A. 12 mV

B. 120 mV

C. 60 mV

D. 600 mV

7) A graph of E_k vs $\log_{10}[K^+]_o$ would be:

A. a straight line.

B. a logarithmic curve.

C. an exponential curve.

D. a sigmoidal curve.

8) In the process of osmosis, the net flow of water molecules into or out of the cell depends primarily on the differences in the:

A. concentration of protein on either side of the cell membrane.

B. concentration of water molecules inside and outside the cell.

C. rate of molecular transport on either side of the cell membrane.

D. rate of movement of ions inside the cell.

9) At inhibitory synapses, a hyperpolarisation of the membrane known as an inhibitory postsynaptic potential is produced rendering V_m more negative. This occurs as a result of:

A. an increase in the postsynaptic membrane's permeability to Na^+ and K^+ ions.

B. an increase in the permeability of the presynaptic membrane to Ca^{2+} ions.

C. the entry of Cl^- ions into the synaptic knob.

D. an increase in the permeability of the postsynaptic membrane to Cl^- ions.

Questions 10–13

The sequence of events during synaptic transmission at the neuromuscular junction can be summarised as follows.

The depolarisation produced by an action potential in the synaptic terminal opens voltage-dependent calcium channels in the terminal membrane. Calcium ions enter the terminal down their concentration and electrical gradients, inducing synaptic vesicles filled with acetylcholine (ACh) to fuse with the plasma membrane facing the muscle cell. The ACh is thereby dumped into the synaptic cleft, and some of it diffuses across the cleft to combine with specific receptors on ACh-activated channels. When ACh is bound, the channel opens and allows sodium and potassium ions to cross the membrane. This depolarises the muscle membrane or *sarcolemma* and triggers an all-or-none action potential in the muscle cell. The action of ACh is terminated by the enzyme acetylcholinesterase, which splits ACh into acetate and choline.

In order to determine how, and under what conditions, ACh works, 2 experiments were done.

10) At the neuromuscular junction, the receptors on the ACh-activated channels are likely located:

- **A.** on the tubule of the T system.
- **B.** in the sarcolemma.
- **C.** on the muscle surface.
- **D.** in the synaptic cleft.

11) A mutation in the gene which codes for acetylcholinesterase would likely inhibit all but which of the following processes?

- **A.** A hyperpolarisation in the postsynaptic membrane
- **B.** A depolarisation in the postsynaptic membrane
- **C.** The passage of a series of nerve impulses along the axon of the postsynaptic neuron
- **D.** The development of an inhibitory postsynaptic potential

Questions 12–13 refer to the following additional information:

Experiment 1

Determining the Effect of the Timing of Calcium Action on Transmitter Release

Calcium ions were removed from the bathing solution of a muscle cell so that release of ACh in response to nerve stimulation was virtually abolished. Calcium ions were then applied to the nerve terminal by ionophoreses, from a micropipette close to the terminal, just before the nerve was stimulated (N), without nerve stimulation, and just after the nerve was stimulated. The results obtained are shown in Figure 1.

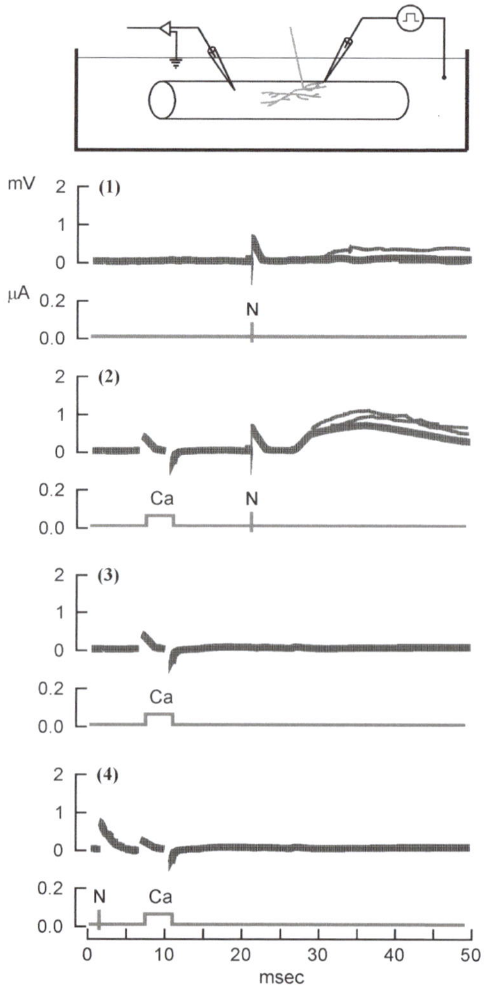

Figure 1

Experiment 2

Determining the Effect of ACh on Neuromuscular Transmission and its Subsequent Action on the Postsynaptic Membrane

Stimulating electrodes were placed on the nerve and a pair of recording electrodes was placed on the muscle. One of the electrodes was placed very close to the end plate region. First curare and then eserine were added to the solution bathing the muscle. The action potentials produced on stimulating the nerve were recorded. The results obtained are shown in Figure 2.

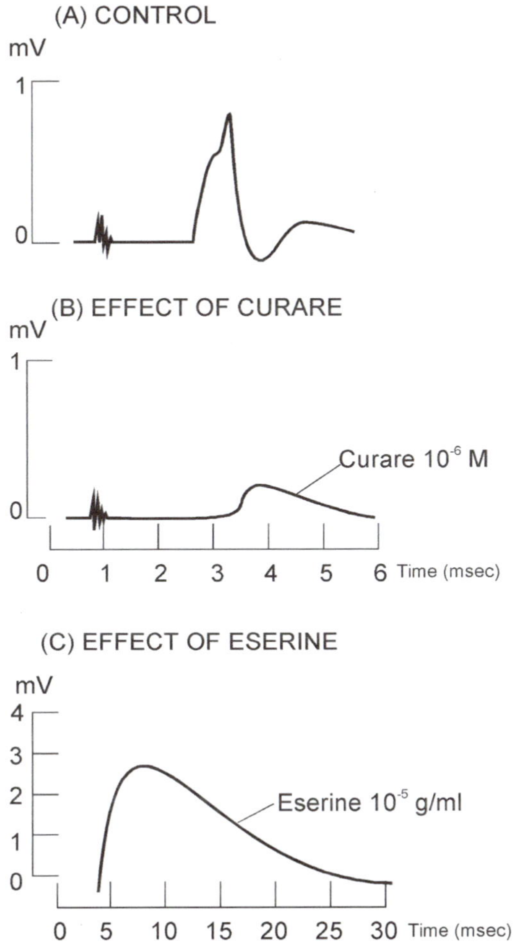

Figure 2

12) According to Figure 1, which of the following conclusions was confirmed by the experiment?

- **A** For transmitter release to occur, calcium ions need only be present after the depolarisation of the presynaptic membrane.
- **B** The presence of calcium ions is the only variable which affects transmitter release at the synapse.
- **C** For transmitter release to occur, calcium ions must be present before and after depolarisation of the presynaptic membrane.
- **D** For transmitter release to occur, calcium ions must be present before depolarisation of the presynaptic membrane.

13) According to Figure 2, all of the following would be correct EXCEPT:

- **A.** the post-stimulation peak in the eserine curve precedes the peak in the curare curve.
- **B.** the curve for the control displays a shorter period of time with negative membrane potential compared to positive.
- **C.** whether eserine or curare had been used in greater concentration cannot be determined from the information provided.
- **D.** stimulating the nerves may create some artifact in the tracings.

High-level Importance

14) A researcher has designed a method to detect skeletal age as a function of infant weight and the measurement of ossification centres of ankle bones (calcaneus and talus) in mm. The results are shown in Figure 1.

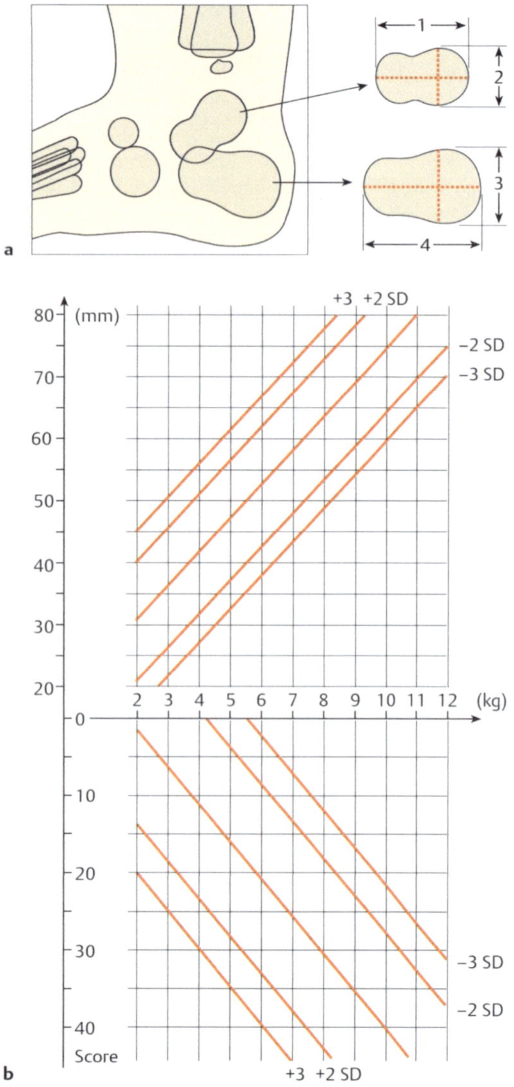

Figure 1: Erasmier method of skeletal age determination. **a** Measurement of the maximum lengths of the calcaneus and talus in mm. **b** Nomogram. Skeletal maturity is found by drawing a vertical line through present body weight (SD = standard deviation away from the normal; ref: Erasmier and Ringertz 1980).

According to Figure 1, what would be a normal measurement of ossification centres of ankle bones for a 6.5 kg infant?

A. 40 mm
B. 50 mm
C. 55 mm
D. More than 60 mm

15) Consider Figure 1.

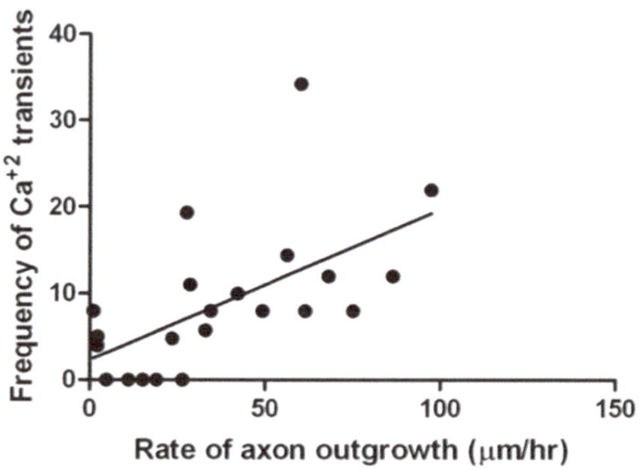

Figure 1: Correlation between the frequency of calcium transients and the rate of axon growth.
Hutchins, B., *Dev Neurobiol.* 2011.

Researchers are investigating the experimental drug NSX-RUV that halves the average required frequency of Ca^{2+} transients for axon growth. What would be the average frequency of Ca^{2+} transients for an axon growth of 50 μm/hr post-administration of NSX-RUV?

A. 1
B. 5
C. 10
D. 20

SPOILER ALERT

Gold Standard has cross-referenced the content in this chapter to examples from ACER's official GAMSAT practice materials. It is for you to decide when you want to explore these questions since you may want to preserve some of ACER's materials for timed mock-exam practice.

Example – Rare, straight assumed knowledge about activating a neuron: Q106 of 5 (presumably, a real past exam question). Note that "Q" is followed by the question number, and, for example, "of 1" refers to booklet number 1 which is referenced in the Spoiler Alert table at the end of Chapter 1. The 15 full-length GAMSAT practice tests by Gold Standard, HEAPS-1 through HEAPS-15, contain specific cross-references to this chapter within the worked solutions. Note that the neuron and muscle cell units in GAMSAT-level practice questions in this chapter come from HEAPS-5 and HEAPS-6.

Chapter Checklist

- ☐ Access your online account to view answers, worked solutions and discussion boards.
- ☐ Reassess your 'learning objectives' for this chapter: Go back to the first page of this chapter and re-evaluate the top 3 boxes and the Introduction.
- ☐ Complete a maximum of 1 page of notes using symbols/abbreviations to represent the entire chapter based on your learning objectives. These are your Gold Notes.
- ☐ Consider your multimedia options based on your optimal way of learning:
    - ☐ Download the free Gold Standard GAMSAT app for your Android device or iPhone.
    - ☐ Create your own, tangible study cards or try the free app: Anki.
    - ☐ Record your voice reading your Gold Notes onto your smartphone (audio files, e.g., *memo* or MP3s) and listen during exercise, transportation, etc.
    - ☐ Try out the Gold Standard GAMSAT online videos at gamsat-prep.com, or you can try other options on YouTube like Khan Academy or Crash Course Biology.
- ☐ Reassess your schedule for your full-length GAMSAT practice tests: ACER and/or HEAPS exams. Ensure that you have scheduled one full day to complete a practice test and 1-2 days for a thorough assessment of worked solutions while adding to your abbreviated Gold Notes.
- ☐ Reassess your progress in scheduling and/or evaluating stress reduction techniques such as regular exercise (sports), yoga, meditation and/or mindfulness exercises (*see* YouTube for suggestions).

NERVOUS AND ENDOCRINE SYSTEMS
Chapter 6

Memorise

* Nervous system: basic structure, major functions
* Basic sensory reception and processing
* Define: endocrine gland, hormone
* Positive and negative feedback

Understand

* Organisation of the nervous system; sensor and effector neurons
* Feedback loop, reflex arc: role of spinal cord, brain
* Endocrine system: specific chemical control at cell, tissue, and organ level
* Cellular mechanisms of hormone action, transport of hormones
* Positive and negative feedback: Concepts, graphs and symbols

Importance

Low level: 1% of GAMSAT Biology questions released by ACER are related to content in this chapter (in our estimation).
* Note that approximately 75% of the questions in GAMSAT Biology are related to just 7 chapters: 1, 2, 3, 4, 7, 12, and 15.

Introduction

The nervous and endocrine systems are composed of a network of highly specialised cells that can communicate information about an organism's surroundings and itself. Thus together, these two systems can process incoming information and then regulate and coordinate responses in other parts of the body.

Although it may not seem that this chapter, overall, has important assumed knowledge, it is part of a process of reading scientific language and becoming familiar with body systems. The GAMSAT-level practice questions at the end of the chapter use reasoning skills that will also be helpful for other Section 3 topics. Instead of trying to remember the names of cranial nerves or hormones, try to observe how various systems work together. Feedback loops (negative and positive, BIO 6.3.6 and 6.3.7) must be considered High-level Importance as they may appear in Physics or many other Biology subtopics. For example, note that in the Introduction to this Masters Series Biology book, we examined feedback in the context of a metabolic pathway (Question 8), and blood clotting (Questions 9-14); in Chapter 10, we will explore feedback in the nephron (Questions 7-10).

Multimedia Resources at GAMSAT-Prep.com

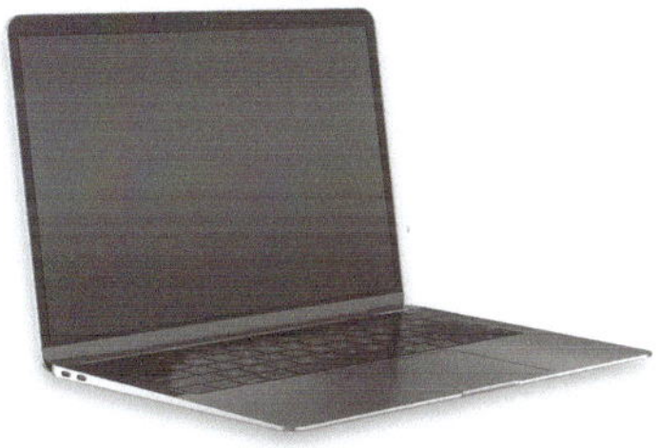

Open Discussion Boards
(*gamsat-prep.com/forum*)

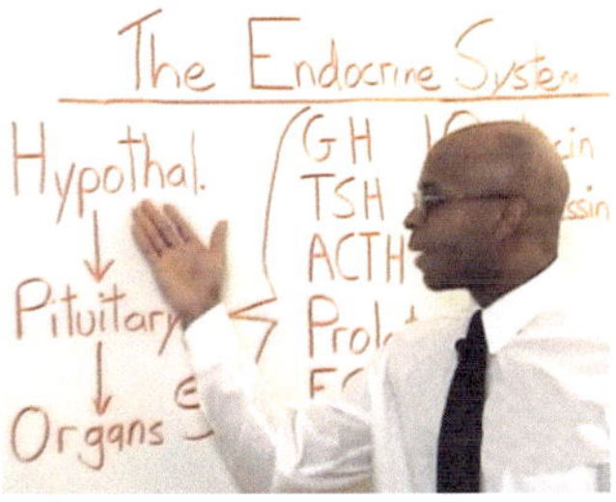

Foundational Videos

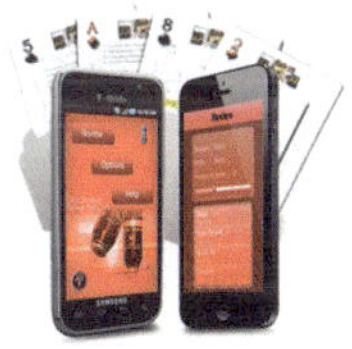

Flashcards

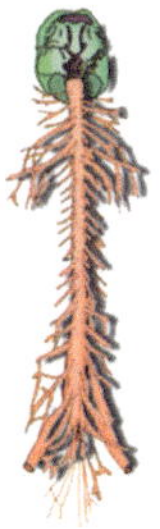

Special Guest

* The real GAMSAT may have advanced-level information presented (i.e. in a passage) but previous knowledge of said information is not required to answer the questions that would follow. Practice questions at the end of this chapter, as well as ACER and GS (HEAPS) practice GAMSATs can help you clarify this point.

6.1 Organisation of the Vertebrate Nervous System

The role of the nervous system is to control and coordinate body activities in a rapid and precise mode of action. The nervous system is composed of central and peripheral nervous systems.

The **central nervous system** (CNS) is enclosed within the cranium (skull) and vertebral (spinal) canal and consists respectively of the brain and spinal cord. The **peripheral nervous system** (PNS) is outside the bony encasement and is composed of peripheral nerves, which are branches or continuations of the spinal or cranial nerves. The PNS can be divided into the **somatic nervous system** and the **autonomic nervous system** which are *anatomically* a portion of both the central and peripheral nervous systems.

The somatic nervous system contains sensory fibers that bring information back to the CNS and motor fibers that innervate skeletal muscles. The autonomic nervous system (ANS) contains motor fibers that innervate smooth muscle, cardiac muscle and glands. The ANS is then divided into *sympathetic* and *parasympathetic* divisions, which generally act against each other. The sympathetic division acts to prepare the body for an emergency situation (fight or flight) while the parasympathetic division acts to conserve energy and restore the body to resting level (rest and digest).

As a rule, a collection of nerve cell bodies in the CNS is called a *nucleus* and outside the CNS it is called a *ganglion*. Neurons that carry information from the environment to the brain or spinal cord are called *afferent neurons*. Neurons that carry motor commands from the brain or spinal cord to the different parts of body are called *efferent neurons*. Neurons that connect sensory and motor neurons in neural pathways are called *interneurons*.

The spinal cord is a long cylindrical structure whose hollow core is called the *central canal*. The central canal is surrounded by a gray matter which is in turn surrounded by a white matter (the reverse is true for the brain: outer gray matter and inner white matter). Basically, the gray matter consists of the cell bodies of neurons whereas the white matter consists of the nerve fibers (axons and dendrites). There are 31 pairs of spinal nerves each leaving the spinal cord at various levels: 8 cervical (neck), 12 thoracic (chest), 5 lumbar (abdomen), 5 sacral and 1 coccygeal (these latter 6 are from the pelvic region). The lower end of the spinal cord is cone shaped and is called the *conus medullaris*.

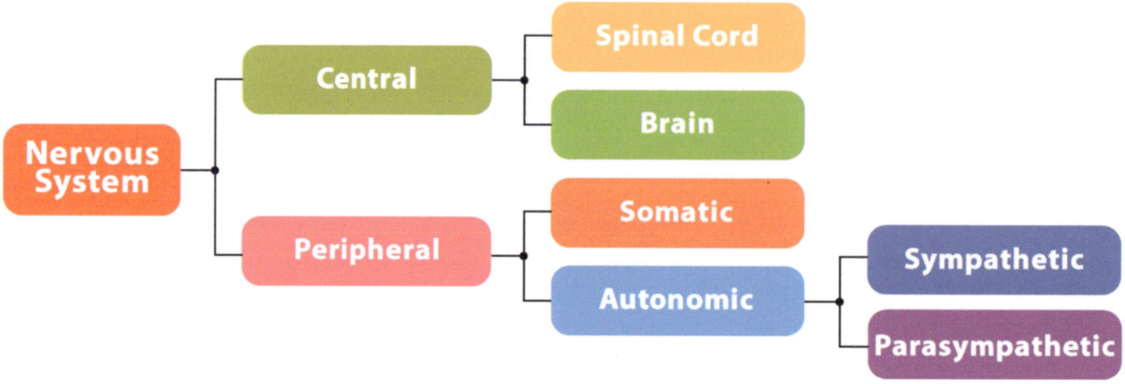

Low-level Importance

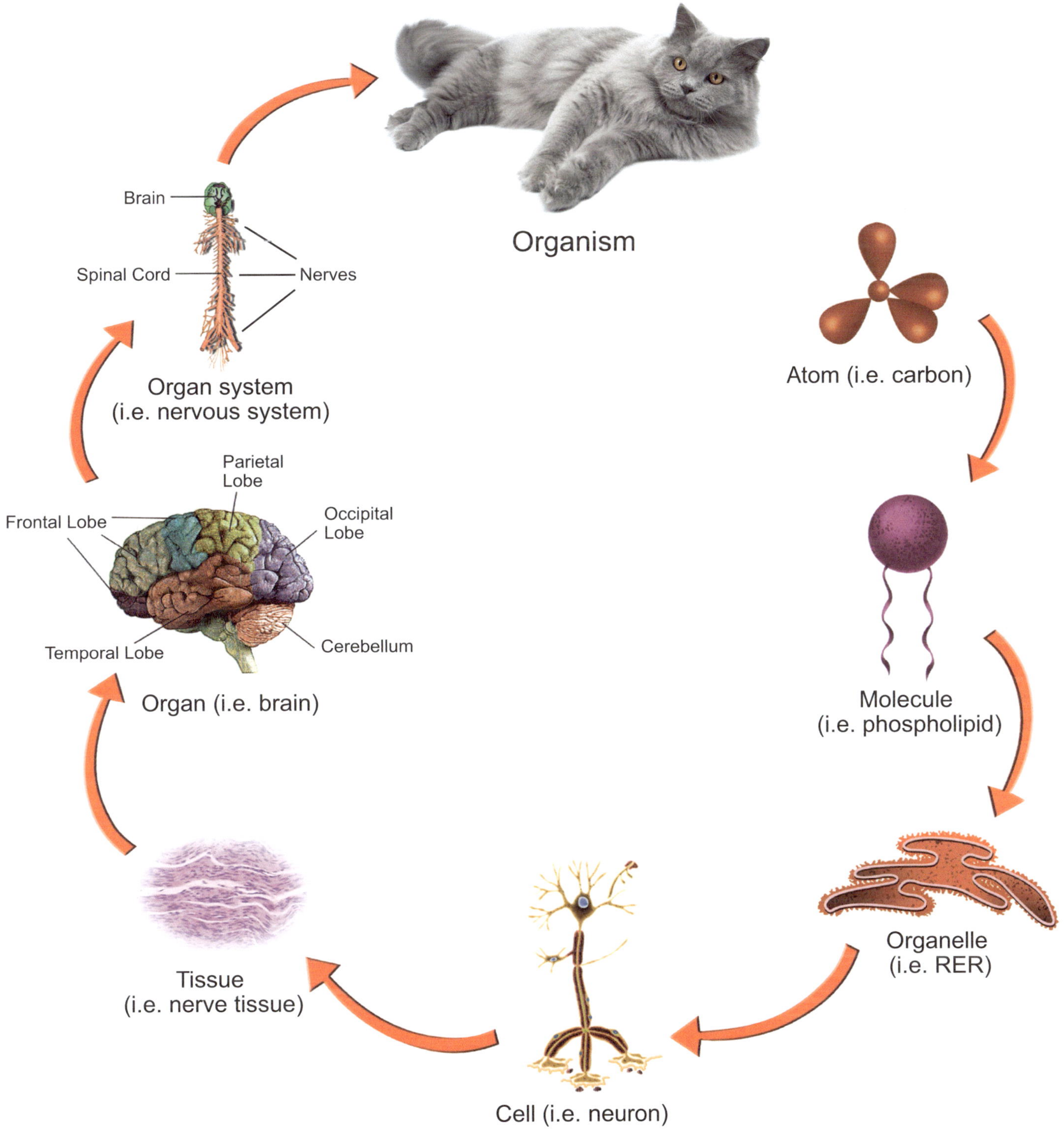

Figure IV.A.6.0: Levels of organisation.

The brain can be divided into three main regions: the forebrain which contains the telencephalon and the diencephalon; the midbrain; and the hindbrain which contains the cerebellum, the pons and the medulla. The **brain stem** includes the latter two structures and the midbrain.

The telencephalon is the **cerebral hemispheres** (cerebrum) which contain an outer surface (cortex) of gray matter. Its function is in higher order processes (i.e. learning, memory, emotions, voluntary motor activity, processing sensory input, etc.). For most people, the left hemisphere specialises in language, while the right hemisphere specialises in patterns and spatial relationships.

Each hemisphere is subdivided into four lobes: *occipital* which receives input from the optic nerve for vision; *temporal* which receives auditory signals for hearing; *parietal* which receives somatosensory information from the opposite side of the body (= heat, cold, touch, pain, and the sense of body movement); and *frontal* which is involved in problem solving and controls voluntary movements for the opposite side of the body.

The diencephalon contains the **thalamus** which is a relay centre for sensory input, and the **hypothalamus** which is crucial for homeostatic controls (heart rate, body temperature, thirst, sex drive, hunger, etc.). Protruding from its base and greatly influenced by the hypothalamus is the **pituitary** which is an endocrine gland. The limbic system, which functions to produce emotions, is composed of the diencephalon and deep structures of the cerebrum (esp. basal ganglia).

The midbrain is a relay centre for visual and auditory input and also regulated motor function.

The hindbrain consists of the cerebellum, the pons and the medulla. The cerebellum plays an important role in coordination and the control of muscle tone. The pons acts as a relay centre between the cerebral cortex and the cerebellum. The medulla controls many vital functions such as breathing, heart rate, arteriole blood pressure, etc.

There are 12 pairs of cranial nerves which emerge from the base of the brain (esp. the brain stem): *olfactory* (I) for smell; *optic* (II) for vision; *oculomotor* (III), *trochlear* (IV) and *abducens* (VI) for eye movements; *trigeminal* (V) for motor (i.e. *mastication* which is chewing) and sensory activities (i.e. pain, temperature, and pressure for the head and face); *facial* (VII) for taste (sensory) and facial expression (motor); *vestibulo-cochlear* (VIII) for the senses of equilibrium (vestibular branch) and hearing (cochlear branch); *glosso-pharyngeal* (IX) for taste and swallowing; *vagus* (X) for speech, swallowing, slowing the heart rate, and many sensory and motor innervations to smooth muscles of the viscera (internal organs) of the thorax and abdomen; *accessory* (XI) for head rotation and shoulder movement; and *hypoglossal* (XII) for tongue movement.

Both the brain and the spinal cord are surrounded by three membranes (= meninges). The outermost covering is called the dura mater, the innermost is called the pia mater (which is in direct contact with nervous tissue), while the middle layer is called the arachnoid mater. {DAP = **d**ura - **a**rachnoid - **p**ia, respectively, from out to in}.

Low-level Importance

6.1.1 The Sensory Receptors

The sensory receptors include any type of nerve ending in the body that can be stimulated by some physical or chemical stimulus either outside or within the body. These receptors include the rods and cones of the eye, the cochlear nerve endings of the ear, the taste endings of the mouth, the olfactory endings in the nose, sensory nerve endings in the skin, etc. Afferent neurons carry sense signals to the central nervous system.

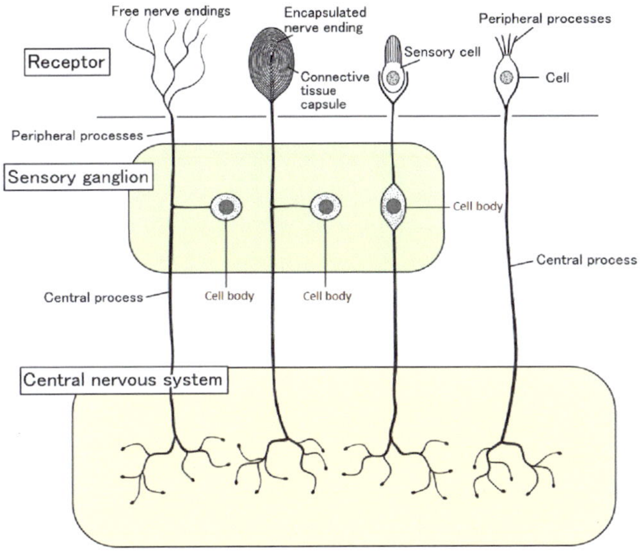

6.1.2 The Effector Receptors

These include every organ that can be stimulated by nerve impulses. An important effector system is skeletal muscle (*see* Figure IV.A.6.1). Smooth muscles of the body and the glandular cells are among the important effector organs. Efferent neurons carry motor signals from the CNS to effector receptors. {The term "effector" in biology refers to an organ, cell or molecule that *acts* in response to a stimulus (cause-effect).}

6.1.3 Reflex Arc

One basic means by which the nervous system controls the functions in the body is the reflex arc, in which a stimulus excites a receptor, appropriate impulses are transmitted into the CNS where various nervous reactions take place, and then appropriate effector impulses are transmitted to an effector organ to cause a reflex effect (i.e. removal of one's hand from a hot object, the knee-jerk reflex, etc.). The preceding can be processed at the level of the spinal cord.

Example of knee-jerk reflex: tapping on the patellar tendon causes the thigh muscle (quadriceps) to stretch. The stretching of muscle stimulates the afferent fibers, which synapse on the motoneuron (= motor neuron; BIO 5.1) in the spinal cord. The activation of the motoneuron causes contraction of the muscle that was stretched. This contraction makes the lower leg extend.

Low-level Importance

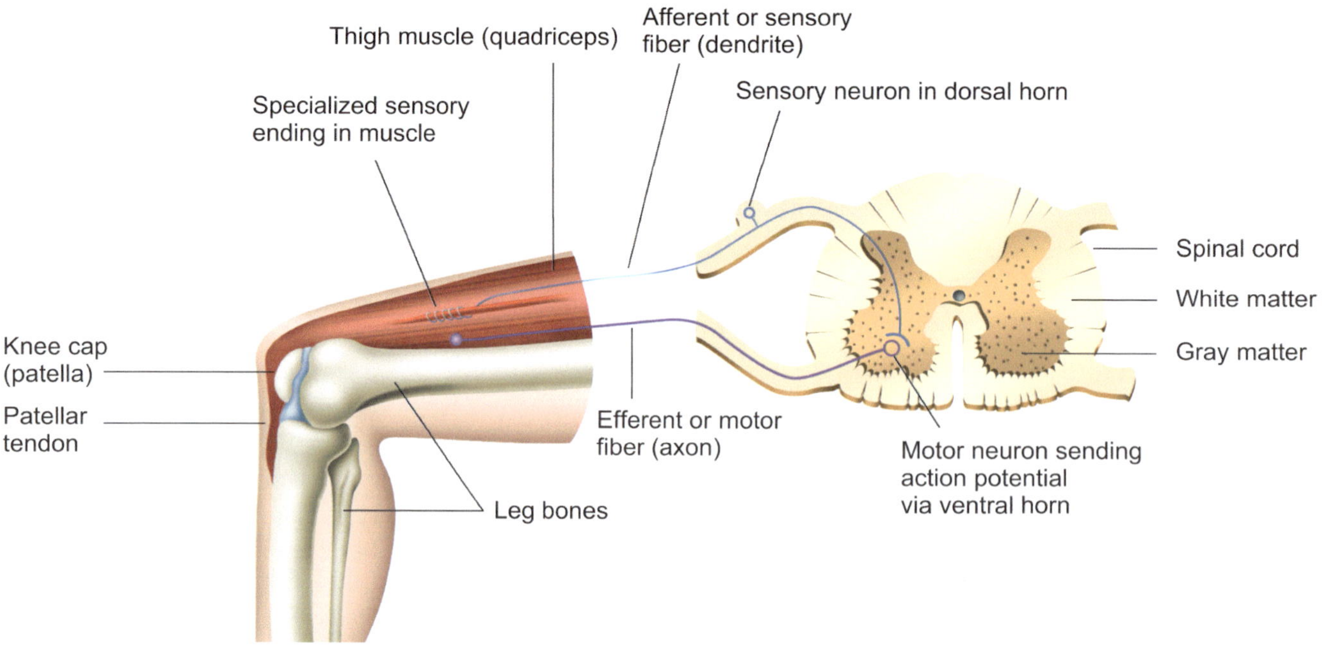

Figure IV.A.6.1: Schematic representation of the basis of the knee jerk reflex.

6.1.4 Autonomic Nervous System

While the Somatic Nervous System controls voluntary activities (i.e. innervates skeletal muscle), the Autonomic Nervous System (ANS) controls involuntary activities. The ANS consists of two components which often antagonise each other: the sympathetic and parasympathetic nervous systems.

The **Sympathetic Nervous System** originates in neurons located in the lateral horns of the gray matter of the spinal cord. Nerve fibers pass by way of anterior (ventral) nerve roots first into the spinal nerves and then immediately into the sympathetic chain. From here fiber pathways are transmitted to all portions of the body, especially to the different visceral organs and to the blood vessels.

The sympathetic nervous system uses norepinephrine as its primary neurotransmitter. This division of the nervous system is crucial in the “fight, fright or flight” responses (i.e. pupillary dilation, increase in breathing, blood pressure and heart rate, increase of blood flow to skeletal muscle, decrease of visceral function, etc.).

Parasympathetic Nervous System: The parasympathetic fibers pass mainly through the *vagus nerves*, though a few fibers pass through several of the other cranial nerves

Low-level Importance

and through the anterior roots of the sacral segments of the spinal cord. Parasympathetic fibers do not spread as extensively through the body as do sympathetic fibers, but they do innervate some of the thoracic and abdominal organs, as well as the pupillary sphincter and ciliary muscles of the eye and the salivary glands.

The parasympathetic nervous system uses acetylcholine as its primary neurotransmitter. This division of the nervous system is crucial for vegetative responses (i.e. pupillary constriction, decrease in breathing, blood pressure and heart rate, increase in blood flow to the gastro-intestinal tract, etc.).

6.1.5 Autonomic Nerve Fibers

The nerve fibers from the ANS are primarily motor fibers. Unlike the motor pathways of the somatic nervous system, which usually include a single neuron between the CNS and an effector, those of the ANS involve *two* neurons. The first neuron has its cell body in the brain or spinal cord but its axon (= *preganglionic fiber*) extends outside of the CNS. The axon enters adjacent sympathetic chain ganglia, where they synapse with the cell body of a second neuron or travel up or down the chain to synapse with that of a remote second neuron (*recall: a ganglion is a collection of nerve cell bodies outside the CNS*). The axon of the second neuron (= *postganglionic fiber*) extends to a visceral effector.

The sympathetic ganglia form chains which, for example, may extend longitudinally along each side of the vertebral column. Conversely, the parasympathetic ganglia are located *near* or *within* various visceral organs (i.e. bladder, intestine, etc.) thus requiring relatively short postganglionic fibers. Therefore, sympathetic nerve fibers are characterised by short preganglionic fibers and long postganglionic fibers while parasympathetic nerve fibers are characterised by long preganglionic fibers and short postganglionic fibers.

Both divisions of the ANS secrete *acetylcholine* from their preganglionic fibers. Most sympathetic postganglionic fibers secrete *norepinephrine* (= nor*adren*alin), and for this reason they are called ***adren**ergic* fibers. The parasympathetic postganglionic fibers secrete acetyl**choline** and are called ***cholin**ergic fibers.*

There are two types of acetylcholine receptors (AChR) that bind acetylcholine and transmit its signal: muscarinic AChRs and nicotinic AChRs, which are named after the agonists muscarine and nicotine, respectively. The two receptors are functionally different; the muscarinic type is a G-protein coupled receptor that mediates a slow metabolic response via second messenger cascades (involving cAMP), while the nicotinic type is a ligand-gated ionotropic channel that mediates a fast synaptic transmission of the neurotransmitter (no use of second messengers).

Low-level Importance

6.2 Sensory Reception and Processing

Each modality of sensation is detected by a particular nerve ending. The most common nerve ending is the free nerve ending. Different types of free nerve endings result in different types of sensations such as pain, warmth, pressure, touch, etc. In addition to free nerve endings, skin contains a number of specialised endings that are adapted to respond to some specific type of physical stimulus.

Sensory endings deep in the body are capable of detecting proprioceptive sensations such as joint receptors which detect the degree of angulation of a joint, Golgi tendon organs which detect the degree of tension in the tendons, and muscle spindles which detect the degree of stretch of a muscle fiber (*see* diagram of reflex with muscle spindle in BIO 6.1.2).

6.2.1 Olfaction

Olfaction (the sense of smell) is perceived by the brain following the stimulation of the olfactory epithelium located in the nostrils. The olfactory epithelium contain large numbers of neurons with chemoreceptors called olfactory cells which are responsible for the detection of different types of smell. Odorant molecules bind to the receptors located on the cilia of olfactory receptor neurons and produce a depolarising receptor potential. Once the depolarisation passes threshold, an action potential is generated and is conducted into CNS. It is believed that there might be seven or more primary sensations of smell which combine to give various types of smell that we perceive in life.

6.2.2 Taste

Taste buds in combination with olfaction give humans the taste sensation. Taste buds are primarily located on the surface of the tongue with smaller numbers found in the roof of the mouth and the walls of the pharynx (throat). Taste buds contain chemoreceptors which are activated once the chemical is dissolved in saliva which is secreted by the salivary glands. Contrary to olfactory receptor cells, taste receptors are not true neurons: they are chemical receptors only.

Four different types of taste buds are known to exist, each of these responding principally to saltiness, sweetness, sourness and bitterness.

When a stimulus is received by either a taste bud or an olfactory cell for the second time, the intensity of the response is diminished. This is called sensory *adaptation*.

6.2.3 Ears: Structure and Function

Ears function in both hearing and balance. It consists of three parts: the *external ear* which receives sound waves; the air-filled *middle ear* which transmits and amplifies sound waves; and the fluid-filled *inner ear* which transduces sound waves into nerve impulse. The vestibular organ, located in the inner ear, is responsible for equilibrium.

The external ear is composed of the external cartilaginous portion, the pinna or *auricle*, and the external auditory meatus or canal. The external auditory meatus connects the auricle and the middle ear or *tympanic cavity*. The tympanic cavity is bordered on the outside by the tympanic membrane, and inside the air-filled cavity are the auditory ossicles - the *malleus* (hammer), *incus* (anvil), and *stapes* (stirrup). The stapes is held by ligaments to a part of inner ear called the *oval window*. The auditory ossicles function in amplifying the sound vibration and transmitting it from the tympanic membrane to the oval window.

The inner ear or *labyrinth* consists of an osseous (= bony) labyrinth containing a membranous labyrinth. The bony labyrinth houses the semicircular canals, the cochlea and the vestibule. The semicircular canals contain the semicircular ducts of the membranous labyrinth, which can detect angular acceleration. The vestibule contains the saccule and utricle, which are sac-like thin connective tissue lined by vestibular hair cells which are responsible for the detection of linear acceleration. Together, the semicircular canals and the vestibule, known as the vestibular system,

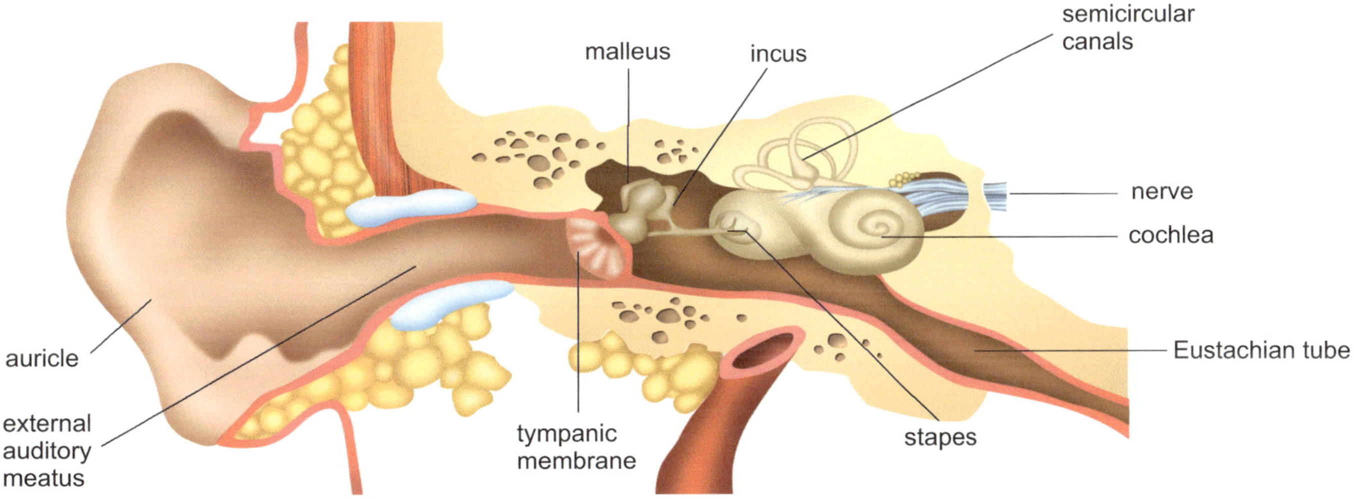

Figure IV.A.6.2: Structure of the external, middle and inner ear.

Low-level Importance

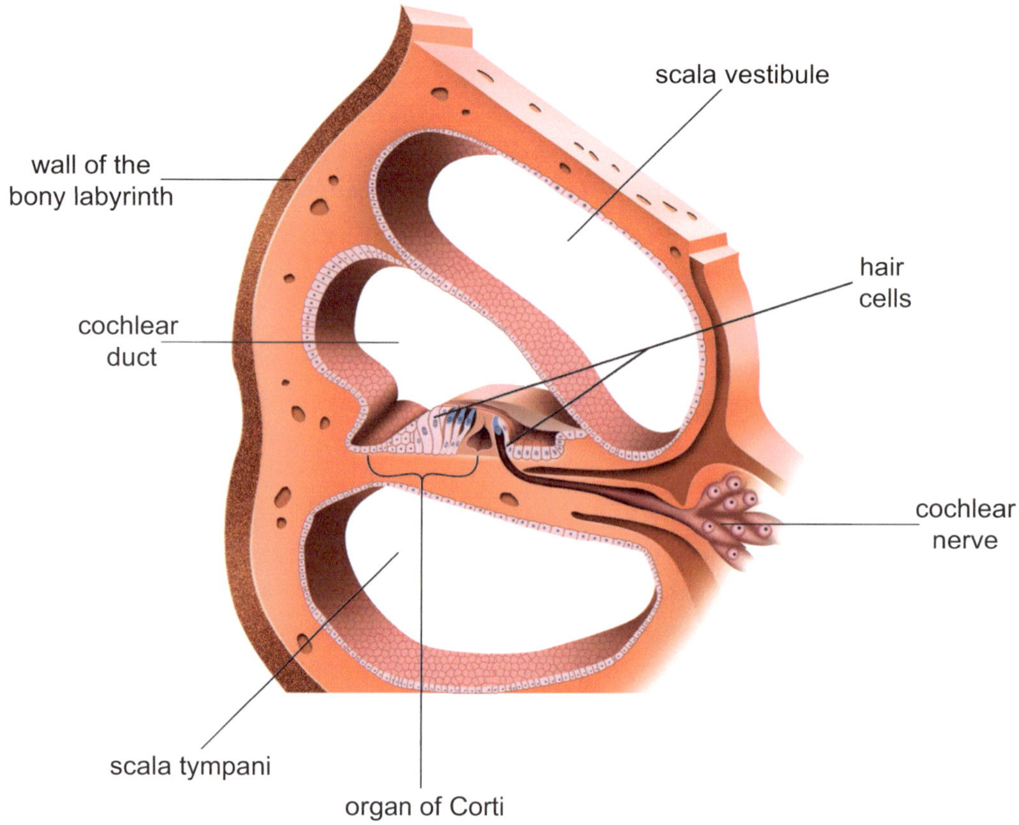

Figure IV.A.6.3: Cross-section of the cochlea.

are responsible for detection of linear and angular acceleration of the head. The cochlea is divided into three spaces: the scala vestibule, scala tympani and the scala media, or cochlear duct. The cochlear duct contains the spiral organ of Corti, which functions in the reception of sound and responds to different sound frequencies.

The eustachian tube connects the middle ear to the pharynx. This tube is important in maintaining equal pressure on both sides of the tympanic membrane. During ascent in an airplane, there is a decrease in cabin air pressure, leading to a relative increase in the pressure of the middle ear. Swallowing or yawning opens the eustachian tube allowing an equalisation of pressure in the middle ear.

Mechanism of hearing: Sound is caused by the compression of waves that travel through the air. Each compression wave is funneled by the external ear to strike the tympanic membrane (ear drum). Thus the sound vibrations are transmitted through the osseous system which consists of three tiny bones (the malleus, incus, and stapes) into the cochlea at the oval window. Movement of the stapes at the oval window causes disturbance in the lymph of cochlea and stimulates the hair cells found in the basilar membrane which is called the *organ of Corti*. Bending of the hair cells causes depolarisation of the basilar membrane. From here the auditory nerves carry the impulses to the auditory area of the brain (*temporal lobe*) where it is interpreted as sound.

6.2.4 Vision: Eye Structure and Function

The eyeball consists of three layers: **i)** an outer fibrous tunic composed of the sclera and cornea; **ii)** a vascular coat (uvea) of choroid, the ciliary body and iris; and **iii)** the retina formed of pigment and sensory (nervous) layers. The anterior chamber lies between the cornea anteriorly (in front) and the iris and pupil posteriorly (behind); the posterior chamber lies between the iris anteriorly and the ciliary processes and the lens posteriorly.

The transparent cornea constitutes the anterior one sixth of the eye and receives light from external environment. The sclera forms

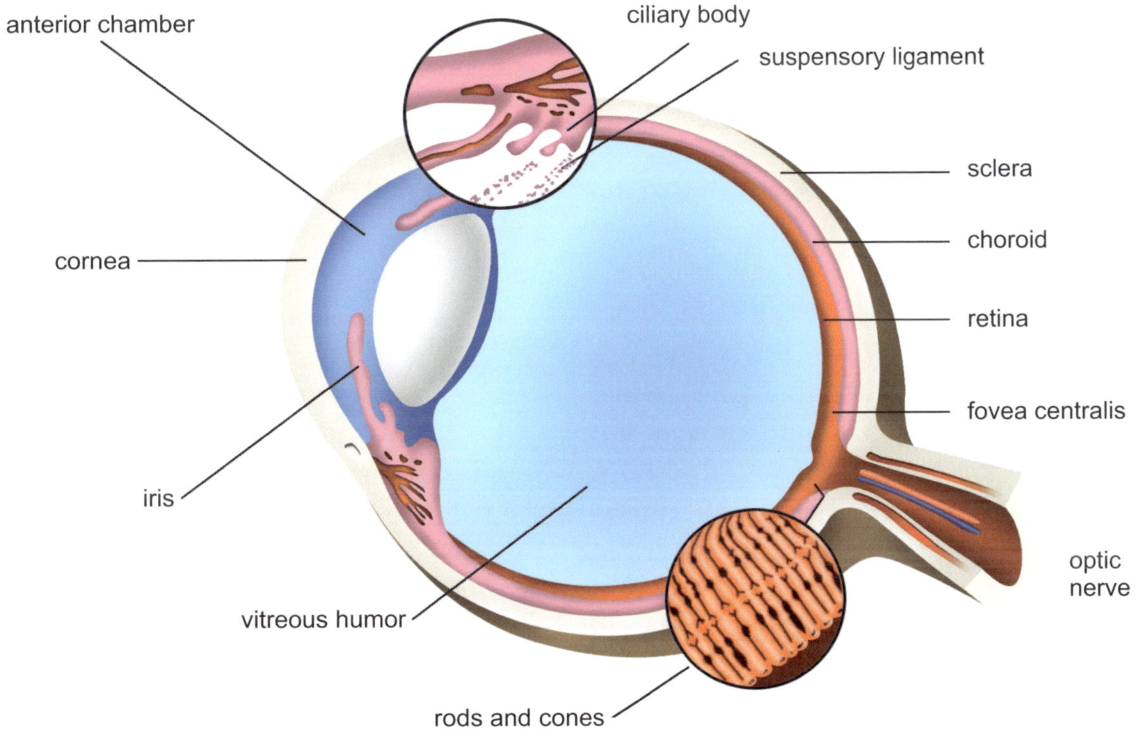

Figure IV.A.6.4: Structure of the eye.

Low-level Importance

the posterior five sixths of the fibrous tunic and is composed of dense fibrous connective tissue. The choroid layer consists of vascular loose connective tissue. The ciliary body is an anterior expansion of the choroid that encircles the lens. The lens can focus light on the retina by the contraction or relaxation of muscles in the ciliary body which transmit tension along suspensory ligaments to the lens.

Contraction of the ciliary muscle makes the lens become more convex, thereby allowing the eye to focus on nearby objects. Relaxation of the ciliary muscle allows the eye to focus on far objects. The iris separates the anterior and the posterior chamber and forms an aperture called the "pupil" whose diameter is continually adjusted by the pupillary muscles. This helps to control the intensity of light impinging on the retina.

The retina is divisible into ten layers. Layers two to five contain the rod and cone receptors of the light pathway.

Rods and Cones: The light sensitive receptors (*photoreceptors*) of the retina are millions of minute cells called rods and cones. The rods (*"night vision"*) distinguish only the black and white aspects of an image and are sensitive to light of low intensity (*"high sensitivity"*). The cones (*"day vision"*) are capable of distinguishing three colours: red, green and blue and are sensitive to light of high intensity (*"low sensitivity"*). From different combinations of these three colours, all colours can be seen.

Photoreceptors contain photosensitive pigments. For example, rods contain the membrane protein *rhodopsin* which is covalently linked to a form of vitamin A. Light causes an isomerisation of *retinal* (an aldehyde form of vitamin A) which can affect Na^+ channels in a manner as to start an action potential.

The central portion of the retina which is called the fovea centralis has only cones, which allows this portion to have very sharp vision, while the peripheral areas, which contain progressively more and more rods, have progressively more diffuse vision. Since acuity and colour vision are mediated by the same cells (cones), visual acuity is much better in bright light than dim light.

Each point of the retina connects with a discrete point in the visual cortex which is in the back of the brain (i.e. the occipital lobe). The image that is formed on the retina is upside down and reversed from left to right. This information leaves the eye via the optic nerve en route to the visual cortex which corrects the image.

Defects of vision

1. Myopia (short-sighted or nearsighted): In this condition, an image is formed in front of the retina because the lens converges light too much since the eyeballs are long. A diverging (concave) lens helps focus the image on the retina and it is used for the correction of myopia.

2. Hyperopia (long-sighted or farsighted): In this condition, an image is formed behind the retina since the eyeballs are too short. A converging (convex) lens helps focus the image on the retina.

3. Astigmatism: In this condition, the curvatures of either the cornea or the lens are different at different angles. A cylindrical lens helps to improve this condition.

4. Presbyopia: This condition is characterised by the inability to focus (especially objects which are closer). This condition, which is often seen in the elderly, is corrected by using a converging lens.

6.3 The Endocrine System

The endocrine system is the set of glands, tissues and cells that secrete hormones directly into circulatory system (ductless). The hormones are transported by the blood system, sometimes bound to plasma proteins, en route to having an effect on the cells of a target organ. Thus hormones control many of the body's functions by acting - predominantly - in one of the following major ways:

1. By controlling transport of substances through cell membranes

2. By controlling the activity of some of the specific genes, which in turn determine the formation of specific enzymes

3. By controlling directly some metabolic systems of cells.

Steroid hormones can diffuse across the plasma membrane and bind to specific receptors in the cytosol or nucleus, thus forming a direct intracellular effect (i.e. on DNA; ORG 12.4.1). Non-steroid hormones do not diffuse across the membrane. They tend to bind plasma membrane receptors, which leads to the production of a second messenger.

Secondary messengers are a component of signal transduction cascades which amplify the strength of a signal (i.e. hormone, growth factors, neurotransmitter, etc.). Examples include cyclic AMP (cAMP), phosphoinositol, cyclic GMP and arachidonic acid systems.

In all four cases, a hormone (= the primary messenger or *agonist*) binds the receptor exposing a binding site for a G-protein (the *transducer*). The G-protein, named for its ability to exchange GDP on its alpha subunit for a GTP (BIO 4.4-4.10), is bound to the inner membrane. Once the exchange for GTP takes place, the alpha subunit of the G-protein transducer breaks free from the beta and gamma subunits, all parts remaining membrane-bound. The alpha subunit is now free to move along the inner membrane and eventually contacts another membrane-bound protein - the *primary effector*.

Low-level Importance

The primary effector has an action which creates a signal that can diffuse within the cell. This signal is the *secondary messenger*.

Calcium ions are important intracellular messengers which can regulate calmodulin and are responsible for many important physiological functions, such as in muscle contraction (BIO 5.2). The enzyme phospholipase C (primary effector) produces diacylglycerol and inositol trisphosphate (secondary messenger), which increases calcium ion (secondary effector) membrane permeability. Active G-protein can also open calcium channels. The other product of phospholipase C, diacylglycerol (secondary messenger), activates protein kinase C (secondary effector), which assists in the activation of cAMP (another second messenger).

The agonist epinephrine (hormone, BIO 6.1.3) can bind a receptor activating the transducer (G-protein) and using a primary effector (adenylyl cyclase) produces a secondary messenger (cAMP) which, in turn, brings about target cell responses that are recognised as the hormone's actions.

Of the following hormones, if there is no mention as to its chemical nature, then it is a non-steroidal hormone (i.e. protein, polypeptide, etc.).

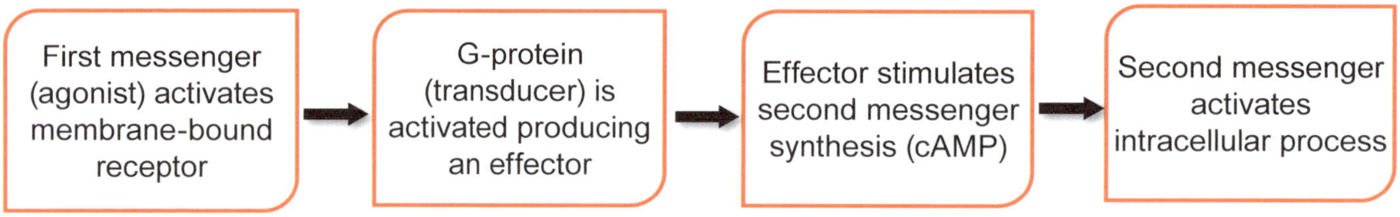

6.3.1 Pituitary Hormones

The **pituitary gland** secretes hormones that regulate a wide variety of functions in the body. This gland is divided into two major divisions: the anterior and the posterior pituitary gland. Six hormones are secreted by the anterior pituitary gland whereas two hormones are secreted by the posterior gland. The **hypothalamus** influences the secretion of hormones from both parts of the pituitary in different ways: **i)** it secretes specific *releasing factors* into special blood vessels (a *portal system* called hypothalamic-hypophysial portal system) which carries these factors (hormones) that affect the cells in the anterior pituitary by either stimulating or inhibiting the release of anterior pituitary hormones; **ii)** the hypothalamus contains neurosecretory cell bodies that synthesise, package and transport their products (esp. the two hormones oxytocin and ADH) down the axons directly into the posterior pituitary where they can be released into circulation.

The hormones secreted by the anterior pituitary gland are as follows:

1. Growth hormone (GH)
2. Thyroid Stimulating Hormone (TSH)
3. Adrenocorticotropic hormone (ACTH)
4. Prolactin
5. Follicle Stimulating Hormone (FSH) or Interstitial Cell Stimulating Hormone (ICSH)
6. Luteinising Hormone (LH)

[N.B. these latter two hormones will be discussed in the section on Reproduction, *see* BIO 14.2, 14.3]

Growth Hormone causes growth of the body. It causes enlargement and proliferation of cells in all parts of the body. Ultimately, the epiphyses of the long bones unite with the shaft of the bones (BIO 11.3.1). After adolescence, growth hormone continues to be secreted lower than the pre-adolescent rate. Though most of the growth in the body stops at this stage, the metabolic roles of the growth hormone continue such as the enhancement of protein synthesis and lean body mass, increasing blood glucose concentration, increasing lipolysis, etc.

Abnormal increase in the secretion of growth hormone at a young age results in a condition called gigantism, while a reduction in the production of growth hormone leads to dwarfism. Abnormal increase in the secretion of growth hormone in adults results in a condition called acromegaly, a disorder characterised by a disproportionate bone enlargement, especially in the face, hands and feet.

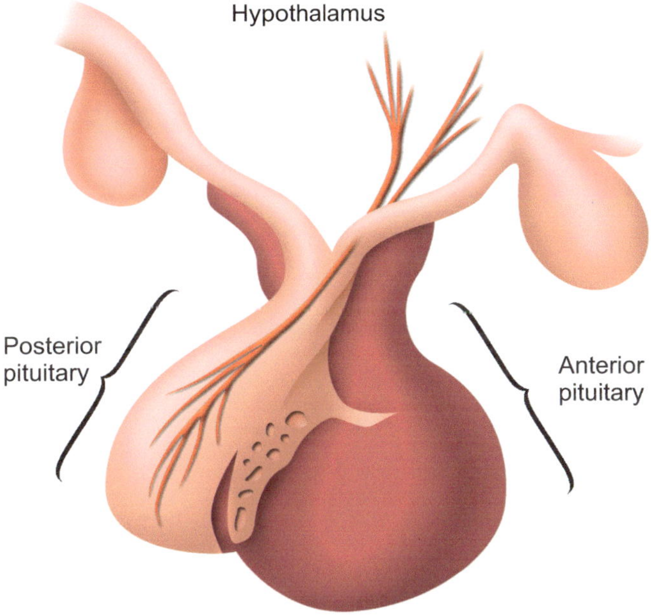

Figure IV.A.6.5: The pituitary gland.

Thyroid Stimulating Hormone stimulates the thyroid gland. The hormones produced by the thyroid gland (*thyroxine:* T_4, *triiodothyronine:* T_3) contain four and three iodine atoms, respectively. They increase the basal metabolic rate of the body (BMR). Therefore, indirectly, TSH increases the overall rate of metabolism of the body.

Adrenocorticotropic Hormone strongly stimulates the production of cortisol by the adrenal cortex, and it also stimulates the production of the other adrenocortical hormones, but to a lesser extent.

Prolactin plays an important role in the development of the breast during pregnancy and promotes milk production in the breast. In addition, a high level of prolactin can inhibit ovulation.

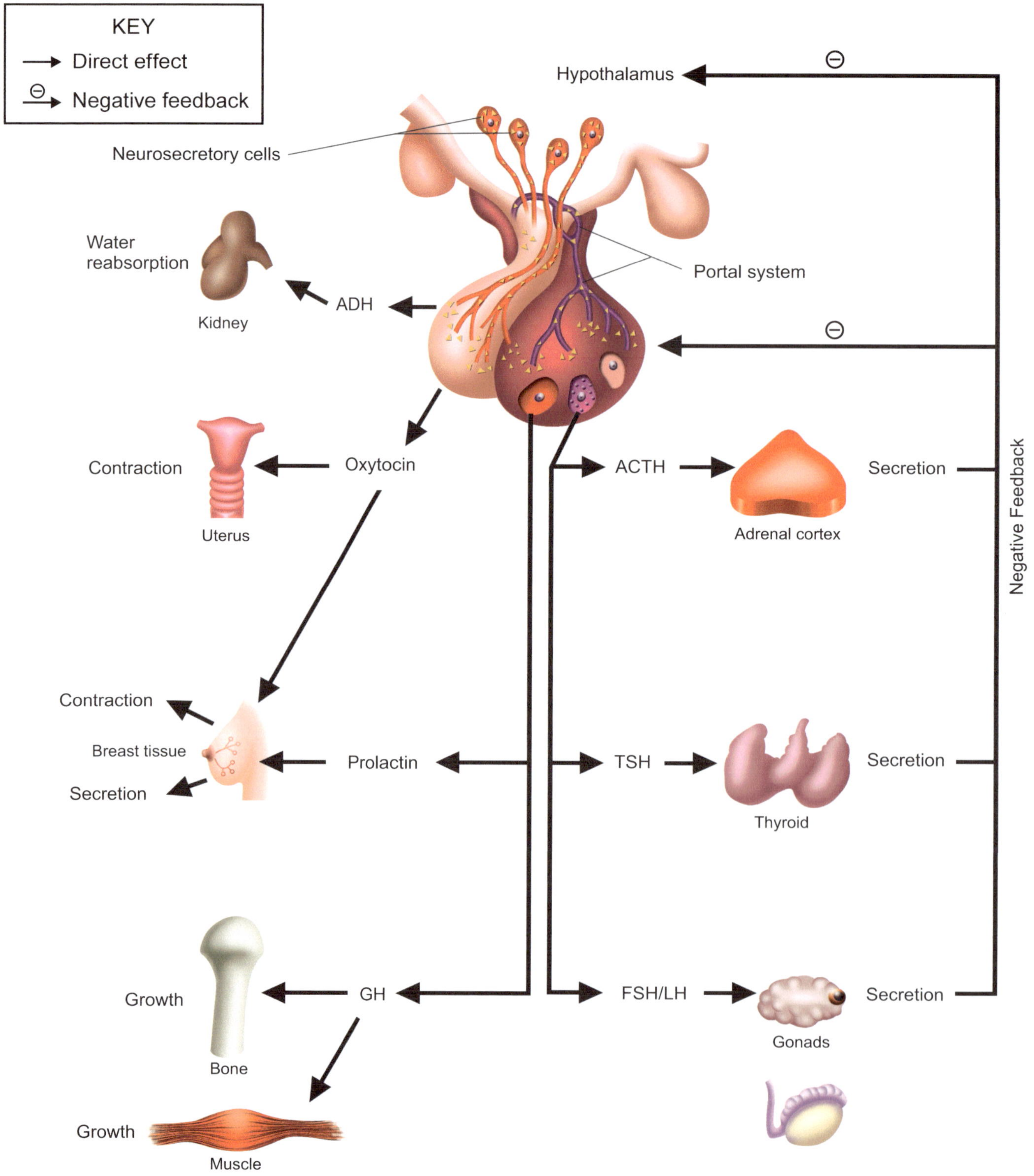

Figure IV.A.6.6: Pituitary hormones and their target organs.

Low-level Importance

Antidiuretic Hormone (ADH) is synthesised by neurosecretory cells in the hypothalamus and then travels down the axons to the posterior pituitary for secretion. Antidiuretic hormone enhances the rate of water reabsorption from the renal tubules leading to the concentration of urine (BIO 10.3). ADH also constricts the arterioles and causes a rise in arterial pressure and hence it is also called *vasopressin*.

Similar to ADH, *oxytocin* originates in the hypothalamus and then travels down the axons to the posterior pituitary for secretion. Oxytocin causes contraction of the uterus and, to a lesser extent, the other smooth muscles of the body. It also stimulates the myoepithelial cells of the breast in a manner that makes the milk flow into the ducts. This is termed milk ejection or milk *let-down*.

6.3.2 Adrenocortical Hormones

On the top of each kidney lies an adrenal gland which contains an inner region (*medulla*) and an outer region (*cortex*). The adrenal cortex secretes three different types of steroid hormones that are similar chemically but vary widely in a physiological manner.

These are:

1. Mineralocorticoids - e.g., Aldosterone
2. Glucocorticoids - e.g., Cortisol, Cortisone
3. Sex Hormones e.g., Androgens, Estrogens

Mineralocorticoids - Aldosterone

The mineralocorticoids influence the electrolyte balance of the body. Aldosterone is a mineralocorticoid which is secreted and then enhances sodium transport from the renal tubules into the peritubular fluids, and at the same time enhances potassium transport from the peritubular fluids into the tubules. In other words, aldosterone causes conservation of sodium in the body and excretion of potassium in the urine. As a result of sodium retention, there is an increased passive reabsorption of chloride ions and water from the tubules. Overproduction of aldosterone will result in excessive retention of fluid, which leads to hypertension.

Glucocorticoids - Cortisol

Several different glucocorticoids are secreted by the adrenal cortex, but almost all of the glucocorticoid activity is caused by cortisol, also called hydrocortisone. Glucocorticoids affect the metabolism of carbohydrates, proteins and lipids. It causes an increase in the blood concentration of glucose by stimulation of gluconeogenesis (generation of glucose from non-carbohydrate carbon substrates). It causes degradation of proteins and causes increased use of fat for energy. Long term use of glucocorticoids suppresses the immune system. It also has an anti-inflammatory effect by inhibiting the release of inflammatory mediators.

Sex hormones

Androgens (i.e. testosterone) are the masculinising hormones in the body. They are responsible for the development of the secondary sexual characteristics in a male (i.e. increased body hair). On the contrary estrogens have a feminising effect in the body and they are responsible for the development of the secondary sexual characteristics in a female (i.e. breast development). The proceeding hormones supplement secretions from the gonads which will be discussed later (*see* "*Reproduction*"; BIO 14.2, 14.3).

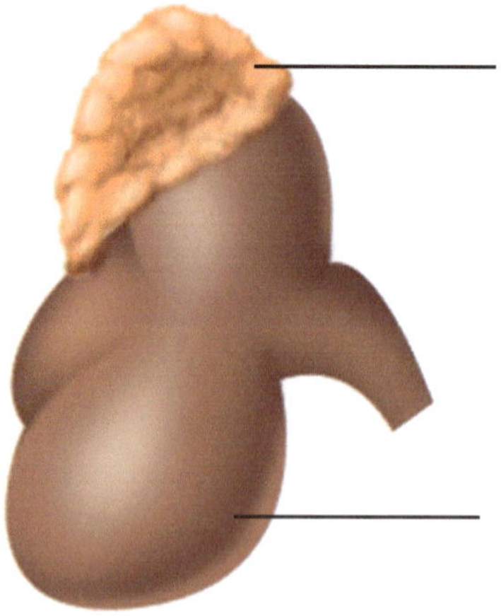

Figure IV.A.6.7: The adrenal gland sits on top of the kidney.

The Adrenal Medulla

The adrenal medulla synthesises epinephrine (= *adrenaline*) and norepinephrine which: **i)** are non-steroidal stimulants of the sympathetic nervous system; **ii)** raise blood glucose concentrations; **iii)** increase heart rate and blood pressure; **iv)** increase blood supply to the brain, heart and skeletal muscle; and **v)** decrease blood supply to the skin, digestive system and renal system.

6.3.3 Thyroid Hormones

The thyroid gland is located anteriorly in the neck and is composed of follicles lined with thyroid glandular cells. These cells secrete a glycoprotein called thyroglobulin. The tyrosine residue of thyroglobulin then reacts with iodine forming monoiodotyrosine (MIT) and diiodotyrosine (DIT). When two molecules of DIT combine, thyroxine (T_4) is formed. When one molecule of DIT and one molecule of MIT combine, tri-iodothyronine (T_3) is formed. The rate of synthesis of thyroid hormone is influenced by TSH from the pituitary.

Once thyroid hormones have been released into the blood stream they combine with several different plasma proteins. Then they are released into the cells from the blood stream. They play a vital role in maturation of CNS as thyroid hormone deficiency leads to irreversible intellectual disability. They increase heart rate, ventilation rate and O_2 consumption. They also increase the size and numbers of mitochondria and these in turn increase the rate of production of ATP, which is a factor that promotes cellular metabolism; glycogenolysis and gluconeogenesis both increase; lipolysis increases; and protein synthesis also increases. The overall effect of thyroid hormone on metabolism is catabolic.

Low-level Importance

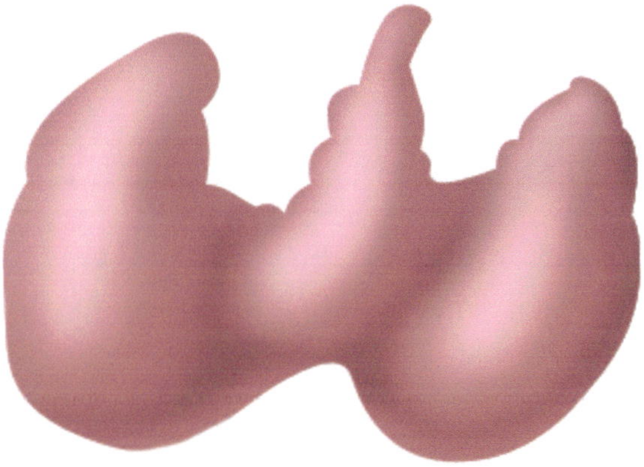

Figure IV.A.6.8: The thyroid gland.

Hyperthyroidism is an excess of thyroid hormone secretion above that needed for normal function. Basically, an increased rate of metabolism throughout the body is observed. Other symptoms include fast heart rate and respiratory rate, weight loss, sweating, tremor, and protruding eyes.

Hypothyroidism is an inadequate amount of thyroid hormone secreted into the blood stream. Generally it slows down the metabolic rate and enhances the collection of mucinous fluid in the tissue spaces, creating an edematous (fluid filled) state called myxedema. Other symptoms include slowed heart rate and respiratory rate, weight gain, cold intolerance, fatigue, and mental slowness.

The thyroid and parathyroid glands affect blood calcium concentration in different ways. The thyroid produces *calcitonin* which inhibits osteoclast activity and stimulates osteoblasts to form bone tissue; thus blood [Ca^{2+}] decreases. The parathyroid glands produce parathormone (= parathyroid hormone = PTH), which stimulates osteoclasts to break down bone, thus raising [Ca^{2+}] and [PO_4^{3-}] in the blood (BIO 5.4.4).

6.3.4 Pancreatic Hormones

The pancreas contains clusters of cells (= *islets of Langerhans*) closely associated with blood vessels. The islets of Langerhans, which perform the endocrine function of the pancreas, contain alpha cells that secrete *glucagon* and beta cells that secrete *insulin*. Glucagon increases blood glucose concentration by promoting the following events in the liver: the conversion of glycogen to glucose (*glycogenolysis*) and the production of glucose from amino acids (*gluconeogenesis*). Insulin decreases blood glucose by increasing cellular uptake of glucose, promoting glycogen formation and decreasing gluconeogenesis. A deficiency in insulin or insensitivity to insulin results in *diabetes mellitus*.

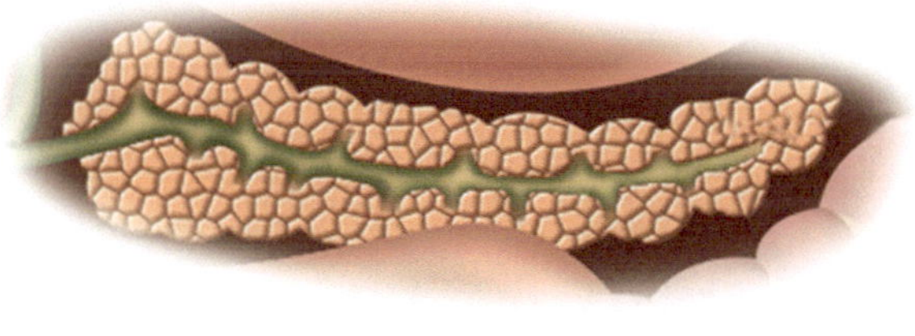

Figure IV.A.6.9: The pancreas.

Low-level Importance

6.3.5 Kidney Hormones

High-level Importance

The kidney produces and secretes *renin*, *erythropoietin* and it helps in the activation of vitamin D. Renin is an enzyme that catalyses the conversion of angiotensinogen to angiotensin I. Angiotensin I is then converted to angiotensin II by angiotensin-converting enzyme (ACE). Angiotensin II acts on the adrenal cortex to increase the synthesis and release of aldosterone, which increases Na^+ reabsorption, and causes vasoconstriction of arterioles leading to an increase in both blood volume and blood pressure. Erythropoietin increases the production of *erythrocytes* by acting on red bone marrow.

Vitamin D is a steroid which is critical for the proper absorption of calcium from the small intestine; thus it is essential for the normal growth and development of bone and teeth. Vitamin D can either be ingested or produced from a precursor by the activity of ultraviolet light on skin cells. It must be further activated in the liver and kidney by hydroxylation.

6.3.6 A Negative Feedback Loop

In order to maintain the internal environment of the body in equilibrium (= *homeostasis*), our hormones engage in various negative feedback loops. Negative feedback is self-limiting: a hormone produces biologic actions that, in turn, directly or indirectly inhibit further secretion of that hormone.

For example, if the body is exposed to extreme cold, the hypothalamus will activate systems to conserve heat (*see Skin as an Organ System*, BIO 13.1) and to produce heat. Heat production can be attained by increasing the basal metabolic rate. To achieve this, the hypothalamus secretes a releasing factor (thyrotropin-releasing hormone - TRH) which stimulates the anterior pituitary to secrete TSH. Thus the thyroid gland is stimulated to secrete the thyroid hormones (T_4/T_3; BIO 6.3.3).

Body temperature begins to return to normal. The high levels of circulating thyroid hormones begin to *inhibit* the production of TRH and TSH (= *negative feedback*) which in turn ensures the reduction in the levels of the thyroid hormones. Thus, although some overshooting is inevitable (*see* Fig. IV.A.6.10), eventually homeostasis is maintained.

The symbols used for negative feedback vary. The symbol is usually self-evident though the meaning may be clarified in the caption, or 'Key' or 'Legend' (*see* Figure IV.A.6.6 and Chapter 6 practice questions). Common symbols include an arrow with a broken line (---►), a normal arrow with an associated negative sign [– or (–) or ⊖], or lines that end as a T or C (e.g., —| or —( ).

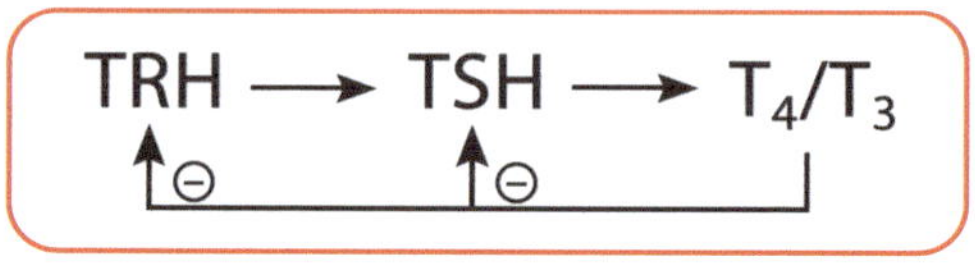

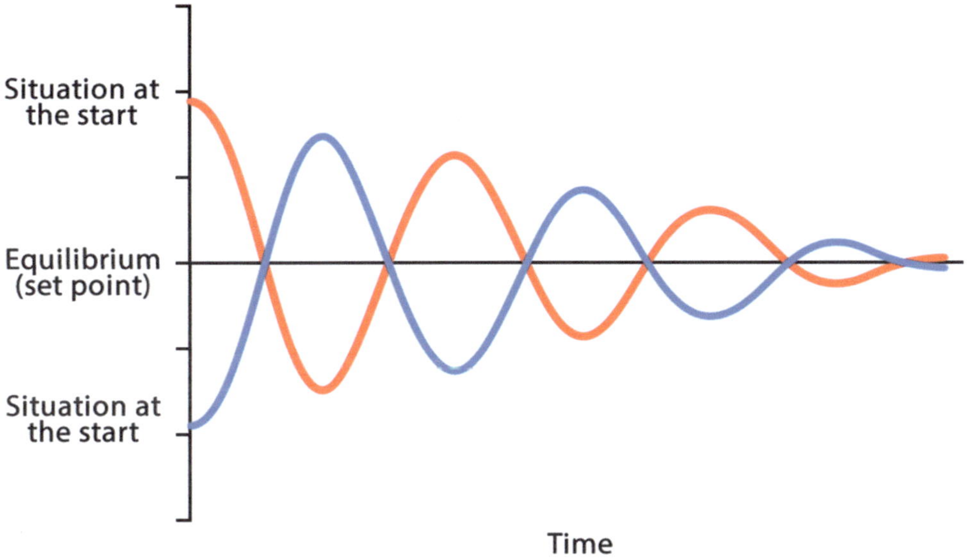

Figure IV.A.6.10: Negative feedback: return to equilibrium (*convergence*) after some degree of overshooting.

6.3.7 A Positive Feedback Loop

As opposed to negative feedback, a positive feedback loop is where the body senses a change and activates mechanisms that accelerate or increase that change. Occasionally this may help homeostasis by working in conjunction with a larger negative feedback loop, but unfortunately it often produces the opposite effect and can be life-threatening.

An example of a beneficial positive feedback loop is seen in childbirth, where stretching of the uterus triggers the secretion of oxytocin (BIO 6.3.1), which stimulates uterine contractions and speeds up labor. Of course, once the baby is out of the mother's body, the loop is broken.

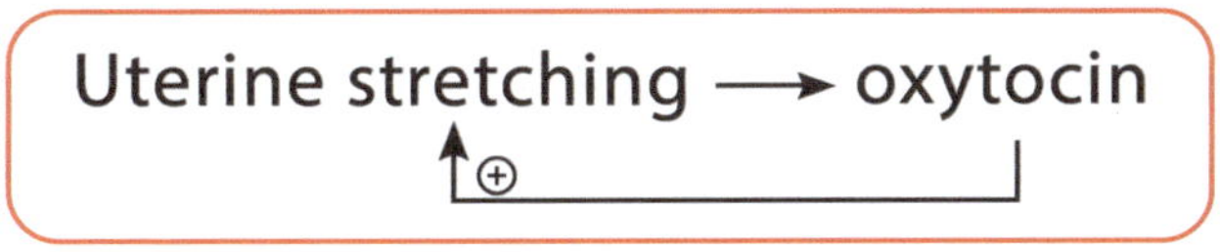

Often, however, positive feedback produces the very opposite of homeostasis: a rapid loss of internal stability with potentially fatal consequences. For example, most human deaths from SARS, the bird flu (H5N1) epidemic, and the COVID-19 pandemic were caused by a "cytokine storm" which is a positive feedback loop between immune cells and cytokines (signalling molecules similar to hormones). Thus, in many cases, it is the body's exaggerated response to infection that is the cause of death rather than the direct action of the original infecting agent. Many diseases involve dangerous positive feedback loops.

The symbols used for positive feedback normally include a simple arrow (→), or an arrow with an associated positive sign [+ or (+) or ⊕]; *see* Figure IV.A.6.6 and chapter practice questions for examples.

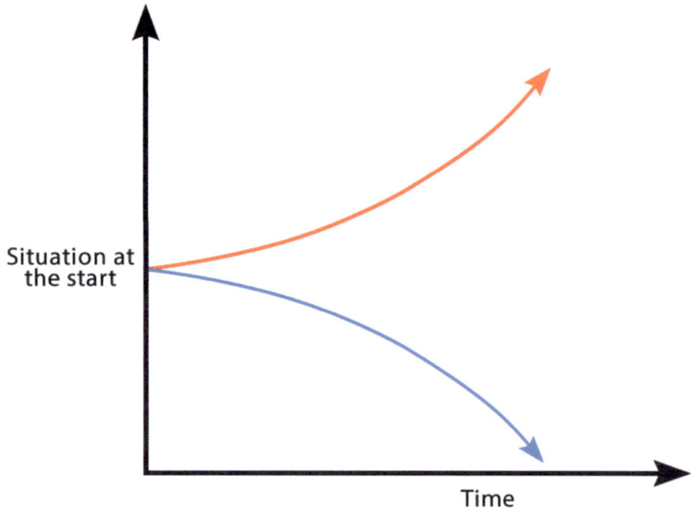

Figure IV.A.6.11: Positive feedback: no equilibrium (*divergence*) with exponential change. Note that the key difference between positive and negative feedback is their response to change: positive feedback amplifies change, while negative feedback reduces change. Positive feedback moves away from a set point (i.e. target), while negative feedback moves towards a set point.

CHAPTER 6: Nervous and Endocrine Systems

GOLD STANDARD FOUNDATIONAL GAMSAT PRACTICE QUESTIONS

1) The structure in the brain responsible for maintaining homeostasis (i.e. body temperature, heart rate, etc.) is the:

A. pituitary.
B. thalamus.
C. hypothalamus.
D. cerebellum.

2) Increased physical activity results in raising the heart rate and blood pressure. The nervous system specifically implicated is:

A. somatic.
B. peripheral.
C. parasympathetic.
D. sympathetic.

3) Which of the following features of a system is unlikely to lead to a stable homeostatic system?

A. Negative feedback
B. Positive feedback
C. Complexity
D. Redundancy

4) Which of the following best represents a possible series of physiological events following the detection by the hypothalamus of a cold environment?

A. heat promoting centre → parasympathetic nerves → adrenal medulla → epinephrine production
B. heat promoting centre → sympathetic nerves → sweat glands → stimulating local secretion
C. heat promoting centre → sympathetic nerves → adrenal medulla → epinephrine production
D. heat promoting centre → parasympathetic nerves → heart → dilated coronary vessels

Low-level Importance

GOLD STANDARD GAMSAT-LEVEL PRACTICE QUESTIONS

5) Hormones occasionally activate intracellular metabolic pathways. Consider the following branched intracellular metabolic pathway.

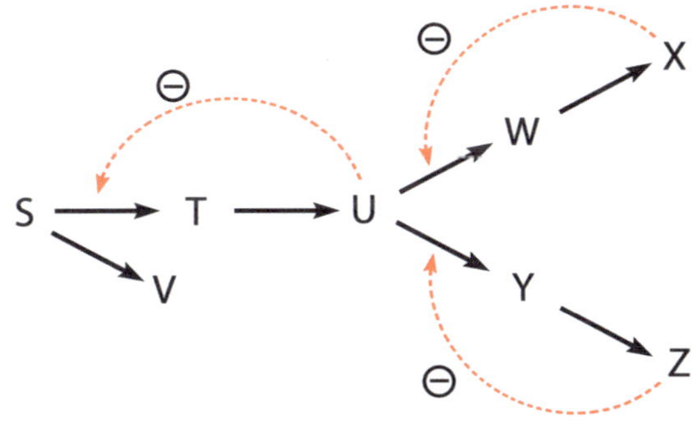

Figure 1: Metabolic pathway under investigation where dashed arrows with minus signs symbolise inhibition of a metabolic step by an end product.

Identify the reaction that would predominate if both X and Z were present in the cell in high concentrations.

A. S → V
B. Y → Z
C. U → W
D. T → U

Questions 6–7

Research suggests that the brain has an "internal clock" that is controlled by the endocrine and nervous systems. This creates a daily rhythm. The hormone ACTH helps to regulate the nervous system and gives the body the ability to respond to changes in sleep patterns. The release of ACTH is suppressed during sleep but increases before a person awakes. The feedback loop in Figure 1 illustrates part of the regulatory hormonal control of the internal clock.

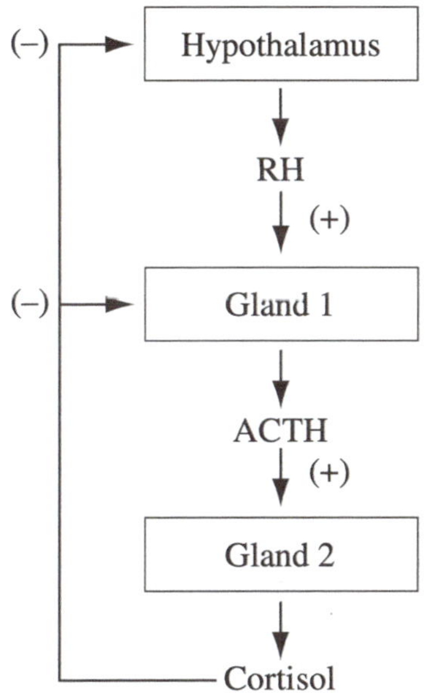

Figure 1

6) The secretion of ACTH is suppressed during sleep as a result of:

A. decreased secretion of RH by the hypothalamus.
B. decreased activity of Gland 2.
C. decreased secretion of cortisol.
D. increased nervous system input to Gland 1.

7) Which of the following is most consistent with positive feedback?

A. Increased RH secretion leads to increased ACTH secretion.
B. Cold temperatures decrease body temperature below normal leading to shivering.
C. Hot temperatures increase body temperature above normal leading to sweating.
D. Blood pressure decreases greatly making blood flow to the heart inadequate which leads to blood pressure decreasing.

Questions 8–11

Aside from diabetes, thyroid disease is the most common glandular disorder. Millions of people are treated for thyroid conditions, often an underactive or overactive gland. Overwhelmingly, women between the ages of 20 and 60 are much more likely than men to succumb to these conditions. The etiology lies in the failure of the immune system to recognise the thyroid gland as part of the body and thus antibodies are sent to attack the gland.

The plasma proteins that bind thyroid hormones are albumin, a prealbumin called thyroxine-binding prealbumin (TBPA), and a globulin with an electrophoretic mobility, thyroxine-binding globulin (TBG). The free thyroid hormones in plasma are in equilibrium with the protein-bound thyroid hormones in the tissues. Free thyroid hormones are added to the circulating pool by the thyroid. It is the free thyroid hormones in plasma that are physiologically active (increasing the metabolic rate) and imbalances in these hormones result in thyroid disease. In thyroid storm, a form of hyperthyroidism, the normal body temperature of 37.5 °C may rise to over 40 °C.

In addition, in humans there are four small parathyroid glands that produce the hormone, parathormone, which is a peptide composed of 84 amino acids. Parathormone and the thyroid hormone calcitonin work antagonistically to regulate the plasma calcium and phosphate levels. Overactive parathyroid glands, *hyperparathyroidism*, can lead to an increase in the level of calcium in plasma and tissues.

Protein	Plasma Level (mg/dl)	Thyroxine Binding Capacity (μg/dl)	Affinity for thyroxine	Amount of thyroxine bound in normal plasma (μg/dl)
Thyroxine binding globulin (TBG)	1.0	20	High	7
Thyroxine binding prealbumin (TBPA)	30.0	250	Moderate	1
Albumin	...	1000	Low	None
Total protein-bound thyroxine in plasma	...	...	...	8

Table 1: Different plasma proteins and their binding capacity and affinity for thyroxine.

8) According to Table 1, it would be expected that:

A. TBG has the highest binding capacity for thyroxine while TBPA has the highest affinity.
B. TBG has the highest binding capacity for thyroxine while albumin has the lowest affinity.
C. albumin has the highest binding capacity for thyroxine while TBPA has the highest affinity.
D. albumin has the highest binding capacity for thyroxine while TBG has the highest affinity.

Question 9 refers to Figure 1.

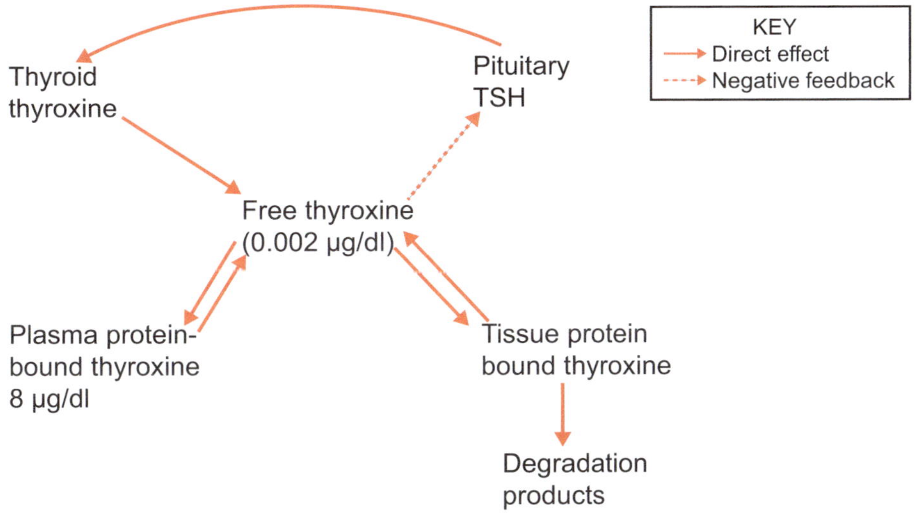

Figure 1

9) According to the equilibrium shown in Figure 1, an elevation in the concentration of free thyroid hormone in the plasma is followed by:

A. an increase in tissue protein-bound thyroxine.

B. an increase in tissue protein-bound thyroxine and plasma protein-bound thyroxine.

C. an increase in the amount of TSH secreted from the pituitary gland.

D. an increase in both the amount of TSH secreted from the pituitary gland and the release of thyroxine from the thyroid gland.

10) Symptoms that can be inferred to be consistent with hypothyroidism and hyperthyroidism, respectively, include:

A. a fine tremor and diminished concentration.

B. brittle nails and kidney stones.

C. rapid heart beat and increased irritability.

D. lethargy and nervous agitation.

11) Which of the following is an example of positive feedback?

A. A body temperature of 39 °C causes a further increase

B. Elevated TSH results in elevated thyroxine

C. Calcitonin and parathormone regulate calcium levels

D. Increased TBG leads to an increase in TSH

High-level Importance

Questions 12–13

Consider Figure 1.

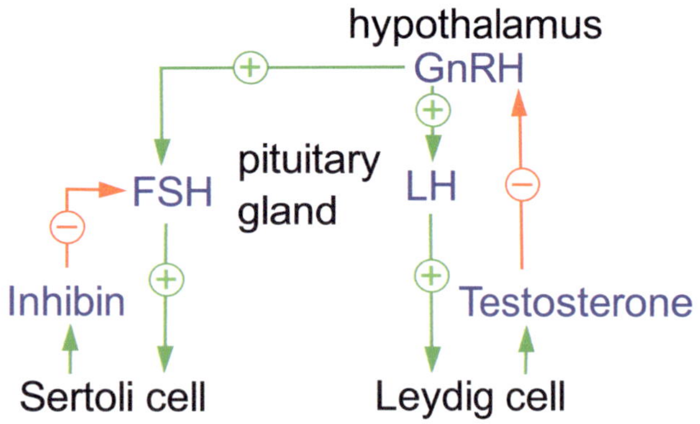

Figure 1: Hypothalamus-pituitary-testicle-hormone-axis

12) Which of the following is a precursor (i.e. a substance that is converted to another) to FSH?

A. GnRH
B. Inhibin
C. Testosterone
D. Neither **A** nor **B** nor **C**.

13) A trial medication, Katai-30, simulates inhibin. Based on Figure 1, if Katai-30 is given to a patient, one would expect an increase in the activity of which of the following?

A. Hypothalamus
B. Pituitary
C. Sertoli cell
D. Leydig cell

Questions 14–15

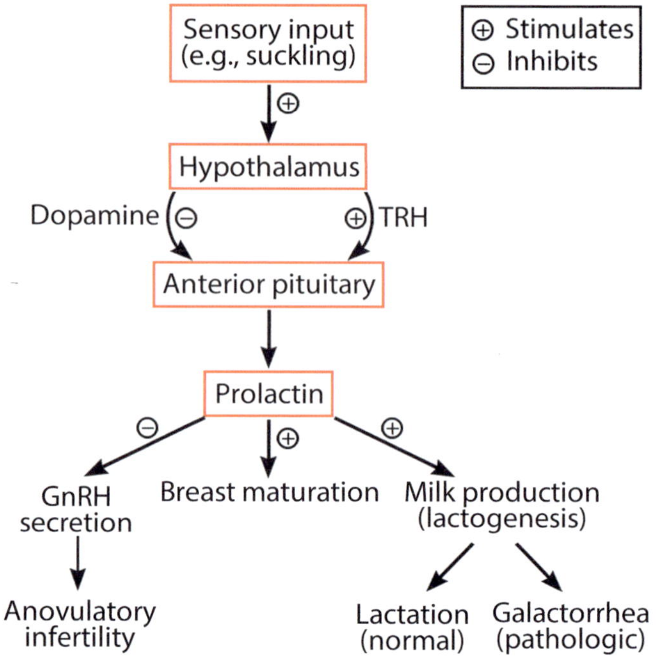

Figure 1

14) An agonist is a substance which initiates a physiological response when combined with a receptor. Bromocriptine is a dopamine agonist. According to Figure 1, if a patient takes bromocriptine, the most immediate effect would be an increase in which of the following?

A. Milk production
B. Dopamine
C. Prolactin
D. GnRH

15) Based on Figure 1, possible clinical uses for bromocriptine would include the treatment of:

A. prolactin-secreting pituitary tumours.
B. galactorrhea.
C. both **A** and **B**.
D. neither **A** nor **B**.

SPOILER ALERT ⚠

Gold Standard has cross-referenced the content in this chapter to examples from ACER's official GAMSAT practice materials. It is for you to decide when you want to explore these questions since you may want to preserve some of ACER's materials for timed mock-exam practice.

Examples – Pathway questions with respect to stomach acid (negative and positive feedback): Q1-5 of 4; is it a precursor? Q17 of 4; a famous graph: Q18 of 5. Note that "Q" is followed by the question number, and, for example, "of 1" refers to booklet number 1 which is referenced in the Spoiler Alert table at the end of Chapter 1. The 15 full-length GAMSAT practice tests by Gold Standard, HEAPS-1 through HEAPS-15, contain specific cross-references to this chapter within the worked solutions. Note that the thyroid hormone unit is from HEAPS-6 and the internal clock unit is from HEAPS-8.

Chapter Checklist

- ☐ Access your online account to view answers, worked solutions and discussion boards.
- ☐ Reassess your 'learning objectives' for this chapter: Go back to the first page of this chapter and re-evaluate the top 3 boxes and the Introduction.
- ☐ Complete a maximum of 1 page of notes using symbols/abbreviations to represent the entire chapter based on your learning objectives. These are your Gold Notes.
- ☐ Consider your multimedia options based on your optimal way of learning:
  - ☐ Download the free Gold Standard GAMSAT app for your Android device or iPhone.
  - ☐ Create your own, tangible study cards or try the free app: Anki.
  - ☐ Record your voice reading your Gold Notes onto your smartphone (audio files, e.g., *memo* or MP3s) and listen during exercise, transportation, etc.
  - ☐ Try out the Gold Standard GAMSAT online videos at gamsat-prep.com, or you can try other options on YouTube like Khan Academy or Crash Course Biology.
- ☐ Reassess your schedule for your full-length GAMSAT practice tests: ACER and/or HEAPS exams. Ensure that you have scheduled one full day to complete a practice test and 1-2 days for a thorough assessment of worked solutions while adding to your abbreviated Gold Notes.
- ☐ Reassess your progress in scheduling and/or evaluating stress reduction techniques such as regular exercise (sports), yoga, meditation and/or mindfulness exercises (*see* YouTube for suggestions).

High-level Importance

THE CIRCULATORY SYSTEM
Chapter 7

Memorise

* Circulatory and lymphatic systems: basic structures and functions
* Basic features of the sigmoidal oxygen dissociation curve for hemoglobin

Understand

* Circulation: structure/function; 4 chambered heart: systolic/diastolic pressure
* Oxygen transport; hemoglobin, oxygen content/affinity, graph and L/R shifts
* Substances transported by blood, lymph
* Source of lymph: diffusion from capillaries by differential pressure

Importance

High level: 19% of GAMSAT Biology questions released by ACER are related to content in this chapter (in our estimation).
* Note that approximately 75% of the questions in GAMSAT Biology are related to just 7 chapters: 1, 2, 3, 4, 7, 12, and 15.

GAMSAT-Prep.com

Introduction

The circulatory system is concerned with the movement of nutrients, gases and wastes to and from cells. The circulatory or cardiovascular system (closed) distributes blood while the lymphatic system (open) distributes lymph.

With respect to Biology assumed knowledge for the GAMSAT, there is no chapter more important than Chapter 7. This is one of the rare chapters in which there are multiple elements that are often helpful for the real exam.

Multimedia Resources at GAMSAT-Prep.com

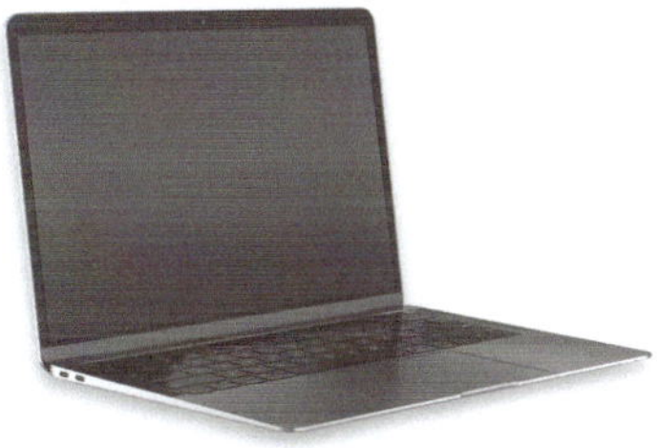

Open Discussion Boards
(*gamsat-prep.com/forum*)

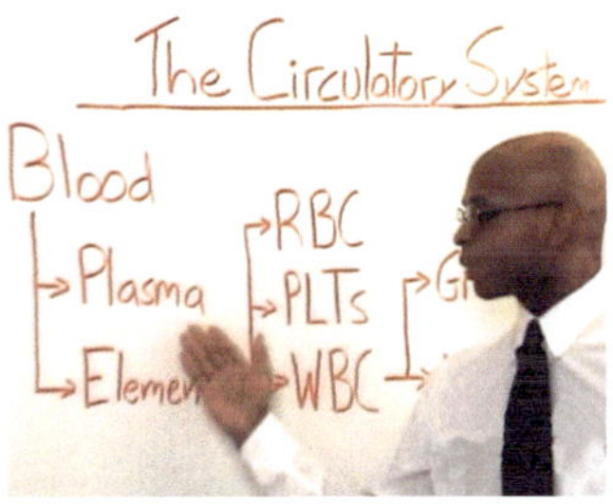

Foundational Videos

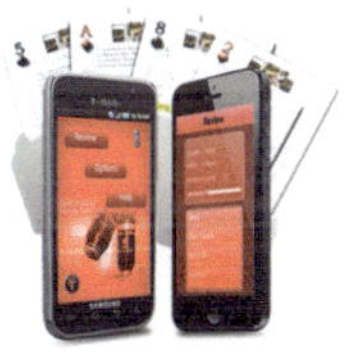

Flashcards

Special Guest

* The real GAMSAT may have advanced-level information presented (i.e. in a passage) but previous knowledge of said information is not required to answer the questions that would follow. Practice questions at the end of this chapter, as well as ACER and GS (HEAPS) practice GAMSATs can help you clarify this point.

7.1 Generalities

High-level Importance

The circulatory system is composed of the heart, blood, and blood vessels. The heart (which acts like a pump) and its blood vessels (which act like a closed system of ducts) are called the *cardiovascular system* which moves the blood throughout the body.

The following represents some important functions of blood within the circulatory system.

* It transports:

- hormones from endocrine glands to target tissues
- molecules and cells which are components of the immune system
- nutrients from the digestive tract (usu. to the liver)
- oxygen from the respiratory system to body cells
- waste from the body cells to the respiratory and excretory systems.

* It aids in temperature control (*thermoregulation*) by:

- distributing heat from skeletal muscle and other active organs to the rest of the body
- being directed to or away from the skin depending on whether or not the body wants to release or conserve heat, respectively.

7.2 The Heart

The heart is a muscular, cone-shaped organ about the size of a fist. The heart is composed of connective tissue (BIO 5.4) and cardiac muscle (BIO 5.2) which includes a region that generates electrical signals (*see* BIO 11.2 for SA node). The heart contains four chambers: two thick muscular walled *ventricles* and two thinner walled *atria*. An inner wall or *septum* separates the heart (and therefore the preceding chambers) into left and right sides. The atria contract or *pump* blood more or less simultaneously and so do the ventricles.

Deoxygenated blood returning to the heart from all body tissues except the lungs (= *systemic circulation*) enters the right atrium through large veins (= *venae cavae*). The blood is then pumped into the right ventricle through the tricuspid valve (which is one of many one-way valves in the cardiovascular system). Next the blood is pumped to the lungs (= *pulmonary circulation*) through semilunar valves (pulmonary valves) and pulmonary arteries {remember: blood in arteries goes away from the heart}.

The blood loses CO_2 and is **oxygenated** in the lungs and returns through pulmonary veins to the left atrium. Now the blood is pumped through the mitral (= bicuspid) valve into the largest chamber of the heart: the left ventricle. This ventricle's task is to return

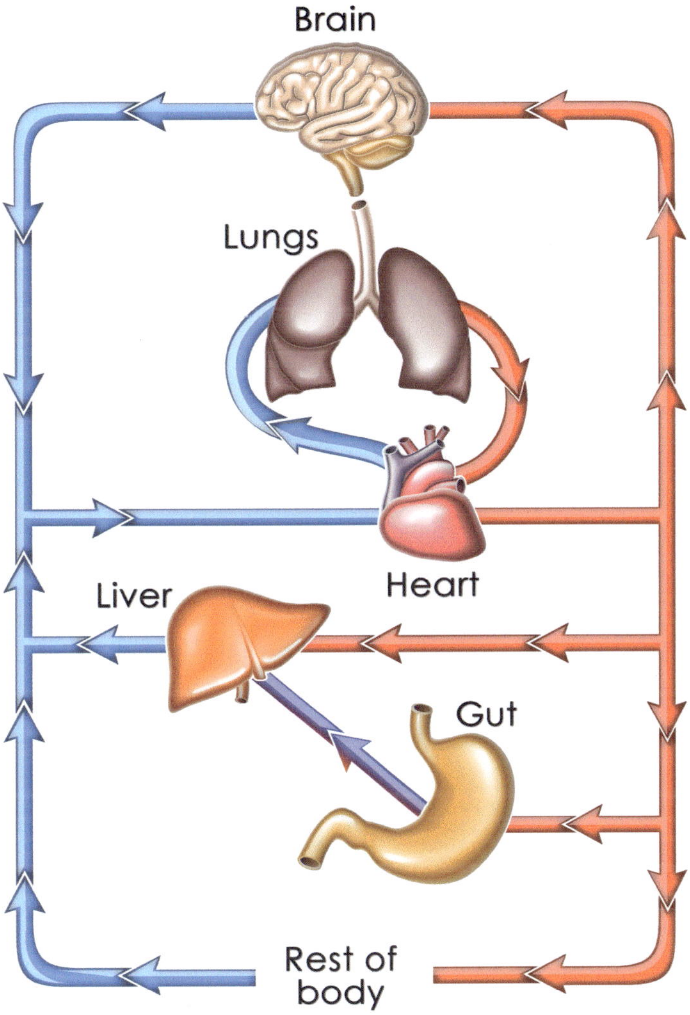

Figure IV.A.7.0: Overview of vascular anatomy.

The vascular anatomy of the human body or for an individual organ is comprised of both in-series and in-parallel vascular components. Blood leaves the heart through the aorta (high in oxygen, red in colour) from which it is distributed to major organs by large arteries, each of which originates from the aorta. Therefore, these major distributing arteries are in parallel with each other. Thus the circulations of the head, arms, gastrointestinal systems, kidneys, and legs are all parallel circulations. There are some exceptions, notably the gastrointestinal (gut) and hepatic (liver) circulations, which are partly in series because the venous drainage from the intestines become the hepatic portal vein which supplies most of the blood flow to the liver. Vessels transporting from one capillary bed to another are called portal veins (besides the liver, note the portal system in the anterior pituitary, BIO 6.3.1).

blood into the systemic circulation by pumping into a huge artery: the *aorta* (its valve is the aortic valve).

The mitral (= bicuspid = 2 leaflets) and tricuspid (tri = 3 leaflets) valves are prevented from everting into the atria by strong fibrous cords (*chordae tendineae*) which are attached to small mounds of muscle (*papillary muscles*) in their respective ventricles. A major cause of heart murmurs is the inadequate functioning of these valves.

7.3 Blood Vessels

Blood vessels include arteries, arterioles, capillaries, venules and veins. Whereas arteries tend to have thick, smooth muscular walls and contain blood at high pressure, veins have thinner walls and low blood pressure. However, veins contain the highest proportion of blood in the cardiovascular system (about 2/3rds). The wall of a blood vessel is composed of an outer adventitia, an inner intima and a *m*iddle *m*uscle layer, the *media*.

Oxygenated blood entering the systemic circulation must get to all the body's tissues. The aorta must divide into smaller and smaller arteries (small artery = **arteriole**) in order to get to the level of the capillary which i) is the smallest blood vessel; ii) often forms branching networks called *capillary beds*; and iii) is the level at which the exchange of wastes and gases (i.e. O_2 and CO_2) occurs by diffusion.

In the next step in circulation, the newly deoxygenated blood enters very small veins (= **venules**) and then into larger and larger veins until the blood enters the venae cavae and then the right atrium. There are two venae cavae: one drains blood from the upper body while the other drains blood from the lower body (*superior* and *inferior* venae cavae, respectively).

Since the walls of veins are thin and somewhat floppy, they are often located in muscles. Thus movement of the leg squeezes the veins, which pushes the blood through 1-way bicuspid valves toward the heart. This is referred to as the *muscle pump.*

Coronary arteries branch off the aorta to supply the heart muscle.

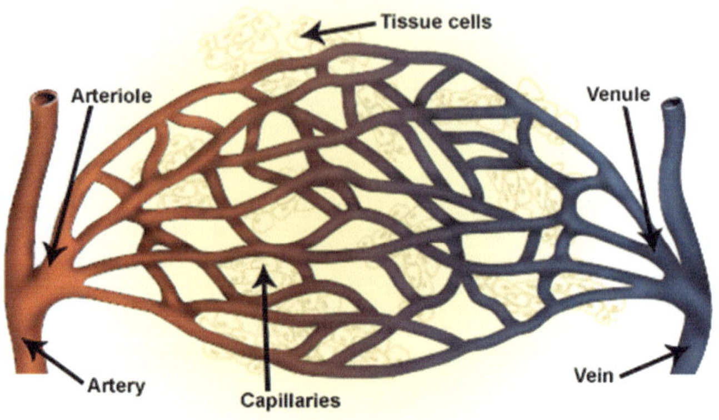

Figure IV.A.7.0b: Overview of small vessel anatomy.

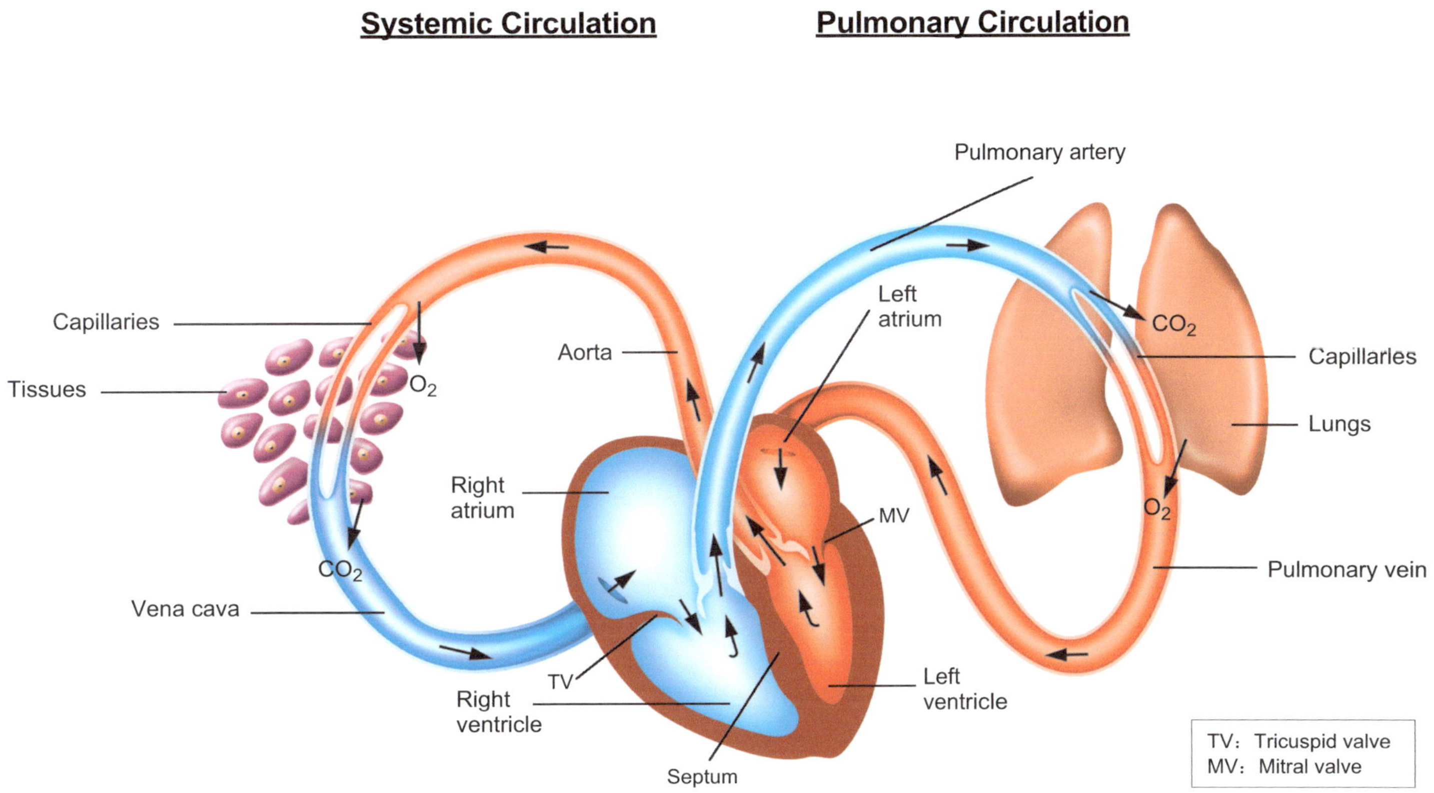

Figure IV.A.7.1: Schematic representation of the circulatory system.

Systemic circulation: transports blood from the left ventricle into the aorta then to all parts of the body and then returns to the right atrium from the superior and inferior venae cavae. *Pulmonary circulation:* transports blood from the right ventricle into pulmonary arteries to the lungs for exchange of oxygen and carbon dioxide and returns blood to the left atrium from pulmonary veins.

7.4 Blood Pressure

Blood pressure is the force exerted by the blood against the inner walls of blood vessels (esp. arteries). Maximum arterial pressure is measured when the ventricle contracts and blood is pumped into the arterial system (= *systolic pressure*). Minimal arterial pressure is measured when the ventricle is relaxed and blood is returned to the heart via veins (= *diastolic pressure*). Pulse pressure is the difference between the systolic pressure and the diastolic pressure. Blood pressure is usually measured in the brachial artery in the arm. A pressure of 120/80 signifies a systolic pressure of 120 mmHg and a diastolic pressure of 80 mmHg. The *pulse pressure* is the difference (i.e. 40 mmHg).

High-level Importance

Peripheral resistance is essentially the result of arterioles and capillaries which resist the flow of blood from arteries to veins (the narrower the vessel, the higher the resistance). Arterioles are the site of the highest resistance in the cardiovascular system. An increase in peripheral resistance causes a rise in blood pressure. As blood travels down the systemic circulation, blood pressure decreases progressively due to the peripheral resistance to blood flow.

7.5 Blood Composition

Blood contains plasma (55%) and *formed elements* (45%). Plasma is a straw coloured liquid which is mostly composed of water (92%), electrolytes, and the following plasma proteins:

* **Albumin** which is important in maintaining the osmotic pressure and helps to transport many substances in the blood

* **Globulins** which include both transport proteins and the proteins which form antibodies

* **Fibrinogen** which polymerises to form the insoluble protein *fibrin* which is essential for normal blood clotting. If you take away fibrinogen and some other clotting factors from plasma you will be left with a fluid called *serum*.

The formed elements of the blood originate from precursors in the bone marrow which produce the following for the circulatory system: 99% red blood cells (= *erythrocytes*), then there are platelets (= *thrombocytes*), and white blood cells (= *leukocytes*). Red blood cells (RBCs) are biconcave cells without nuclei (*anucleate*) that circulate for 110-120 days before their components are recycled by macrophages. Interestingly, mature RBCs do not possess most organelles such as mitochondria, Golgi nor ER because RBCs are packed with hemoglobin. The primary function of hemoglobin is the transport of O_2 and CO_2 to and from tissue.

Platelets are cytoplasmic fragments of large bone marrow cells (*megakaryocytes*) which are involved in blood clotting by adhering to the collagen of injured vessels, releasing mediators which cause blood vessels to constrict (= *vasoconstriction*), etc.

Calcium ions (Ca^{2+}) are also important in blood clotting because they help in signaling platelets to aggregate.

White blood cells help in the defense against infection; they are divided into *granulocytes* and *agranulocytes* depending on whether or not the cell does or does not contain granules, respectively.

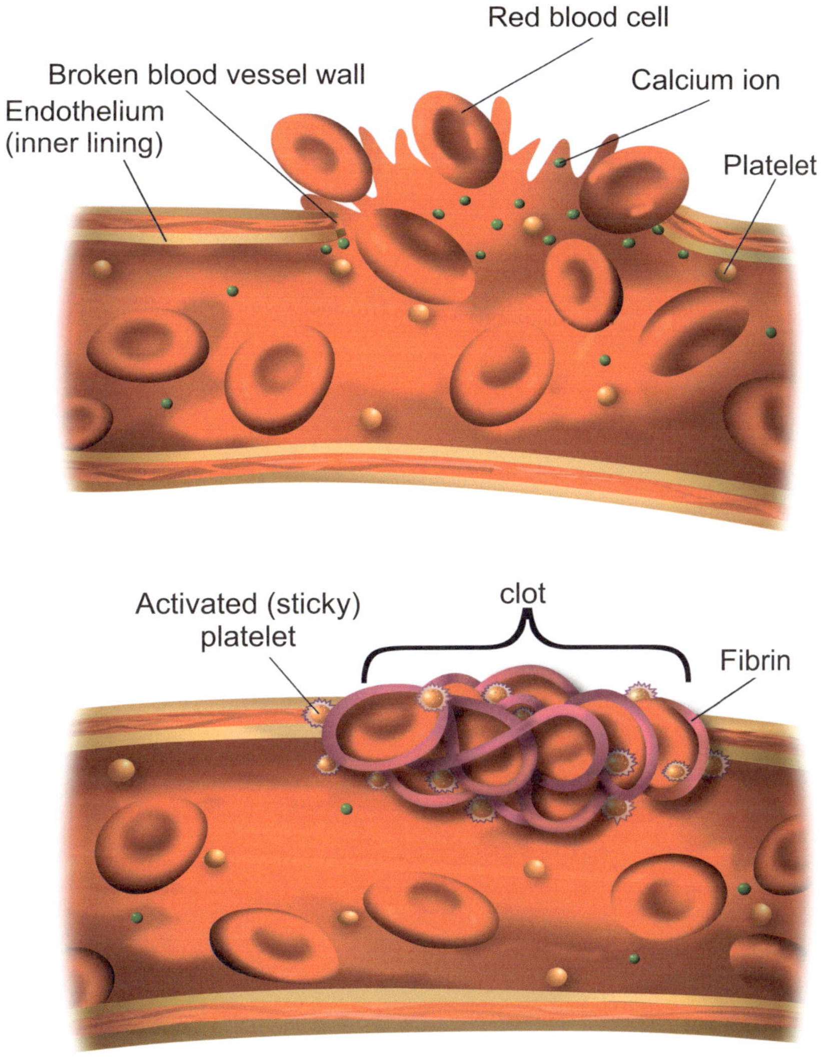

Figure IV.A.7.1.1: Schematic representation of blood clotting.

Granulocytes (= *polymorphonuclear leukocytes*) possess varying number of azurophilic (burgundy when stained) granules and are divided into: i) neutrophils which are the first white blood cells to respond to infection, they are important in controlling bacterial infection by phagocytosis - killing and digesting bacteria - and are the main cellular constituent of pus; ii) eosinophils which, like neutrophils, are phagocytic and also participate in allergic reactions and the destruction of parasites; iii) basophils which can release both anticoagulants (heparin) and substances important in hypersensitivity reactions (histamine).

High-level Importance

Agranulocytes (= *mononuclear leukocytes*) lack specific granules and are divided into: **i)** *lymphocytes* which are vital to the immune system (*see Immune System*, chapter 8); **ii)** *monocytes* (often called *phagocytes* or *macrophages* when they are outside of the circulatory system) which can phagocytose large particles.

The hematocrit measures how much space (volume) in the blood is occupied by red blood cells and is expressed as a percentage. Normal hematocrit in adults is about 45%.

{*See* BIO 15.2 *for ABO Blood Types*}

7.5.1 Hemoglobin

Each red blood cell carries hundreds of molecules of a substance which is responsible for their red colour: **hemoglobin**. Hemoglobin (Hb) is a complex of *heme*, which is an iron-containing porphyrin ring, and *globin*, which is a tetrameric (= has 4 subunits) protein consisting of two α-subunits and two β-subunits. The iron from the heme group is normally in its reduced state (Fe^{2+}); however, in the presence of O_2, it can be oxidised to Fe^{3+}.

In the lungs, oxygen concentration or *partial pressure* is high, thus O_2 dissolves in the blood; oxygen can then quickly and reversibly combine with the iron in Hb forming bright red *oxyhemoglobin*. The binding of oxygen to hemoglobin is cooperative. In other words, each oxygen that binds to Hb facilitates the binding of the next oxygen. Consequently, the dissociation curve for oxyhemoglobin is sigmoidal as a result of the change in affinity of hemoglobin as each O_2 successively binds to the globin subunit (*see* BIO 4.3).

Examine Figure IV.A.7.2 carefully. Notice that at a PO_2 of 100 mmHg (e.g. arterial blood), the percentage of saturation of hemoglobin is almost 100%, which means all four heme groups on the four hemoglobin subunits are bound with O_2. At a PO_2 of 40 mmHg (e.g. venous blood), the percentage of saturation of hemoglobin is about 75%, which means three of the four heme groups on the four hemoglobin subunits are bound with O_2. At a PO_2 of 27 mmHg, the percentage of saturation of hemoglobin is only 50%, which means half of the four heme groups on the four hemoglobin subunits are bound with O_2. The partial pressure of oxygen (PO_2) at 50% saturation is called P50.

The curve can: **(i)** <u>shift to the left</u> which means that for a given PO_2 in the tissue capillary there is decreased unloading (release) of oxygen and that the affinity of hemoglobin for O_2 is increased; or **(ii)** <u>shift to the right</u> which means that for a given PO_2 in the tissue capillary there is increased

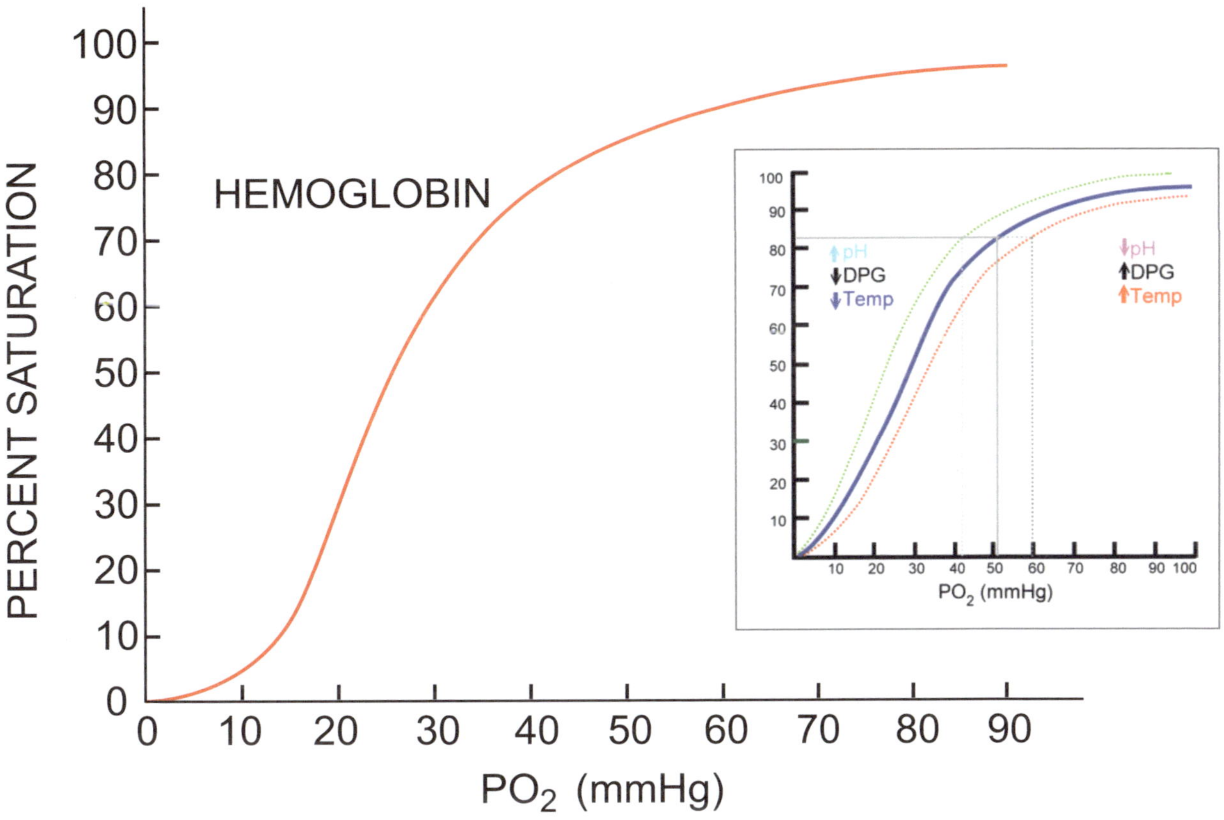

Figure IV.A.7.2: Oxygen dissociation curve: percent O_2 saturation versus O_2 partial pressure. Inset: Blue dissociation curve; left shift in green; right shift in red.

unloading of oxygen and that the affinity of hemoglobin for O_2 is decreased. The latter occurs when the tissue (i.e. muscle) is very active and thus requires more oxygen.

Thus a right shift occurs when the muscle is hot (↑ temperature during exercise), acid (↓ pH due to lactic acid produced in exercising muscle, *see* BIO 4.4. and 4.5), hypercarbic (↑CO_2 as during exercise, tissue produces more CO_2, *see* BIO 4.4. and 12.4.1), or contains high levels of organic phosphates (esp. increased synthesis of 2,3-DPG in red blood cells as a means to adapt to chronic hypoxemia). {Mnemonic: "CADET, face Right!" Right shift with increased: **C**O_2, **A**cid, 2,3-**D**PG, **E**xercise, and **T**emperature.}

In the body tissues where the partial pressure of O_2 is low and CO_2 is high, O_2 is released and CO_2 combines with the protein component of Hb forming the darker coloured *carbaminohemoglobin* (also called: deoxyhemoglobin). The red colour of muscle is due to a different heme-containing protein concentrated in muscle called myoglobin. Myoglobin is a monomeric protein containing one heme prosthetic group. The O_2 binding curve for myoglobin is hyperbolic, which means that it lacks cooperativity (*see* BIO 4.3).

7.5.2 Capillaries: A Closer Look

High-level Importance

Capillary fluid movement can occur as a result of two processes: diffusion (dominant role) and filtration (secondary role but critical for the proper function of organs, especially the kidney; BIO 10.3). Osmotic pressure (BIO 1.1.1, CHM 5.1.3) due to proteins in blood plasma is sometimes called colloid osmotic pressure or oncotic pressure. The Starling equation is an equation that describes the role of hydrostatic and oncotic forces (= Starling forces) in the movement of fluid across capillary membranes as a result of filtration.

When blood enters the arteriole end of a capillary, it is still under pressure produced by the contraction of the ventricle. As a result of this pressure, a substantial amount of water (hydrostatic) and some plasma proteins filter through the walls of the capillaries into the tissue space. This fluid, called interstitial fluid (BIO 7.6), is simply blood plasma minus most of the proteins.

Interstitial fluid bathes the cells in the tissue space and substances in it can enter the cells by diffusion (mostly) or active transport. Substances, like carbon dioxide, can diffuse out of cells and into the interstitial fluid.

Near the venous end of a capillary, the blood pressure is greatly reduced. Here another force comes into play. Although the composition of interstitial fluid is similar to that of blood plasma, it contains a smaller concentration of proteins than plasma and thus a somewhat greater concentration of water. This difference sets up an osmotic pressure. Although the osmotic pressure is small, it is greater than the blood pressure at the venous end of the capillary. Thus the fluid reenters the capillary here.

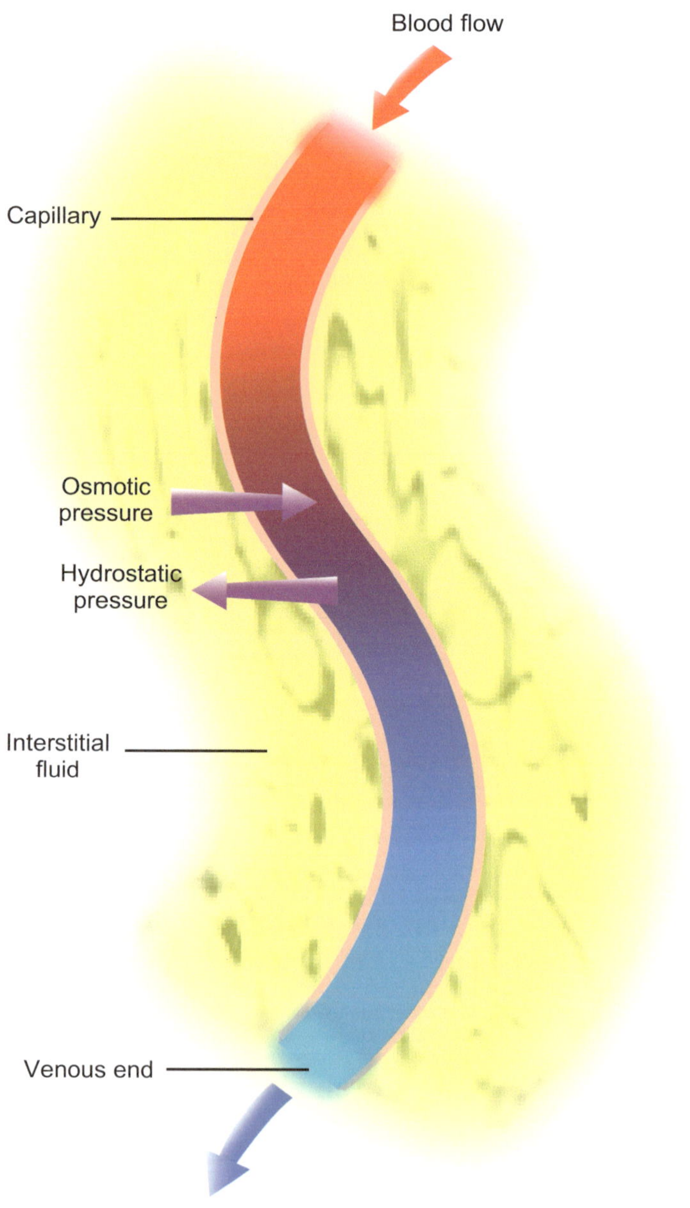

Figure IV.A.7.2b: Circulation at the level of the capillary. The exchange of water, oxygen, carbon dioxide, and many other nutrient and waste chemical substances between blood and surrounding tissues occurs at the level of the capillary.

To summarise: when the blood pressure is greater than the osmotic pressure, filtration is favored and fluid tends to move out of the capillary; when the blood pressure is less than the osmotic pressure, reabsorption is favored and fluid tends to enter into the capillary.

7.6 Introduction to the Lymphatic System

Body fluids can exist in blood vessels (intravascular), in cells (intracellular) or in a 3rd space which is intercellular (between cells) or extracellular (outside cells). Such fluids are called interstitial fluids. The **lymphatic system** is a network of vessels which can circulate fluid from the 3rd space to the cardiovascular system.

Aided by osmotic pressure, interstitial fluids enter the lymphatic system via small closed-ended tubes called *lymphatic capillaries* (in the small intestine they are called *lacteals*). Once the fluid enters it is called **lymph**. The lymph continues to flow into larger and larger vessels propelled by muscular contraction (esp. skeletal) and one-way valves. Then the lymph will usually pass through *lymph nodes* and then into a large vessel (esp. *the thoracic duct*) which drains into one of the large veins which eventually leads to the right atrium.

Lymph functions in important ways. Most protein molecules which leak out of blood capillaries are returned to the bloodstream by lymph. Also, microorganisms which invade tissue fluids are carried to lymph nodes by lymph. Lymph nodes contain *lymphocytes* and macrophages which are components of the immune system.

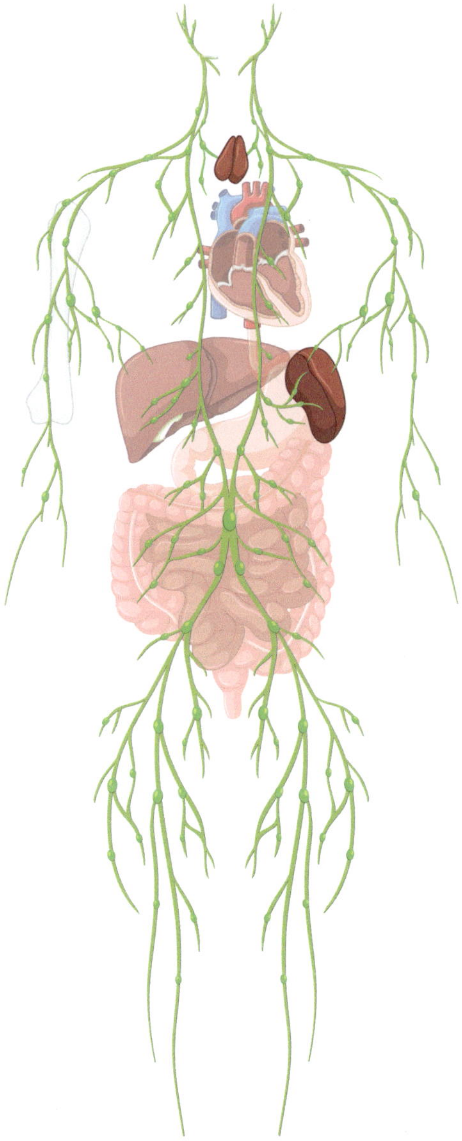

Figure IV.A.7.2c: A simplification of human lymphatic vessels. Note the lymphatic vessels in green which are dotted by green lymph nodes.

High-level Importance

CHAPTER 7: The Circulatory System

GOLD STANDARD FOUNDATIONAL GAMSAT PRACTICE QUESTIONS

1) In humans, which of the following orders of blood circulation is correct?

A. vena cava → right atrium → right ventricle → pulmonary arteries → pulmonary veins → left atrium.
B. vena cava → left atrium → left ventricle → pulmonary veins → pulmonary arteries → right ventricle.
C. vena cava → right ventricle → left ventricle → pulmonary veins → pulmonary arteries → left atrium.
D. vena cava → left atrium → left ventricle → pulmonary vein → pulmonary artery → right atrium.

2) Mitral valve stenosis is a disorder in which the valve opening between the left atrium and the left ventricle is narrowed enough to cause a decreased blood flow between those two chambers of the heart. As a result of mitral valve stenosis, blood pressure would be elevated in all of the following structures EXCEPT the:

A. aorta.
B. left atrium.
C. pulmonary arteries.
D. pulmonary capillaries.

3) Blood in the pulmonary veins is rich in:

A. myoglobin.
B. carbaminohemoglobin.
C. oxyhemoglobin.
D. lymph.

4) Hemoglobin found in humans is composed of four chains that can each bind one oxygen molecule. Given a fully saturated hemoglobin molecule, the sigmoidal shape of the oxygen saturation curve in humans is an indication of which of the following?

A. The first oxygen molecule dissociates from the heme component, while the next three dissociate from the globin component.
B. It becomes easier to lose the second and third oxygen molecules.
C. It becomes more difficult to lose the second and third oxygen molecules.
D. The fourth oxygen molecule dissociates from the heme component, while the previous three dissociate from the globin component.

GOLD STANDARD GAMSAT-LEVEL PRACTICE QUESTIONS

Questions 5–6

A Sankey diagram of the human circulatory system provides approximate relative percentages of cardiac output delivered to major organ systems as can be seen in Figure 1. Note that cardiac output is the amount of blood pumped from the heart over time.

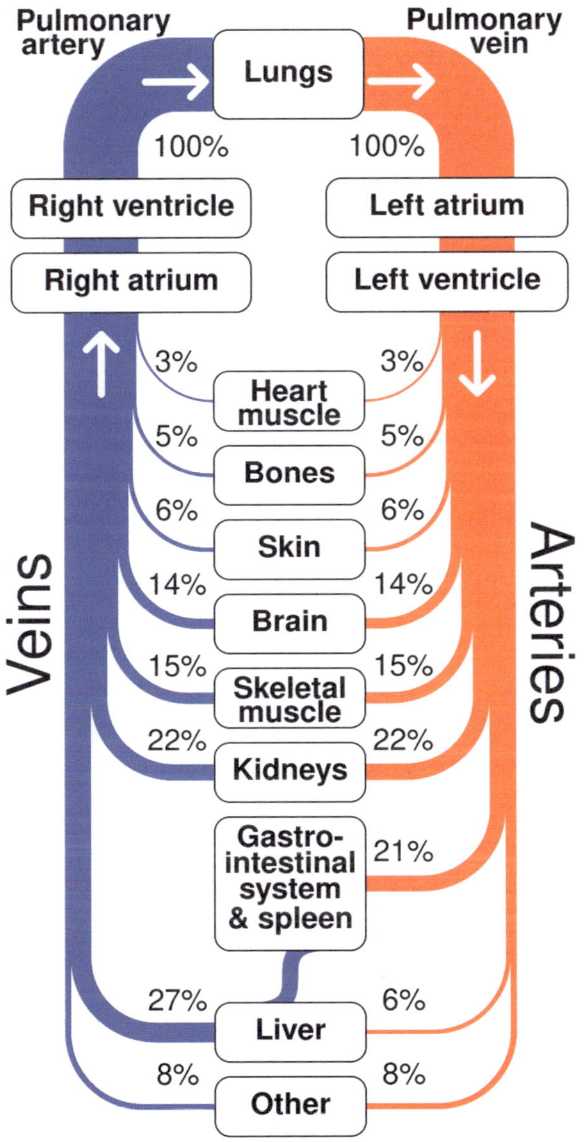

Figure 1

5) According to Figure 1, where is the largest percentage of oxygenated blood received?

A. Kidneys
B. Liver
C. Lungs
D. A combination of brain and bones

6) Based on Figure 1, what percent of the total amount of blood coming to the liver originates from the gastro-intestinal system and spleen?

A. 6%
B. 21%
C. 27%
D. 78%

7) Estimate the average number of heart beats over a lifetime for a person.

A. 2.9×10^{11}
B. 2.9×10^{9}
C. 2.9×10^{7}
D. 2.9×10^{5}

High-level Importance

Questions 8–10

The following represents normal values for arterial blood in humans: pH 7.4, bicarbonate 24 mmol/L, pCO_2 40 (please note: the first 2 questions of this unit are also in GAMSAT Maths, GM 3.9).

Consider the following diagram.

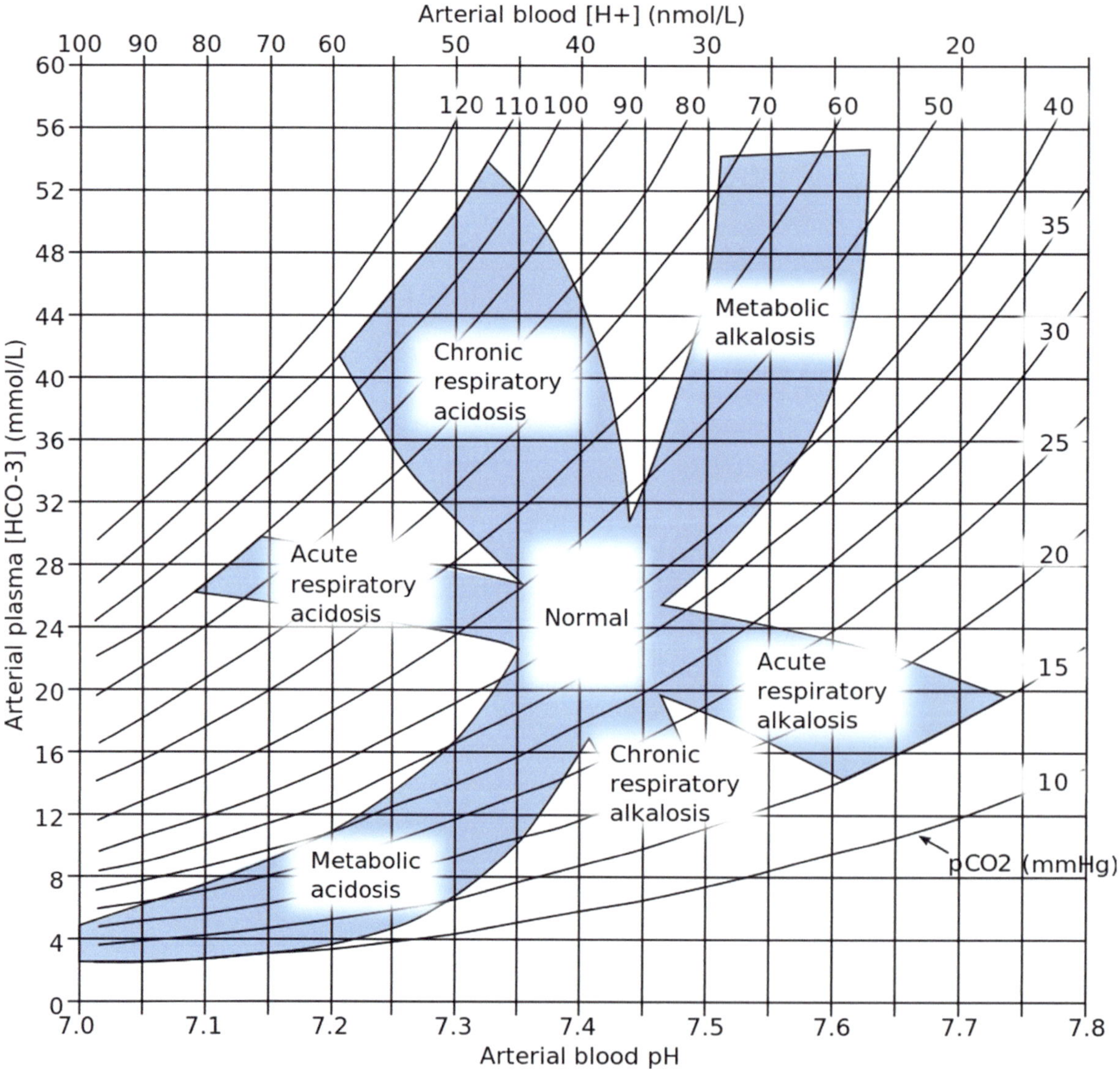

Figure 1

8) According to Figure 1, an arterial blood pH of 7.5 with a pCO_2 of 25, corresponds best with which of the following?

A. Metabolic alkalosis
B. Acute respiratory alkalosis
C. Chronic respiratory alkalosis
D. Chronic respiratory acidosis

9) Consider a patient with metabolic alkalosis. Based on Figure 1, which of the following would be most consistent with returning the patient back to normal?

A. Increase in arterial $[H^+]$, decrease arterial bicarbonate
B. Increase arterial pH, increase arterial bicarbonate
C. Decrease pCO_2, decrease arterial $[H^+]$
D. Increase pCO_2, decrease arterial bicarbonate

10) Based on Figure 1, which of the following is directly correlated with an increasing severity of metabolic acidosis?

A. Arterial blood pH
B. Arterial bicarbonate
C. Arterial $[H^+]$
D. pCO_2

Questions 11–12

The cardiac cycle refers to the sequence of mechanical and electrical events that repeats with every heartbeat. It includes the phase of relaxation diastole and the phase of contraction systole. The frequency of the cardiac cycle is described by the heart rate, which is typically expressed as beats per minute (bpm).

Consider Figure 1.

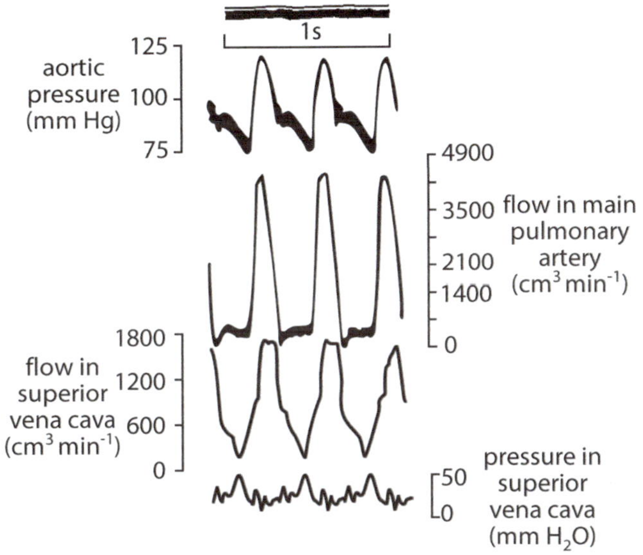

Figure 1: Simultaneous records of aortic pressure, pulmonary artery flow, and superior vena cava flow and pressure. [Brecher (1956). *Venous return*. Grune and Stratton Inc., New York.]

11) Which of the following is most consistent with the heart rate in Figure 1?

A. Less than 80 bpm
B. 80-110 bpm
C. 111-145 bpm
D. Over 145 bpm

12) According to the information provided, determine the approximate volume of blood in litres that is carried by the main pulmonary artery in one day.

A. 2.9×10^3 litres
B. 7.9×10^3 litres
C. 2.9×10^6 litres
D. 7.9×10^6 litres

Questions 13–15

Consider Figure 1 which demonstrates the oxygen dissociation curves for the hemoglobin (Hb) in muscle capillaries for various mammals. The partial pressure of oxygen (pO_2) in mammalian pulmonary (lung) tissue is approximately 100 mm Hg, while in the capillaries it is approximately 40 mm Hg. The partial pressure of carbon dioxide (pCO_2) is 40 and 50 mm Hg, respectively.

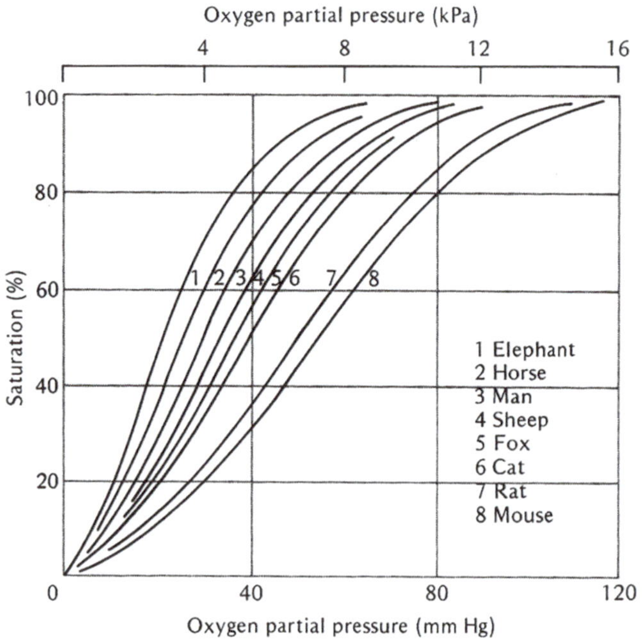

Figure 1: Oxygen dissociation curves for Hb in various mammals
(ref: blc.arizona.edu/courses/schaffer)

13) Which conclusion can be drawn from Figure 1?

- **A.** The hemoglobin of smaller mammals will retain oxygen at a lower pO_2 than that of larger mammals.
- **B.** The activity of the mammal is directly proportional to the ability of its hemoglobin to release oxygen.
- **C.** The hemoglobin of larger mammals will release oxygen at a higher pO_2 than that of smaller mammals.
- **D.** The size of the mammal is inversely proportional to the ability of its hemoglobin to release oxygen.

14) At an oxygen partial pressure of 40 kPa, one might expect that:

- **A.** most mammals would have a Hb saturation of 50% or higher.
- **B.** the Hb of approximately half of mammals would be fully saturated.
- **C.** the Hb of all mammals would be less that 50% saturation.
- **D.** the Hb of all mammals would be fully saturated.

15) The goat is closely related to sheep but scientifically in a different family. A male sheep is a ram. A ram is susceptible to Bengi fever which causes sepsis resulting in an increase in its metabolic rate. A septic ram would likely have an oxygen dissociation curve most consistent with which of the following?

- **A.** Man
- **B.** Sheep
- **C.** Fox
- **D.** All of the above

SPOILER ALERT ⚠

Gold Standard has cross-referenced the content in this chapter to examples from ACER's official GAMSAT practice materials. It is for you to decide when you want to explore these questions since you may want to preserve some of ACER's materials for timed mock-exam practice.

Examples – Structure and function of the circulatory system: Q1-5 of 1, and Q1-4 of 5; interstitial fluid: Q10 of 1; oxygen dissociation curves in mammals: Q52-54 of 3; percent cardiac output to the liver Q72 of 4; percent oxygen and circulation puzzle: Q31-34 of 5. Note that "Q" is followed by the question number, and, for example, "of 1" refers to booklet number 1 which is referenced in the Spoiler Alert table at the end of Chapter 1. The 15 full-length GAMSAT practice tests by Gold Standard, HEAPS-1 through HEAPS-15, contain specific cross-references to this chapter within the worked solutions. Note that the cardiac cycle graph is from HEAPS-3, and the oxygen dissociation curves in mammals is from HEAPS-8. HEAPS-1 to 5 are laden with Chapter 7 practice questions. If you go to YouTube and search for ACER GAMSAT Pink Booklet by Gold Standard unit 1, we do a slow step-by-step analysis of the order of the blood vessels in the diagram in BIO 7.3 before discussing ACER's unit. This video is also available for free in your gamsat-prep.com account.

Chapter Checklist

- ☐ Access your online account to view answers, worked solutions and discussion boards.
- ☐ Reassess your 'learning objectives' for this chapter: Go back to the first page of this chapter and re-evaluate the top 3 boxes and the Introduction.
- ☐ Complete a maximum of 1 page of notes using symbols/abbreviations to represent the entire chapter based on your learning objectives. These are your Gold Notes.
- ☐ Consider your multimedia options based on your optimal way of learning:
  - ☐ Download the free Gold Standard GAMSAT app for your Android device or iPhone.
  - ☐ Create your own, tangible study cards or try the free app: Anki.
  - ☐ Record your voice reading your Gold Notes onto your smartphone (audio files, e.g., *memo* or MP3s) and listen during exercise, transportation, etc.
  - ☐ Try out the Gold Standard GAMSAT online videos at gamsat-prep.com, or you can try other options on YouTube like Khan Academy or Crash Course Biology.
- ☐ Reassess your schedule for your full-length GAMSAT practice tests: ACER and/or HEAPS exams. Ensure that you have scheduled one full day to complete a practice test and 1-2 days for a thorough assessment of worked solutions while adding to your abbreviated Gold Notes.
- ☐ Reassess your progress in scheduling and/or evaluating stress reduction techniques such as regular exercise (sports), yoga, meditation and/or mindfulness exercises (*see* YouTube for suggestions).

THE IMMUNE SYSTEM

Chapter 8

Memorise	Understand	Importance
* Roles in immunity: Antigens vs antibodies	* Concepts of antigen, antibody, interaction * Structure of a standard antibody molecule * Mechanism of stimulation by antigen	**Medium level: 6% of GAMSAT Biology** questions released by ACER are related to content in this chapter (in our estimation). * Note that approximately 75% of the questions in GAMSAT Biology are related to just 7 chapters: 1, 2, 3, 4, 7, 12, and 15.

Introduction

The immune system protects against disease. Many processes are used in order to identify and kill various microbes (*see* Microbiology, Chapter 2, for examples) as well as tumor cells (more detail when you get into medical school!). There are 2 acquired responses of the immune system: cell-mediated and humoral.

Multimedia Resources at GAMSAT-Prep.com

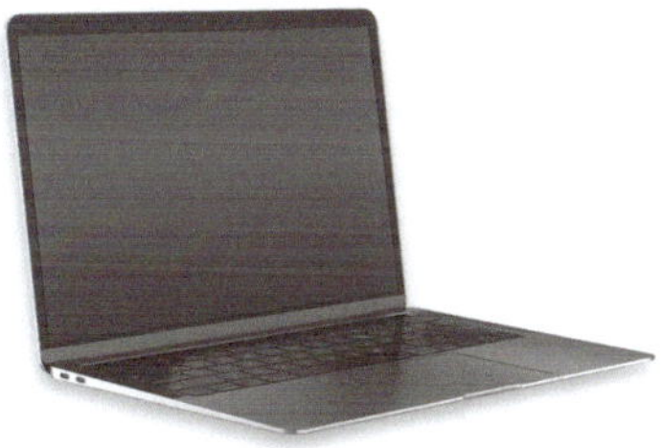

Open Discussion Boards
(*gamsat-prep.com/forum*)

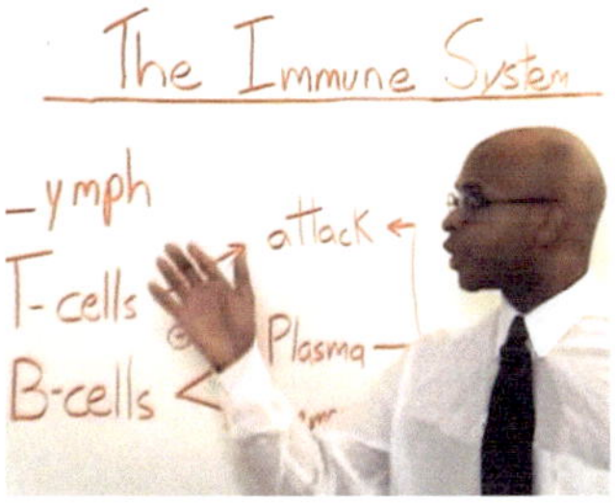

Foundational Videos

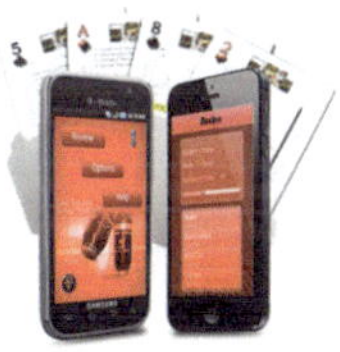

Flashcards

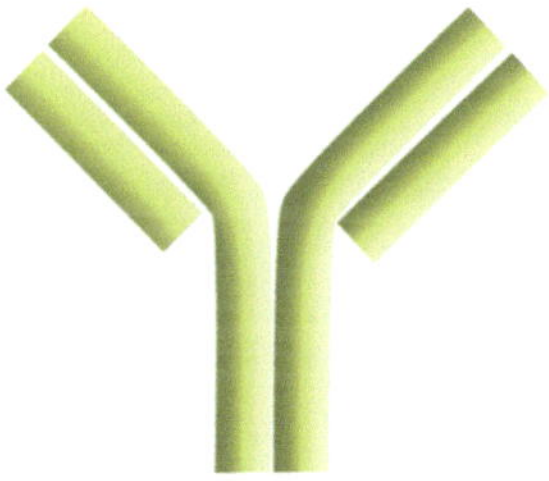

Special Guest

* The real GAMSAT may have advanced-level information presented (i.e. in a passage) but previous knowledge of said information is not required to answer the questions that would follow. Practice questions at the end of this chapter, as well as ACER and GS (HEAPS) practice GAMSATs can help you clarify this point.

8.1 Overview

The immune system is composed of various cells and organs which defend the body against pathogens (e.g. viruses, bacteria), toxins or any other foreign agents. Substances (usu. proteins) on the foreign agent causing an immune response are called **antigens**. There are two acquired responses to an antigen: **(1)** the **cell mediated response** where T-lymphocytes are the dominant force and act against microorganisms, tumors, and virus infected cells; and **(2)** the **humoral response** where B-lymphocytes are the dominant force and act against specific proteins present on foreign molecules.

8.2 Cells of the Immune System

Medium-level Importance

B-lymphocytes originate in the bone marrow. Though T-lymphocytes also originate in the bone marrow, they go on to mature in the thymus gland. T-lymphocytes learn with the help of macrophages to recognise and attack only foreign substances (i.e. antigens) in a direct cell to cell manner (= *cell-mediated* or *cellular immunity*). T-lymphocytes have two major subtypes: T-helper cells and T-cytotoxic cells. The latter T-cells (T_8, T_C, or T *c*ytotoxic) mediate the apoptosis of foreign cells and virus-infected cells. The former T-cells (T_4, T_H or T *h*elper) mediate the cellular response by secreting substances to activate macrophages, other T-cells and even B-cells. {T_H-cells are specifically targeted and killed by the HIV virus in AIDS patients}

B-lymphocytes act indirectly against the foreign agent by producing and secreting <u>antigen-specific</u> proteins called **antibodies**, which are sometimes called immunoglobulins (= *humoral immunity*). Antibodies are "designer" proteins which can specifically attack the antigen for which it was designed. The antibodies along with other proteins (i.e. complement proteins) can attack the antigen-bearing particle in many ways:

- **Opsonisation** which is the altering of cell membranes so the pathogen is more susceptible to phagocytosis by neutrophils and macrophages
- **Neutralisation** which is the blocking of parts of the surface of a pathogen to render its attack ineffective (rarely this can lead to *lysis*, the digesting of a plasma membrane)
- **Agglutination** which is the clumping of antigen-bearing cells
- **Chemotaxis** which is the attracting of other cells (i.e. phagocytes) to the area which can lead to *inflammation*, which includes the migration of cells, release of fluids and dilatation of blood vessels.

The activated antibody secreting B-lymphocyte is called a *plasma cell*. After the first or *primary* response to an antigen, both T- and B-cells produce *memory cells* which are formed during the initial response to an antigenic challenge. These memory cells remain in the circulation and will make the next or secondary response much faster and much greater. {Note: though lymphocytes are vital to the immune system, it is the neutrophil which responds to injury first; BIO 7.5}

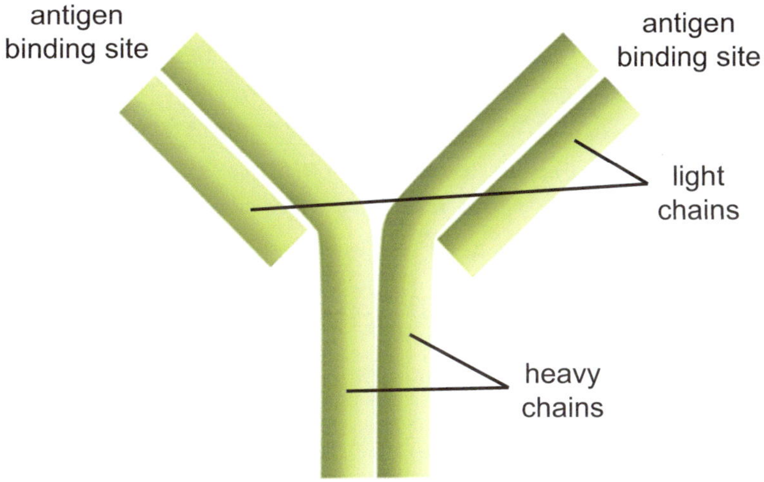

Figure IV.A.8.1: Schematic representation of an antibody. Antibodies are composed of disulfide bond-linked heavy and light chains. The unique part of the antigen recognised by an antibody is called the epitope. The antigen binding site on the antibody is extremely variable (= hypervariable). At the base of the 'Y' is the 'Fc region' where the antibody communicates with other components of the immune system (*see* Figure IV.A.8.2).

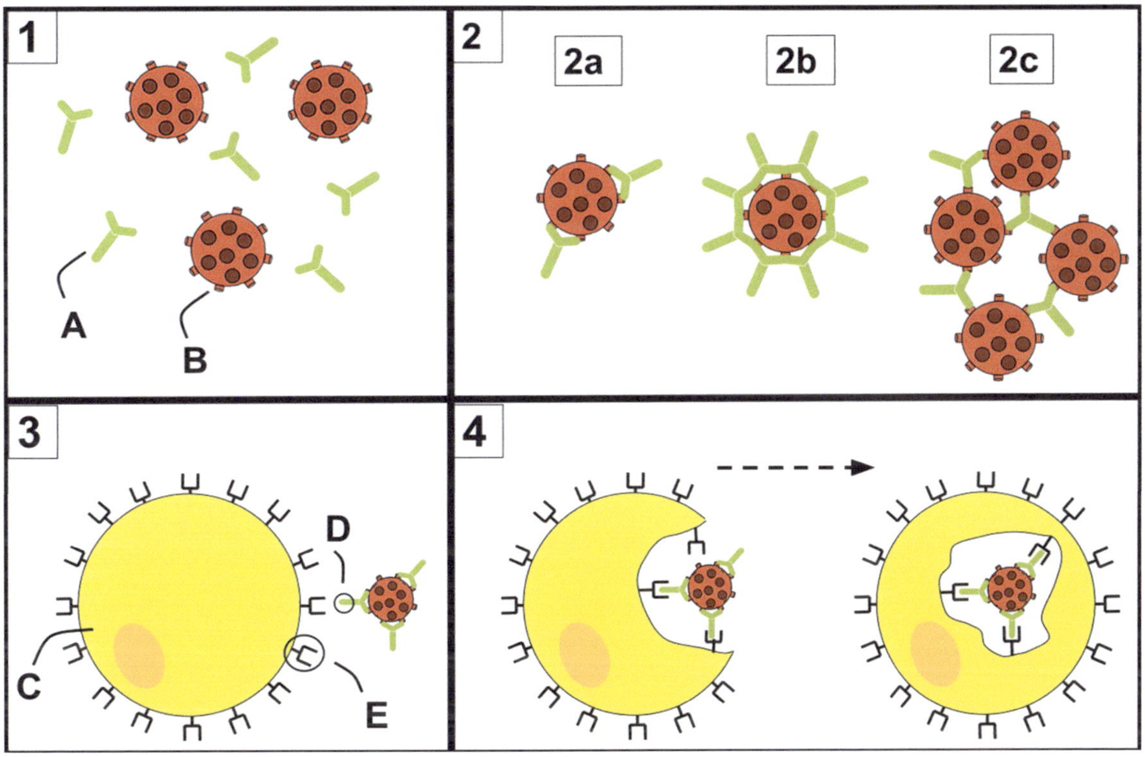

Figure IV.A.8.2: Antibody-antigen interaction. **1)** Antibodies (A) and pathogens (B; e.g. viruses or bacteria) freely roam in the blood. **2)** The antibodies bind to pathogens, and can do so in different formations such as: opsonisation **(2a)**, neutralisation **(2b)**, and agglutination **(2c)**. **3)** A phagocyte (C) approaches the pathogen, and the Fc region (D) of the antibody binds to one of the Fc receptors (E) of the phagocyte. **4)** Phagocytosis occurs as the pathogen is ingested and, hopefully, destroyed! (ref: α)

T-cells cannot recognise, and therefore react to, 'free' floating antigen. T-cells can only recognise an antigen that has been processed and presented by cells in association will a special cell surface molecule called the major histocompatibility complex (MHC). In fact, "antigen presenting cells", through the use of MHC, can teach both B-cells and T-cells which antigens are safe (*self*) and which are dangerous and should be attacked (*nonself*). MHC Class I molecules present to T_C cells while MHC Class II molecules present to T_H cells.

Antibody (= Immunoglobulin = Ig)	Description
IgA, Dimer 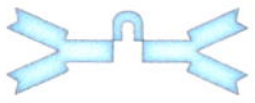	Found in saliva, tears and breast milk. Found in mucosal areas, such as the GI, respiratory and urogenital tracts thus prevents colonisation by pathogens.
IgD, Monomer 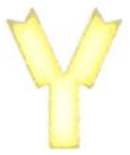	Functions mainly as an antigen receptor on B-cells that have not been exposed to antigens. Activates mast cells and basophils (BIO 7.5) to produce antimicrobial factors.
IgE, Monomer 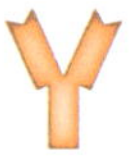	Binds to particles that induce allergic reactions (= allergens) and triggers histamine release from mast cells and basophils. Also protects against parasitic worms.
IgG, Monomer 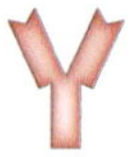	In its four forms, provides the majority of antibody-based immunity against invading germs or pathogens. The only antibody capable of crossing the placenta (BIO 14.6) to give passive immunity to the fetus.
IgM, Pentamer 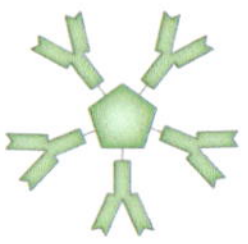	Expressed on the surface of B-cells (monomer) and in a secreted form (pentamer = complex of 5 monomers). Eliminates pathogens in the early stages of B-cell mediated (humoral) immunity before there is sufficient IgG.

Table IV.A.8.1: Antibody isotypes of mammals. Antibodies are grouped into different "isotypes" based on which heavy chain they possess. The five different antibody isotypes known in mammals are displayed in the table. (ref: β)

8.3 Tissues of the Immune System

The important tissues of the immune system are the bone marrow, and the lymphatic organs which include the thymus, the lymph nodes and the spleen. The roles of the bone marrow and the thymus have already been discussed. It is of value to add that the thymus secretes a hormone (= *thymosin*) which appears to help stimulate the activity of T-lymphocytes.

Lymph nodes are often the size of a pea and are found in groups or chains along the paths of the larger lymphatic vessels. Their functions can be broken down into three general categories: i) a non-specific filtration of bacteria and other particles from the lymph using the phagocytic activity of macrophages;

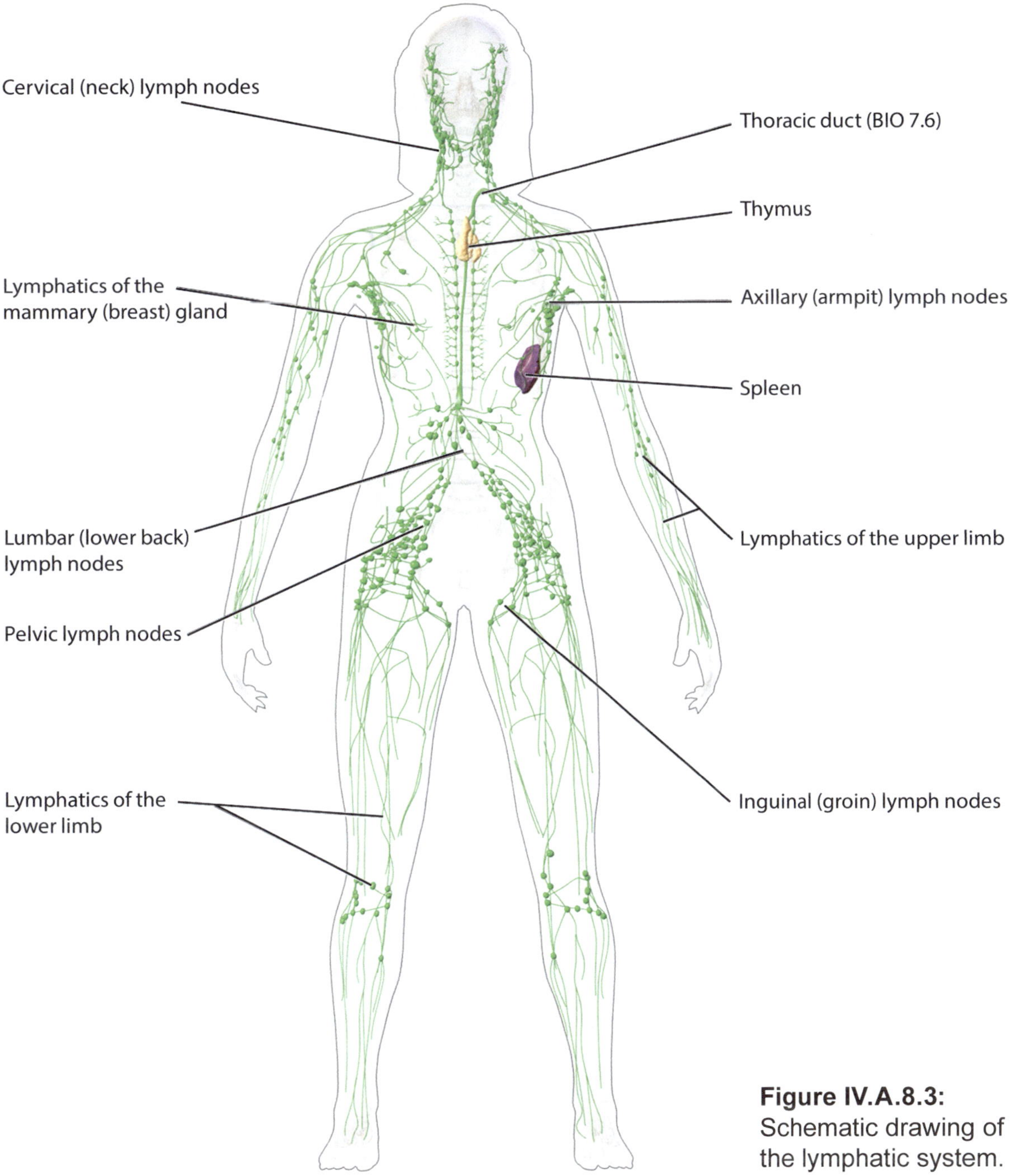

Figure IV.A.8.3: Schematic drawing of the lymphatic system.

ii) the storage and proliferation of T-cells, B-cells and antibody production; iii) initiate immune response on the recognition of antigen.

The **spleen** is the largest lymphatic organ and is situated in the upper left part of the abdominal cavity. Within its lobules it has tissue called red and white pulp. The white pulp of the spleen contains all of the organ's lymphoid tissue (T-cells, B-cells, macrophages, and other antigen presenting cells) and is the site of active immune responses via the proliferation of T- and B-lymphocytes and the production of antibodies by plasma cells. The red pulp is composed of several types of blood cells including red blood cells, platelets and granulocytes. Its main function is to filter the blood of antigen and phagocytose damaged or aged red blood cells (the latter has a lifespan of approximately 110-120 days). In addition, the red pulp of the spleen is a site for red blood cell storage (i.e. a blood storage organ).

8.4 Advanced Topic: ELISA

ELISA, enzyme-linked immunosorbent serologic assay, is a rapid test used to determine if a particular protein is in a sample and, if so, to quantify it (= assay). ELISA relies on an enzymatic conversion reaction and an antibody-antigen interaction which would lead to a detectable signal – usually a colour change. Consequently, ELISA has no need of any radioisotope nor any radiation-counting apparatus.

There are 2 forms of ELISA: (1) direct ELISA uses monoclonal antibodies to detect antigen in a sample; (2) indirect ELISA is used to find a specific antibody in a sample (i.e. HIV antibodies in serum). {Notice the similarity with the concept of "direct" and "indirect" immunofluorescence, BIO 1.5.1}

Medium-level Importance

CHAPTER 8: The Immune System

GOLD STANDARD FOUNDATIONAL GAMSAT PRACTICE QUESTIONS

1) Antigens are consistent with which of the following?

A. Proteins released during an inflammatory response
B. Proteins found in the blood that cause foreign blood cells to clump
C. Proteins embedded in B-cell membranes
D. Foreign molecules that trigger the generation of antibodies

2) When a pathogen (i.e. a bacterium, virus, or other microorganism that can cause disease) invades the body, it will trigger an immune response due to unique molecules called X. These will lead to the formation of very specific, matching Y in response to the X. The letters X and Y, respectively, likely represent:

A. antigens and antibodies.
B. antibodies and antigens.
C. T-cells and macrophages.
D. macrophages and T-cells.

GOLD STANDARD GAMSAT-LEVEL PRACTICE QUESTIONS

Questions 3–5

Helper T cells play a vital function in the immune system, and aid in a variety of roles depending on the subset they belong to. The development of Th1 and Th2 cells are influenced by the activities of several cytokines, all of which are carefully modulated by a complex system of signal transduction pathways.

The figure below gives a simplified overview of the molecules and proteins involved in helper T cell differentiation, and how they interact.

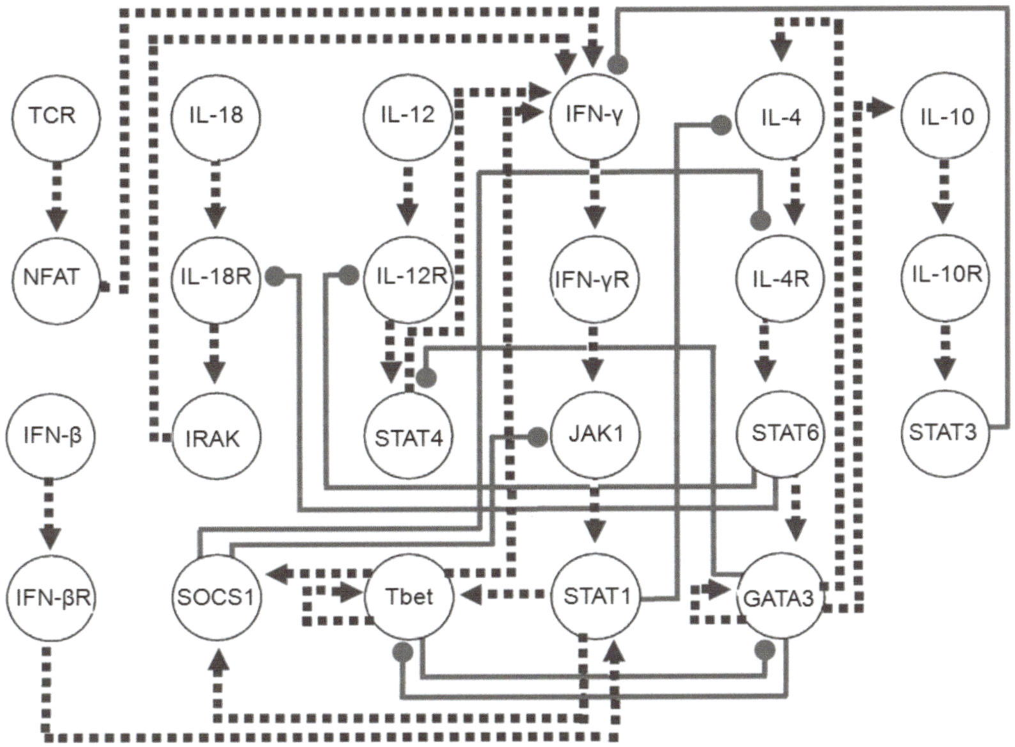

Figure 1: Regulatory pathway of proteins involved in T helper cell differentiation. Positive interactions are shown with dashed lines, while negative interactions are shown as solid lines.
Adapted from Mendoza L, Xenarios I, "A method for the generation of standardised qualitative dynamical systems of regulatory networks," *Theor Biol Med Model* (2006).

3) An overexpression of GATA3 would most likely lead to:

- **A.** an increase in Tbet activity.
- **B.** the reduction in the conversion of STAT4 to IFN-γ.
- **C.** a decrease in IL-4R activity.
- **D.** a decrease in IFN-γ activity.

4) Mouse experiments have shown that SOCS1 knockouts, where SOCS1 is not active, are lethal, with 100% mortality rates by the third week. The mutation causes a number of effects, likely to include:

- **A.** decreased IL-4R activity.
- **B.** overexpression of T-bet.
- **C.** overexpression of IL-12.
- **D.** deactivation of STAT6.

5) If not for negative feedback, the production of all of the following would likely lead to disease and death except:

A. GATA3.
B. Tbet.
C. IL-4.
D. None of the above

Questions 6–8

Viral hepatitis type B (serum hepatitis) is an infection of humans that primarily damages the liver. The causative agent is a virus called HBV, which is transmitted in much the same way as the HIV virus.

If HBV could be cultivated in the laboratory in unlimited amounts, it could be injected into humans as a vaccine to stimulate immunity against hepatitis type B. Unfortunately, it is not yet possible to grow HBV in laboratory culture. However, the blood of chronically infected people contains numerous particles of a harmless protein component of the virus. This protein, called HBsAg, can be extracted from the blood, purified, and treated chemically to destroy any live virus that might also be present. When HBsAg particles are injected into humans, they stimulate immunity against the complete infectious virus.

Of late, a new source of HBsAg particles have become available. Thanks to genetic engineering, a technique for cloning the gene for HBsAg into cells of the common bread yeast *Saccharomyces cerevisiae* has been developed. The yeast expresses the gene and makes HBsAg particles that can be extracted after the cells are broken. Since yeast cells are easy to propagate, it is now possible to obtain unlimited amounts of HBsAg particles.

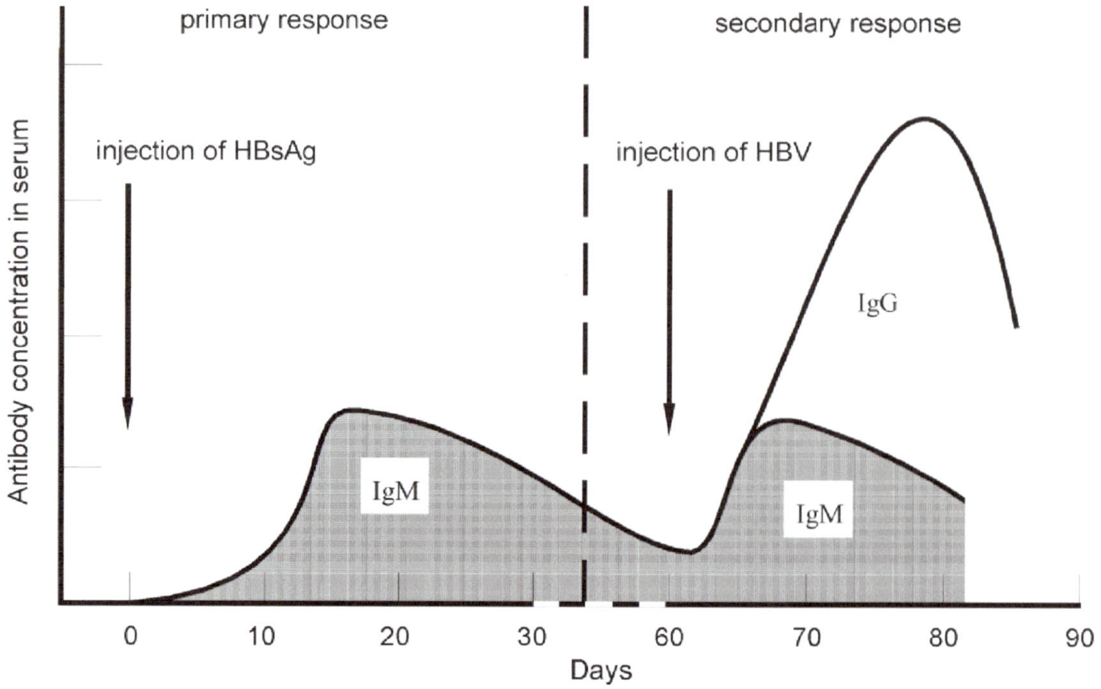

Figure 1

6) Before being injected into humans, the HBV virus would first have to:

A. be cloned in yeast cells to ensure that enough of the virus had been injected to elicit an immune response.
B. have its protein coat removed.
C. be purified.
D. be inactivated.

7) Figure 1 shows the immune response for an initial injection of HBsAg and a subsequent injection of the HBV virus. Which of the following best explains the differences in the two responses?

A. During the initial response, the immune response was carried out primarily by macrophages and B-lymphocytes.
B. During the secondary response, T-cells possessing membrane receptors, recognised and attacked the viral antigens.
C. Memory cells produced by T- and B-cells during the first exposure made the second response faster and more intense.
D. Memory cells produced by macrophages during the first infection recognised the viral antigens more quickly during the second infection, causing antibody production to be increased.

8) According to Figure 1, all of the following are correct EXCEPT:

A. if the slope of the curve was taken at any time t, the units could be in mg/day.
B. the time difference between the peak IgM and IgG secondary responses is less than the delay in the IgM primary response.
C. the peak IgM primary response has a delay similar in duration to the peak IgG secondary response.
D. the difference between peak IgG and peak IgM concentrations is greater than the peak IgM concentration.

9) A study characterising chronic wasting disease in moose was conducted by comparing the antibody-signal ratios of various animals in Norway. In Figure 1, numbers on the x-axis indicate the animal sample type: 1, scrapie; 2, CH1641; 3, CH1641-like; 4, BSE; 5, reindeer; 6, L-type atypical BSE; 7, moose no. 1; 8, moose no. 2.

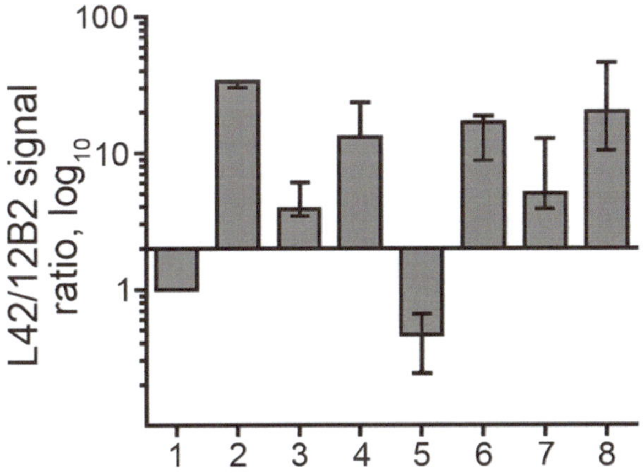

Figure 1: Bar graph of antibody signal ratios used to evaluate chronic wasting disease in moose. Bars represent mean values; error bars represent the range of observed values.
(modified from: Tran, Rolandsen; 10.3201/eid2412.180702)

Figure 1 shows that the L42/12B2 antibody-signal ratio of moose no. 2 is greater than that of reindeer, by approximately what factor?

A. 2x
B. 4x
C. 20x
D. 40x

GOLD STANDARD GAMSAT-LEVEL PRACTICE QUESTIONS (cont'd)

Questions 10–12

Antigens are chemical substances (usually proteins) that when introduced into the body cause an immune response. Lymphocytes are responsible for much of the body's immunity; they differentiate into B cells and T cells. Some B cells differentiate into antibody producing plasma cells. Antibodies combine with antigens to form an antibody-antigen complex.

Some T cells differentiate into cytotoxic T cells which engulf and destroy antibody-antigen complexes.

Three experiments were performed to study the effect of the thymus gland on the development of immune system cells in mice.

Experiment 1

The thymuses of newborn mice were radiolabeled and transplanted into unradiolabeled newborns whose thymuses had been removed. Within one week, 90% of the radiolabel was located in the lymphatic tissue (connective tissue that contains large numbers of lymphocytes; functions in the surveillance and defense from foreign materials) of the transplant recipient mice.

Experiment 2

Thymus cells were removed from nine day old and fifteen day old mice. The cells were grown in culture, and checked every day for T cell development. T cells only developed in the fifteen day old mice.

Experiment 3

A thymectomy (thymus removal) was performed on both newborn and adult mice. The table below shows the results on both sample groups following the procedure.

	newborns	adults
Able to produce some T cells	no	yes
Able to produce all T cells	no	yes
Able to produce some antibodies	yes	yes
Able to produce all antibodies	no	yes
Able to reject foreign tissue	no	yes

10) Which of the following experiments directly supports the conclusion that the immune system of newborn mice is compromised by the removal of the thymus?

A. 1 only
B. 3 only
C. 1 and 3 only
D. 2 and 3 only

11) Thymectomy would least affect the development of immune system cells of which group?

A. Newborn mice
B. Day old mice
C. 15 day old mice
D. Adult mice

12) All of the following could explain the rejection of foreign tissue by the bodies of adult mice, EXCEPT:

A. uncontrolled cell growth at the site of tissue transplantation.
B. antibody-antigen complex formation.
C. phagocytosis by neutrophils.
D. phagocytosis by macrophages.

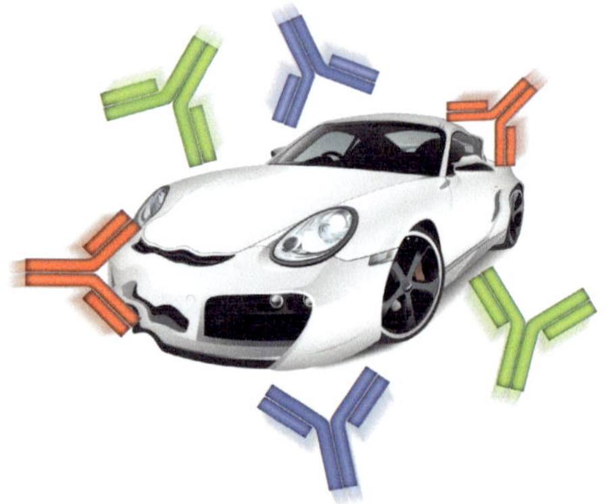

Autoimmunity!

Figure IV.A.8.4: Actually, "autoimmunity" refers to a disease process where the immune system attacks one's own cells and tissues as opposed to one's own car.

SPOILER ALERT

Gold Standard has cross-referenced the content in this chapter to examples from ACER's official GAMSAT practice materials. It is for you to decide when you want to explore these questions since you may want to preserve some of ACER's materials for timed mock-exam practice.

Examples – Graph-based reasoning with antibodies and antigens: Q79-82 of 3. Note that "Q" is followed by the question number, and, for example, "of 1" refers to booklet number 1 which is referenced in the Spoiler Alert table at the end of Chapter 1. The 15 full-length GAMSAT practice tests by Gold Standard, HEAPS-1 through HEAPS-15, contain specific cross-references to this chapter within the worked solutions. Note that the helper T-cell pathway unit is a rare sample from HEAPS-1; the viral hepatitis unit is from HEAPS-6; and thymectomy from HEAPS-8.

Chapter Checklist

- ☐ Access your online account to view answers, worked solutions and discussion boards.
- ☐ Reassess your 'learning objectives' for this chapter: Go back to the first page of this chapter and re-evaluate the top 3 boxes and the Introduction.
- ☐ Complete a maximum of 1 page of notes using symbols/abbreviations to represent the entire chapter based on your learning objectives. These are your Gold Notes.
- ☐ Consider your multimedia options based on your optimal way of learning:
  - ☐ Download the free Gold Standard GAMSAT app for your Android device or iPhone.
  - ☐ Create your own, tangible study cards or try the free app: Anki.
  - ☐ Record your voice reading your Gold Notes onto your smartphone (audio files, e.g., *memo* or MP3s) and listen during exercise, transportation, etc.
  - ☐ Try out the Gold Standard GAMSAT online videos at gamsat-prep.com, or you can try other options on YouTube like Khan Academy or Crash Course Biology.
- ☐ Reassess your schedule for your full-length GAMSAT practice tests: ACER and/or HEAPS exams. Ensure that you have scheduled one full day to complete a practice test and 1-2 days for a thorough assessment of worked solutions while adding to your abbreviated Gold Notes.
- ☐ Reassess your progress in scheduling and/or evaluating stress reduction techniques such as regular exercise (sports), yoga, meditation and/or mindfulness exercises (*see* YouTube for suggestions).

References

α: Figure IV.A.8.2
Antibody-antigen interaction: Images adapted from Maher33, Wikimedia Commons.

β: Table IV.A.8.1
Antibody isotypes of mammals: Images in the first column of the table by Martin Brändli, brandlee86, Wikimedia Commons.

THE DIGESTIVE SYSTEM
Chapter 9

Memorise

* Major organs of the GI tract
* Stomach: low pH, acidic gastric juice

Understand

* Basic function of the upper GI and lower GI tracts; the importance of surface area
* Bile: storage in gallbladder, function
* Pancreas: production of enzymes; transport of enzymes to small intestine
* Small intestine: production of enzymes, site of digestion, neutralise stomach acid
* Peristalsis; structure and function of villi

Importance

Medium level: 6% of GAMSAT Biology questions released by ACER are related to content in this chapter (in our estimation).
* Note that approximately 75% of the questions in GAMSAT Biology are related to just 7 chapters: 1, 2, 3, 4, 7, 12, and 15.

GAMSAT-Prep.com

Introduction

The digestive system is involved in the mechanical and chemical break down of food into smaller components with the aim of absorption into, for example, blood or lymph. Thus digestion is a form of catabolism. The presence of intestinal folds, villi and microvilli on the surface of intestinal cells (*enterocytes*) increase the absorptive area. Peristalsis - progressive wavelike contractions - helps to move intestinal contents while changes in motility increase the contact time between nutrients and the absorptive surface.

Although there is not much assumed knowledge for the GAMSAT in this chapter, you can become familiar with the basics and then the practice questions will deliver a full-course meal: a gastric metabolic pathway (flow chart), log-scale graphs, and the famous ternary diagram. The latter is a special, triangular nomogram that has been reported to pop up on real exams for years and can be found in ACER's Pink Booklet. If you have no experience reading such graphs, go to GAMSAT Maths Chapter 3 (logs: GM 3.8; ternary: GM 3.9). Again, unless you are quite comfortable with basic algebra, then a study of GAMSAT Maths is advisable prior to attempting graph-based questions.

Multimedia Resources at GAMSAT-Prep.com

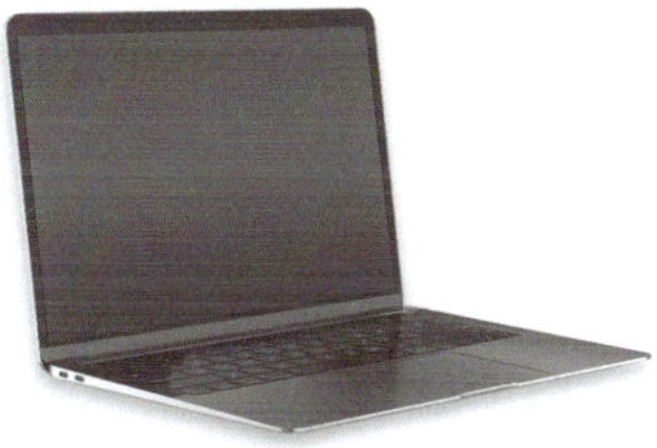

Open Discussion Boards
(*gamsat-prep.com/forum*)

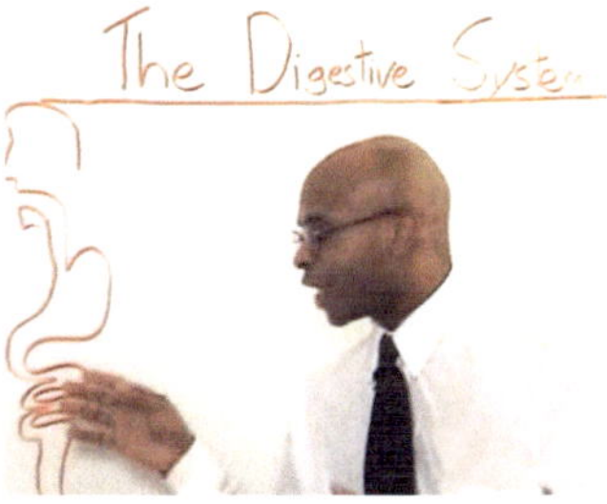

Foundational Videos

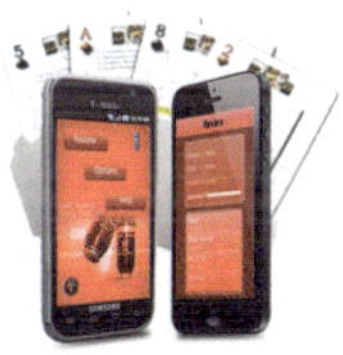

Flashcards

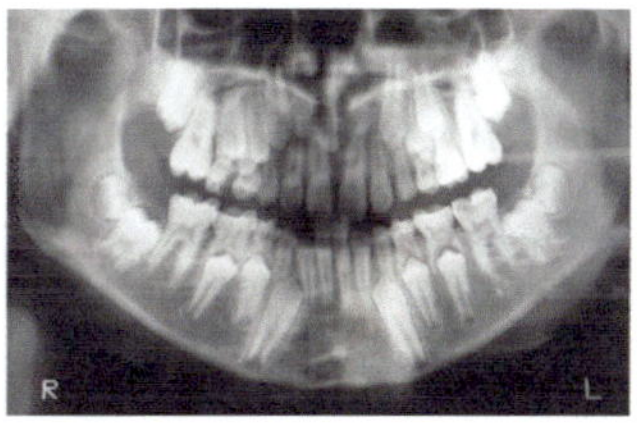

Special Guest

* The real GAMSAT may have advanced-level information presented (i.e. in a passage) but previous knowledge of said information is not required to answer the questions that would follow. Practice questions at the end of this chapter, as well as ACER and GS (HEAPS) practice GAMSATs can help you clarify this point.

9.1 Overview

The digestive or *gastrointestinal* (= GI) system is principally concerned with the intake and reduction of food into subunits for absorption. These events occur in five main phases which are located in specific parts of the GI system: **i) ingestion** which is the taking of food or liquid into the mouth; **ii) fragmentation** which is when larger pieces of food are *mechanically* broken down; **iii) digestion** where macromolecules are *chemically* broken down into subunits which can be absorbed; **iv) absorption** through cell membranes; and **v) elimination** of the waste products. The GI system secretes enzymes and hormones that facilitate in the process of ingestion, digestion, absorption as well as elimination.

The GI tract (gut or *alimentary canal*) is a muscular tract about 9 metres long covered by a layer of mucosa which has definable characteristics in each area along the tract. The GI tract includes the oral cavity (mouth), pharynx, esophagus, stomach, small intestine, large intestine, and anus. The GI system includes the accessory organs which release secretions into the tract: the salivary glands, gallbladder, liver, and pancreas (*see Figure IV.A.9.1*).

Medium-level Importance

9.2 The Oral Cavity and Esophagus

Ingestion, fragmentation and digestion begin in the oral cavity. Teeth are calcified, hard structures in the oral cavity used to fragment food (= *mastication*). Children have twenty teeth (= *deciduous*) and adults have thirty-two (= *permanent*). From front to back, each quadrant (= *quarter)* of the mouth contains: two incisors for cutting, one cuspid (= *canine*) for tearing, two bicuspids (= *premolars*) for crushing, and three molars for grinding.

Digestion of food begins in the oral cavity when the 3 pairs of salivary glands (*parotid*, *sublingual*, and *submandibular*) synthesise and secrete saliva. Saliva lubricates the oral cavity, assists in the process of deglutition, controls bacterial flora and initiates the process of digestion. Its production is unique in that it is increased by both sympathetic and parasympathetic innervation. Major components of saliva include salivary amylase, lysozyme, lingual lipase and mucus. Amylase is an enzyme which starts the initial digestion of carbohydrates by splitting starch and glycogen into disaccharide subunits. Lipase is an enzyme which starts the initial digestion of triglyceride (fats). The mucous helps to bind food particles together and lubricate it as it is swallowed.

Swallowing (= *deglutition*) occurs in a coordinated manner in which the tongue and pharyngeal muscles propel the bolus of food into the esophagus while at the same time the upper esophageal sphincter relaxes to permit food to enter. The epiglottis is a small flap of

Basic Dental Anatomy and Pathology

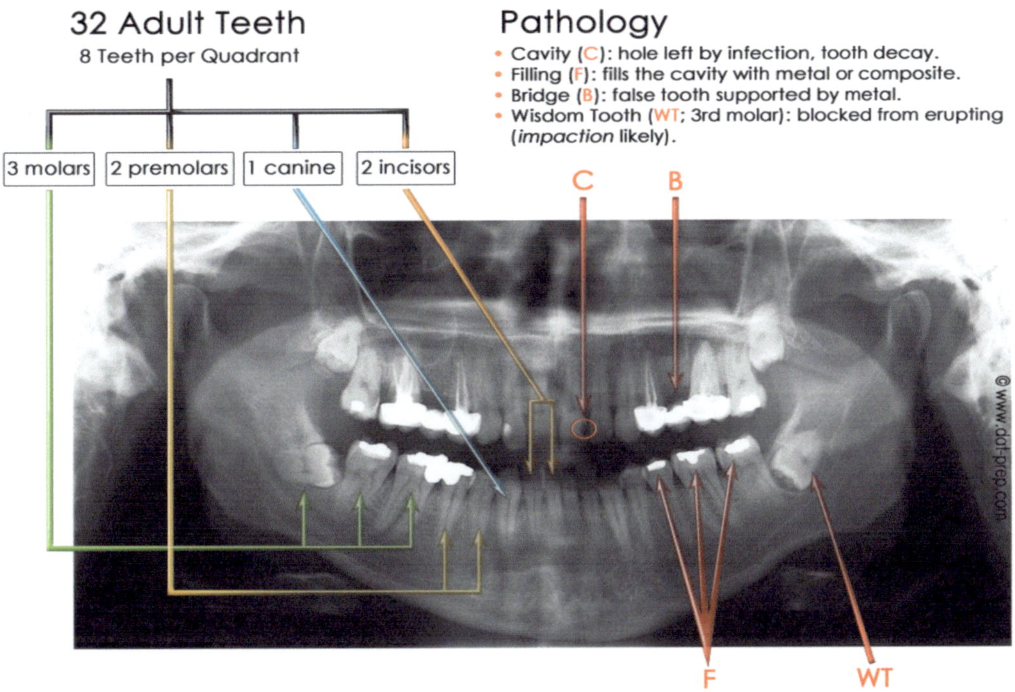

Figure IV.A.9.0a: Dental X-ray of an adult. The pathology of teeth is not prerequisite knowledge for the GAMSAT and is only presented for your interest (and as a minor contribution to the future studies of those of you who are studying GAMSAT for dentistry!).

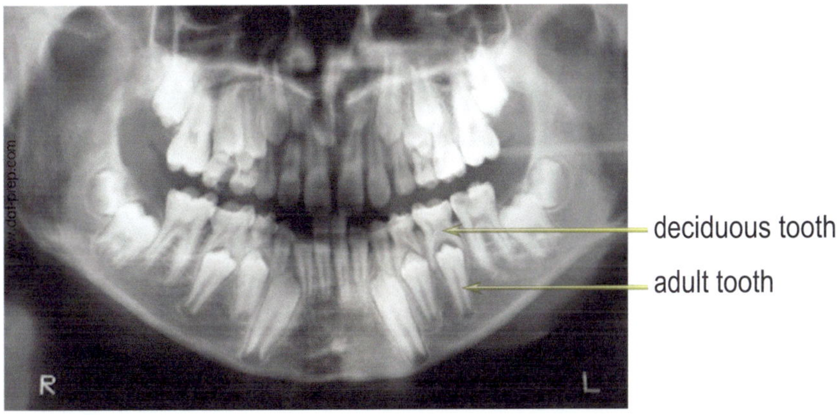

Figure IV.A.9.0b: Dental X-ray of a child showing deciduous (AKA: baby, primary, milk, temporary) teeth and emerging adult (permanent) teeth. Note the "R" on the X-ray indicates the right side of the patient who is facing the observer.

Medium-level Importance

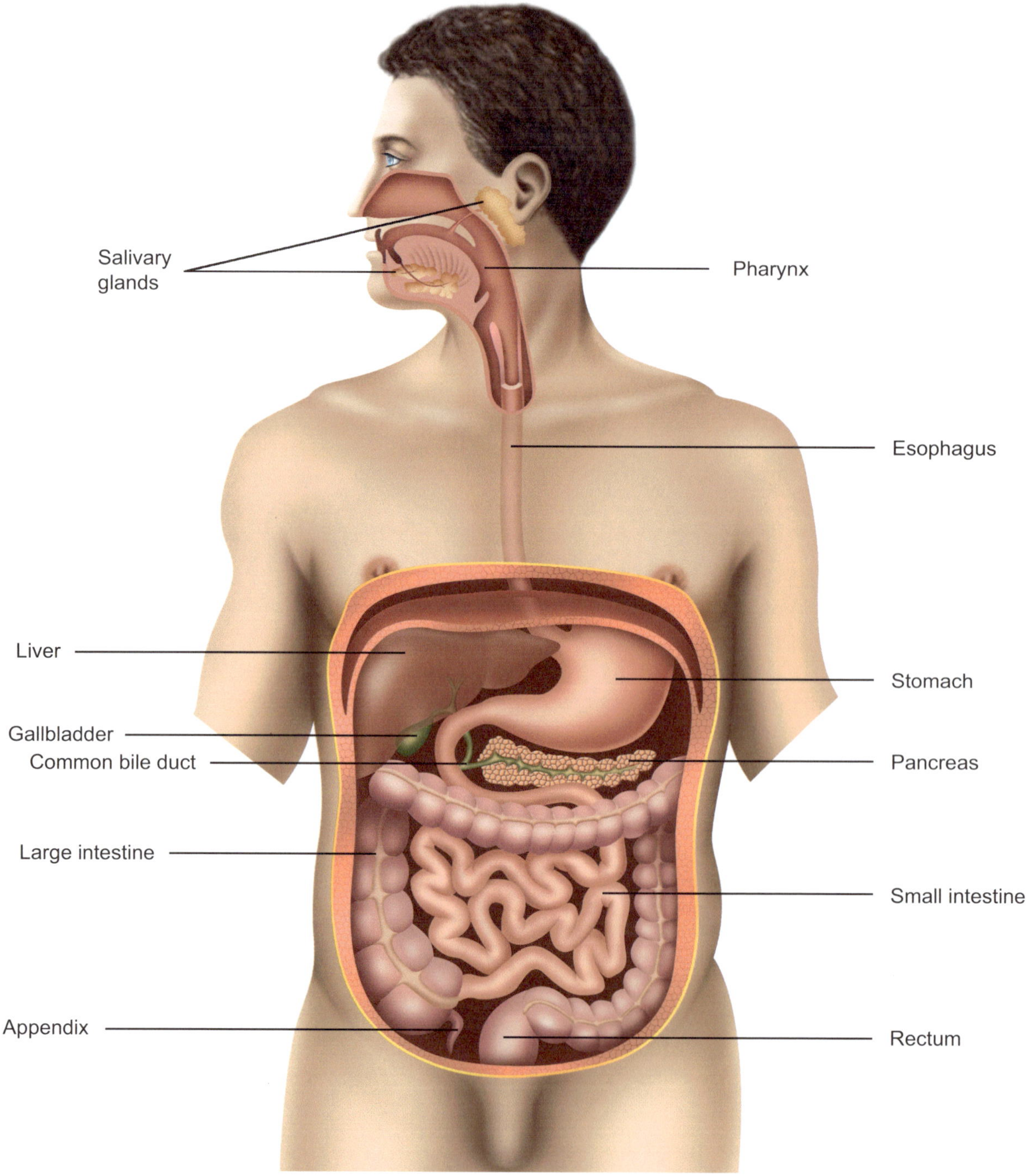

Figure IV.A.9.1: Schematic drawing of the major components of the digestive system.

tissue which covers the opening to the airway (= *glottis*) while swallowing. Gravity and peristalsis help bring the food through the esophagus to the stomach.

The GI system is supplied by both extrinsic innervation and intrinsic innervation. The extrinsic innervation includes the sympathetic and parasympathetic nervous system. The parasympathetic nervous system, mediated by the vagus and pelvic nerves, usually stimulates the functions of the GI tract while the sympathetic nervous system usually inhibits the functions of the GI tract. The intrinsic innervation located in the gut wall includes the *myenteric nerve plexus* and *submucosal nerve plexus* which control GI tract motility including peristalsis.

Peristalsis, which is largely the result of two muscle layers in the GI tract (i.e. the **i**nner c**i**rcular and **o**uter l**o**ngitudinal layers), is the sequential wave-like muscular contractions which propell food along the tract. The rate, strength and velocity of muscular contractions are modulated by the ANS.

9.3 The Stomach

The stomach continues in fragmenting and digesting the food with its strong muscular activity and its acidic gastric juice, which consists of various digestive enzymes including pepsin. The walls of the stomach are lined by thick mucosa which contains goblet cells. These goblet cells of the GI tract protect the lumen from the acidic environment by secreting mucous.

The important components of gastric juice are: **i)** HCl which keeps the pH low (approximately = 2) to kill microorganisms, to aid in partial hydrolysis of proteins, and to provide the environment for **ii)** *pepsinogen*, an inactive form of enzyme (= *zymogen*) secreted by gastric chief cells, which is later converted to its active form *pepsin* in the presence of a low pH. Pepsin is involved in the breakdown of proteins. Both the hormone gastrin, which is produced in the stomach, and parasympathetic impulses can increase the production of gastric juice.

The preceding events turns food into a semi-digested fluid called chyme. Chyme is squirted through a muscular sphincter in the stomach, the *pyloric sphincter*, into the first part of the small intestine, the *duodenum*. Many secretions are produced by exocrine glands in the liver and pancreas and enter the duodenum via the *common bile duct*. Exocrine secretions eventually exit the body through ducts. For example, *goblet cells*, which are found in the stomach and throughout the intestine, are exocrine secretory cells which produce mucus which lines the epithelium of the gastrointestinal tract.

9.4 The Exocrine Roles of the Liver and Pancreas

9.4.1 The Liver

Medium-level Importance

The liver occupies the upper right part of the abdominal cavity. It has many roles including: the conversion of glucose to glycogen; the synthesis of glucose from non-carbohydrates; the production of plasma proteins; the destruction of red blood cells; the deamination of amino acids and the formation of urea; the conversion of toxic ammonia to much less toxic urea (the urea cycle); the storage of iron and certain vitamins; the alteration of toxic substances and most medicinal products (*detoxification*); and its exocrine role - the production of **bile** by liver cells (= *hepatocytes*).

Bile is a yellowish - green fluid mainly composed of water, cholesterol, pigments (from the destruction of red blood cells) and salts. It is the **bile salts** which have a digestive function by the emulsification of fats. Emulsification is the dissolving of fat globules into tiny droplets called *micelles* which have hydrophobic interiors and hydrophilic exteriors (cf. Plasma Membrane, BIO 1.1). Bile salts orient themselves around those lipid droplets with their hydrophilic portions towards the aqueous environment and their hydrophobic portions towards the micelle interior and keep them dispersed. Emulsification also helps in the absorption of the fat soluble vitamins A, D, E, and K.

Thus bile is produced by the liver, stored and concentrated in a small muscular sac, the **gallbladder**, and then secreted into the duodenum via the common bile duct.

9.4.2 The Pancreas

The pancreas is close to the duodenum and extends behind the stomach. The pancreas has both endocrine (*see Endocrine Systems; BIO 6.3.4*) and exocrine functions. It secretes pancreatic juice, which consists of alkaline fluid and digestive enzymes, into the pancreatic duct that joins the common bile duct. Pancreatic juice is secreted both due to parasympathetic and hormonal stimuli. The hormones *secretin* and *CCK* are produced and released by the duodenum in response to the presence of chyme. Secretin acts on the pancreatic ductal cells to stimulate HCO_3^- secretion, whose purpose is to neutralise the acidic chyme. CCK acts on pancreatic acinar cells to stimulate the exocrine pancreatic secretion of digestive enzymes. These enzymes are secreted as enzymes or proenzymes (= *zymogens*; BIO 4.3) that must be activated in the intestinal lumen. The enzymes include pancreatic amylase, which can break down carbohydrates into monosaccharides; pancreatic lipase, which can break down fats into fatty acids and monoglycerides; and nuclease, which can break down nucleic acids. The protein enzymes (proteases) include trypsin, chymotrypsin, carboxypeptidase, which can break down proteins into amino acids, dipeptides or tripeptides.

9.5 The Intestines

The **small intestine** is divided into the duodenum, the jejunum, and the ileum, in that order. It is this part of the GI system that completes the digestion of chyme, absorbs the nutrients (i.e. monosaccharides, amino acids, nucleic acids, etc.), and passes the rest onto the large intestine. Peristalsis is the primary mode of transport. Contraction behind the bolus and simultaneous relaxation in front of the bolus propel chyme forward. Segmentation also aids in small intestine movement - it helps to mix the intestinal contents without any forward movement of chyme. Of course, parasympathetic impulses increase intestinal smooth muscle contraction while sympathetic impulses decrease intestinal smooth muscle contraction.

Absorption is aided by the great surface area involved including the finger-like projections **villi** and **microvilli** (*see the Generalised Eukaryotic Cell*, BIO 1.1F and 1.2). Intestinal villi, which increase the surface area ten-fold, are evaginations into the lumen of the small intestine and contain blood capillaries and a single lacteal (lymphatic capillary). Microvilli, which increase the surface area twenty-fold, contain a dense bundle of actin microfilaments cross-linked by proteins fimbrin and villin.

Absorption of carbohydrates, proteins and lipids is completed in the small intestine. Carbohydrates must be broken down into glucose, galactose and fructose for absorption to occur. In contrast, proteins can be absorbed as amino acids, dipeptides and tripeptides. Specific transporters are required for amino acids and peptides to facilitate the absorption across the luminal membrane. Lipids are absorbed in the form of fatty acids, monoglycerides and cholesterol. In the intestinal cells, they are re-esterified to triglycerides, cholesterol ester and phospholipids.

The lacteals absorb most fat products into the lymphatic system while the blood capillaries absorb the rest taking these nutrients to the liver for processing via a special vein - the *hepatic portal vein* [A portal vein carries blood from one capillary bed to another; BIO 7.3]. Goblet cells secrete a copious amount of mucus in order to lubricate the passage of material through the intestine and to protect the epithelium from abrasive chemicals (i.e. acids, enzymes, etc.).

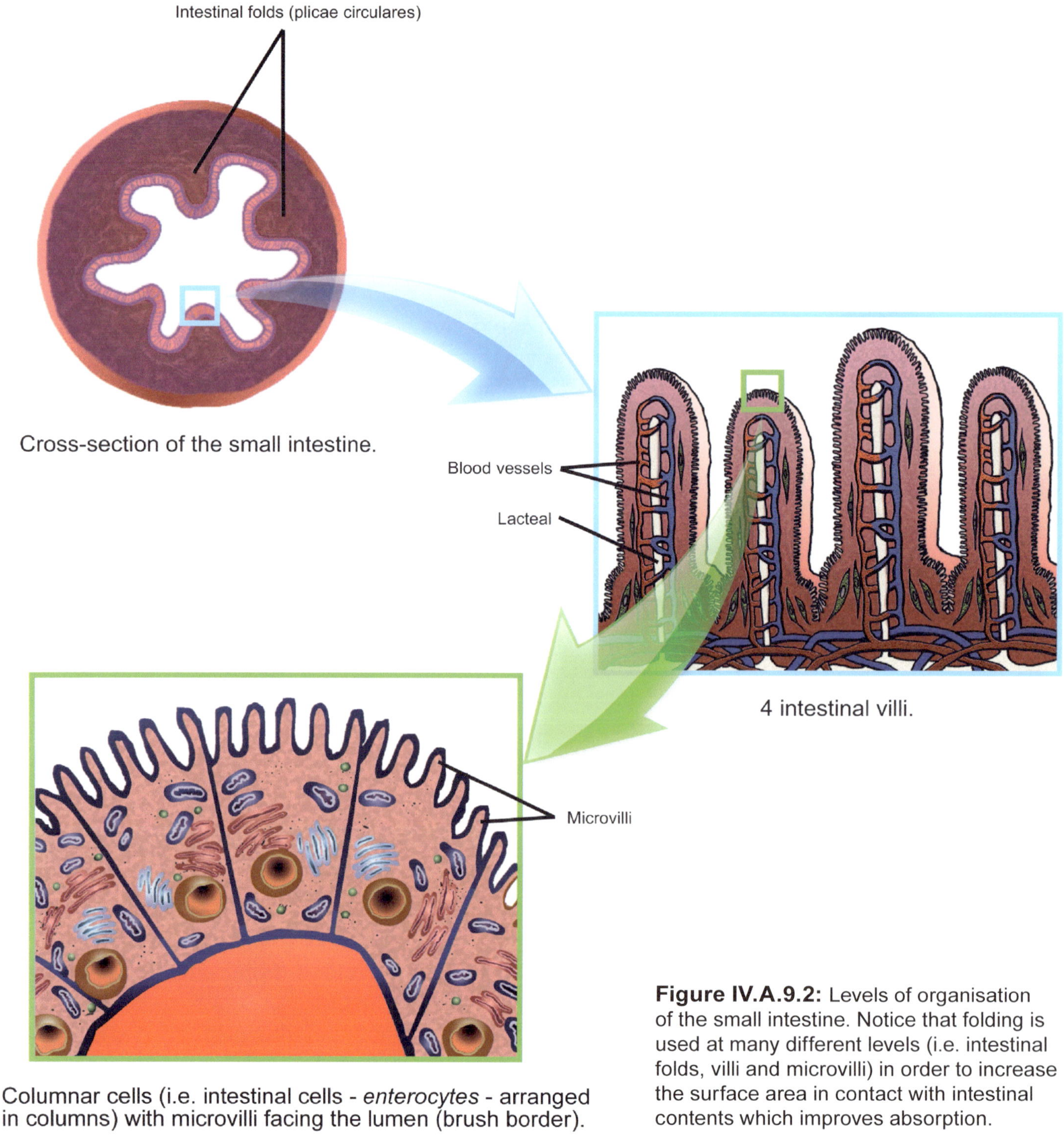

Figure IV.A.9.2: Levels of organisation of the small intestine. Notice that folding is used at many different levels (i.e. intestinal folds, villi and microvilli) in order to increase the surface area in contact with intestinal contents which improves absorption.

9.5.1 The Large Intestine

The large intestine is divided into: the cecum which connects to the ileum and projects a closed-ended tube - the appendix; the colon which is subdivided into ascending, transverse, descending, and sigmoid portions; the rectum which can store feces; and the anal canal which can expel feces (*defecation*) through the anus with the relaxation of the anal sphincter and the increase in abdominal pressure. The large intestine has little or no digestive functions. It absorbs water and electrolytes from the residual chyme and it forms feces. Feces is mostly water, undigested material, mucous, bile pigments (responsible for the characteristic colour) and bacteria (= gut flora = 60% of the dry weight of feces).

Essentially, the relationship between the gut and bacteria is mutualistic and symbiotic (BIO 2.2). Though people can survive with no bacterial flora, these microorganisms perform a host of useful functions, such as fermenting unused energy substrates, training the immune system, preventing growth of harmful species, producing vitamins for the host (i.e. vitamin K), and bile pigments.

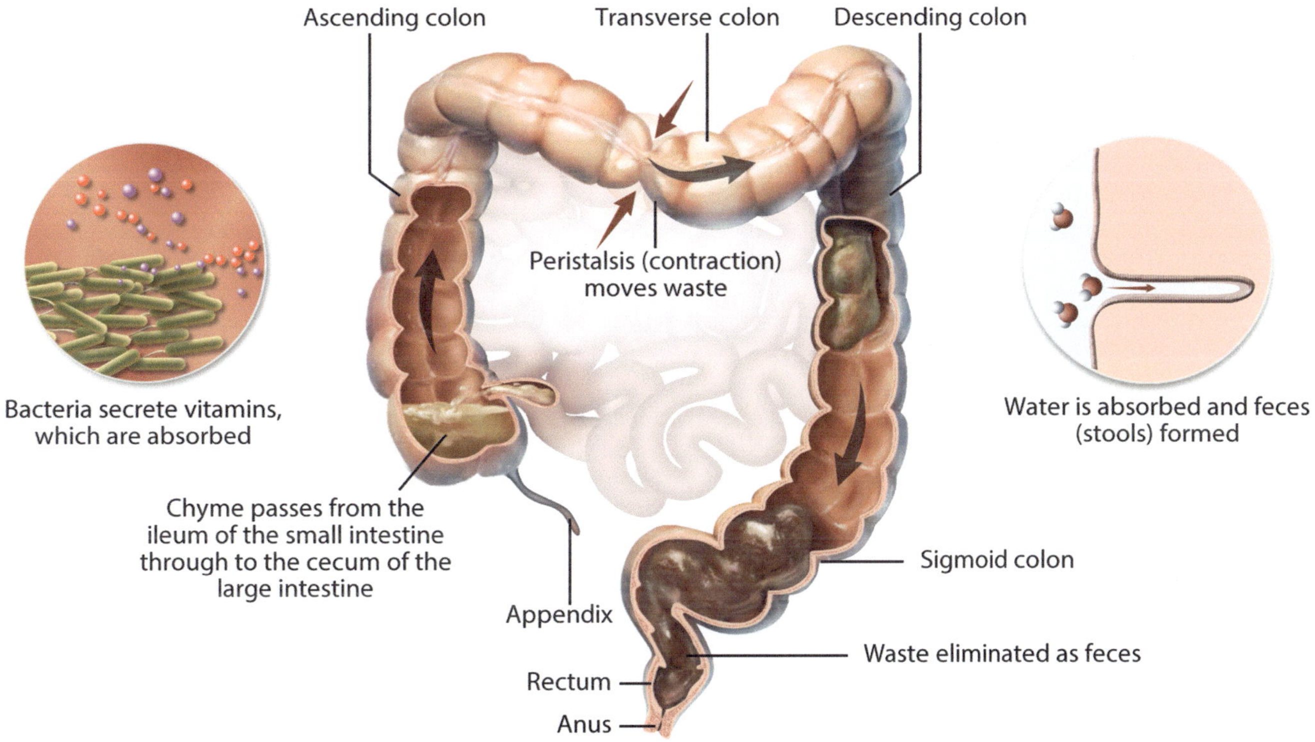

Figure IV.A.9.3: Schematic drawing including the major components of the large intestines.

High-level Importance

CHAPTER 9: The Digestive System

GOLD STANDARD GAMSAT-LEVEL PRACTICE QUESTIONS

Please note: Although we normally begin with foundational questions, in order to be sure that you do not need to turn pages back and forth in order to answer graph-based units, we have moved the foundational questions to 7, 8 and 9. You may choose to begin there.

Questions 1–6

The most common type of gallstone is the cholesterol gallstone which occurs when cholesterol crystals form due to an imbalance between the 3 main components in the lipid portion of bile.

The latter is composed of bile salts, phospholipid (i.e. lecithin), and cholesterol, and the triangle (i.e. the ternary graph, Figure 1) represents all possible ratios of the three lipid constituents. Each point within the triangle corresponds to a particular composition of the three components, which can be read off the graph as indicated; each point on one of the sides corresponds to a particular composition of just two components.

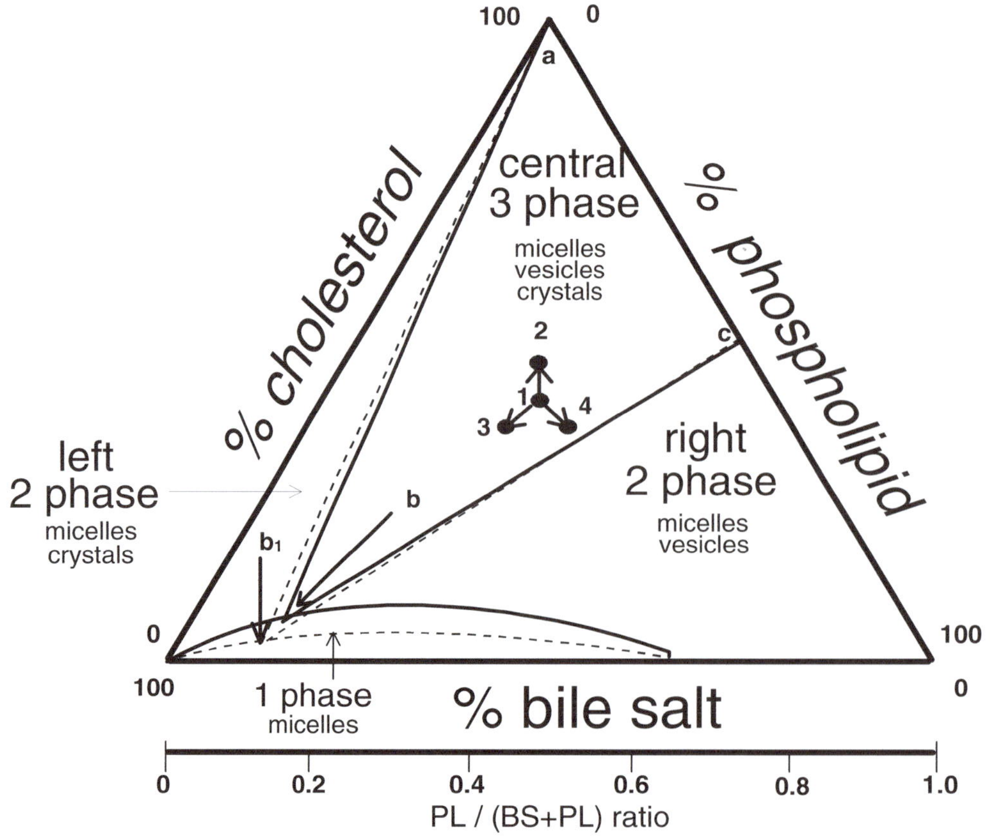

Figure 1: Ternary graph showing the balance between the 3 lipid components of bile implicated in the development of cholesterol gallstones.
[Moschetta et al., Cholesterol crystallisation in model biles, Journal of Lipid Research Volume 42, 2001]

To determine the percentage composition in the lipid component of bile for a given point, i.e., point b_1 in the 1 phase micelles section of the graph, consider straight lines from b_1:

- parallel to the bile salt side to determine the cholesterol percentage (= 5% cholesterol).
- parallel to the cholesterol side to determine the phospholipid percentage (= 10% phospholipid, PL).
- parallel to the phospholipid side to determine the bile salt percentage (= 85% bile salt, BS).

Below the ternary graph is a simple linear axis displaying the PL / (BS + PL) ratio. The 3 corners of the central 3 phase triangle are labelled a, b and c. Note that point b represents approximately 0.18 PL / (BS + PL) ratio.

1) Which of the following is most consistent with Figure 1?

   A. A cholesterol concentration of 40% or more is possible with a PL / (BS + PL) ratio of 0.2 or less.
   B. Knowing the composition of any 2 of the lipid components of bile makes it possible to calculate the third component.
   C. A cholesterol concentration of 30% or greater results in gallstone formation.
   D. Phospholipid content in bile is directly associated with gallstone formation.

2) Which of the following LEAST accurately represents the point labelled 4 within the central 3 phase triangle?

   A. Its composition will lead to the production of gallstones.
   B. Its PL / (BS + PL) ratio is approximately 0.5.
   C. It has the same cholesterol composition as point 3.
   D. It has the same phospholipid composition as point 2.

3) According to Figure 1, if an equal mixture of all 3 components (i.e. cholesterol, phospholipid, and bile salt) would make Mix Alpha, and then all of the phospholipid would be removed from Mix Alpha to make Mix Beta, which of the following would be true?

   A. Mix Alpha was 1 phase
   B. Mix Beta is 1 phase
   C. Mix Alpha was left 2 phase
   D. Mix Beta is left 2 phase

4) Label 1 within the central 3 phase triangle contains which of the following?

   A. 50% bile salt, 20% phospholipid, 30% cholesterol
   B. 30% bile salt, 30% phospholipid, 40% cholesterol
   C. 25% bile salt, 25% phospholipid, 50% cholesterol
   D. 40% bile salt, 10% phospholipid, 50% cholesterol

High-level Importance

The next 2 questions are based on the following additional information.

Numbers of large cholesterol (ChM) crystals and small cholesterol crystals were examined during a 10-day incubation period in supersaturated model systems containing TDC, TC or TUDC and plotting in the left two-phase zone.

(●) TDC; (◆) TC; (■) TUDC

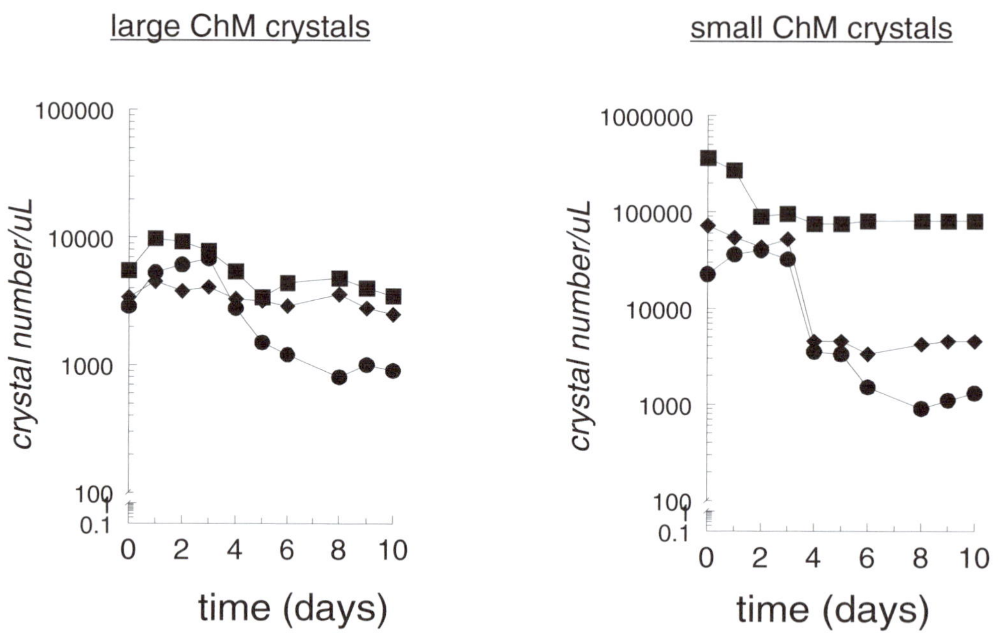

Figure 2

5) According to Figure 2, the greatest change in total crystal number/μL (including large and small crystals) during the 10-day trial contained:

A. TDC
B. TC
C. TUDC
D. Both **A** and **B** are within the margin of error.

6) According to Figure 2, after 48 hours into the experiment, the difference in small crystal number/μL between TDC and TUDC is best approximated by which of the following?

A. Less than 10%
B. Between 10% and 20%
C. Between 20% and 30%
D. None of the above

GOLD STANDARD FOUNDATIONAL GAMSAT PRACTICE QUESTIONS

7) The diagram below constitutes a schematic of events involved as energy is ultimately released from food. Note that *pepsinogen* is a substance which is secreted by the stomach wall and converted into the enzyme *pepsin* by gastric acid.

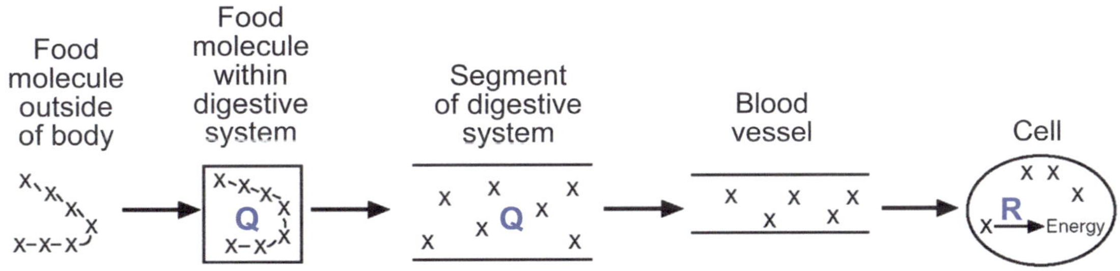

The chain of X's and the letters Q and R in the diagram likely represent which of the following?

	X-X-X-X-X-X-X	Q and R
A.	pepsinogen	antibodies
B.	pepsinogen	hormones
C.	nutrient	wastes
D.	nutrient	enzymes

8) Pepsin is a gastric enzyme that initiates the digestion of proteins (long chains of amino acids) to polypeptides and peptides (shorter chains of amino acids). Which of the following likely represents the curve for the rate of activity of pepsin?

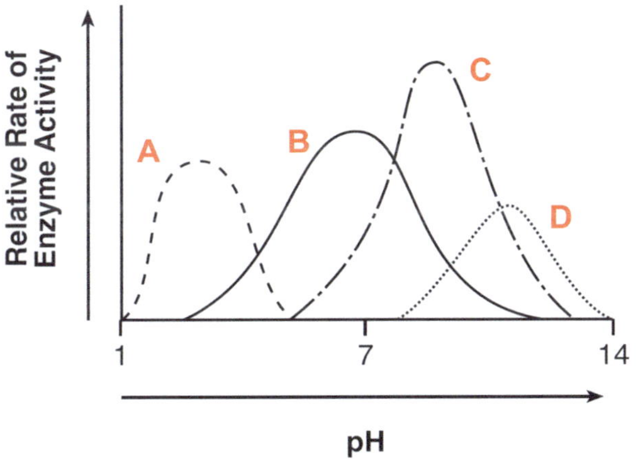

9) Enterocytes, or intestinal absorptive cells, are columnar cells which line the inner surface of the small and large intestines. Select the most accurate statement(s) about the absorptive area of the human intestine.

I. The presence of intestinal folds, villi and microvilli on the surface of enterocytes increase the absorptive area.

II. An autoimmune disorder that leads to the destruction of enterocytes - without affecting motility - would most likely lead to constipation.

A. **I** only
B. **II** only
C. **I** and **II**
D. Neither **I** nor **II**

Medium-level Importance

GOLD STANDARD GAMSAT-LEVEL PRACTICE QUESTIONS (cont'd)

Questions 10–12

The main regulatory molecules for acid secretion in the human stomach include three that stimulate acid secretion (acetylcholine, histamine, gastrin) and one that inhibits acid secretion (somatostatin). Acetylcholine is a neurotransmitter that can be released by enteric neurons via vagal stimulation. Histamine is a paracrine that is released from ECL (enterochromaffin-like) cells. Gastrin is a hormone that is released by G cells located in the gastric epithelium. Somatostatin, which can act as a paracrine or a hormone, is secreted by D cells of the gastric epithelium. The main interactions are summarised in Figure 1.

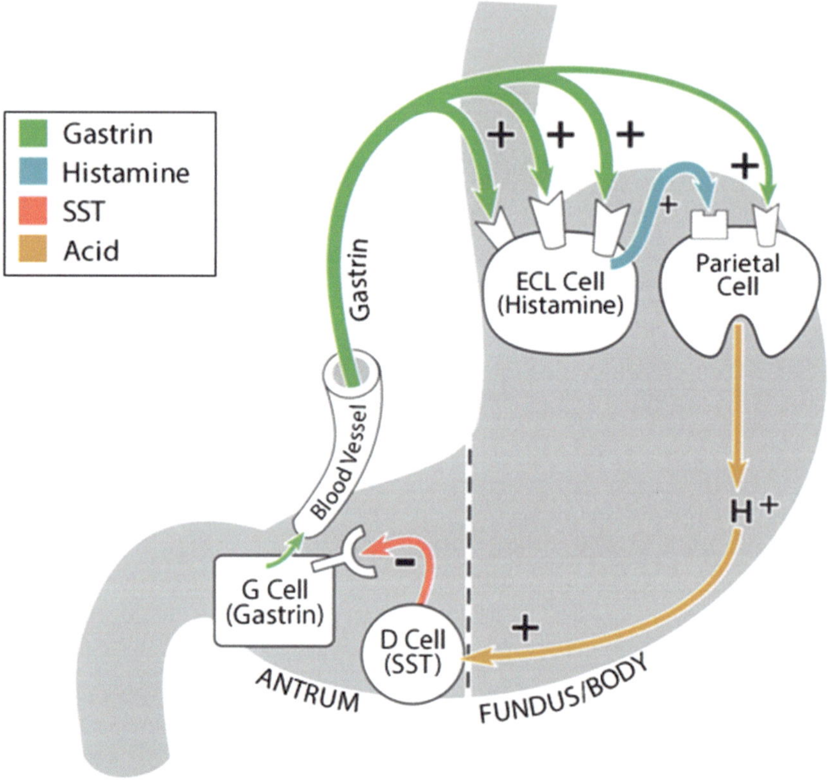

Figure 1: Regulation of gastric acid secretion by gastrin, histamine, somatostatin (SST), and acid in the gastric lumen. From the collection of Professor Mitchell L. Schubert, with the acknowledgment of Mary Beatty-Brooks (medical illustrator)

Cimetidine (Tagamet) was among the first of the rational drug-design structures, and the process began by assessing the structure of histamine. Cimetidine is now a popular, inexpensive antacid that can reduce the incidence of gastritis, reflux, and peptic ulcer disease. Major steps in the design of cimetidine include (1) using a histamine receptor model (H2) that led to the development of burimamide; (2) improving on the efficacy and safety of burimamide (*see* the following image of its structure) by replacing sulfur with nitrogen with an additional functional group to reduce the protonated form of this antacid, which eventually resulted in the production of cimetidine.

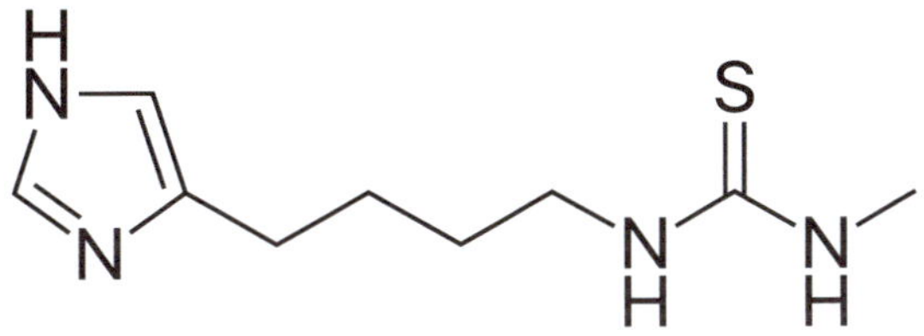
Burimamide

10) Chief cells (not shown in Figure 1) release the zymogen, pepsinogen, when stimulated by gastrin or cholinergic activity from the vagus nerve and are inhibited by somatostatin. Breakdown products of proteins are known to stimulate G cells. The most direct consequence of the production of acid by parietal cells would be that the production of:

A. somatostatin would decrease.
B. pepsinogen would decrease.
C. histamine would increase.
D. acid would increase.

11) In addition to stimulating gastric chief cells, cholinergic activity from the vagus nerve increases acid production by stimulating parietal cells. Yet another action of the cholinergic activity from the vagus, consistent with the information provided, would likely be which of the following?

A. Sensitising ECL cells to gastrin
B. Sensitising parietal cells to somatostatin
C. Desensitising ECL cells to gastrin
D. Desensitising parietal cells to histamine

12) Cimetidine likely functions by:

A. not binding to the histamine receptor and acting as an agonist.
B. not binding to the histamine receptor and acting as an antagonist.
C. binding to the histamine receptor and acting as an agonist.
D. binding to the histamine receptor and acting as an antagonist.

SPOILER ALERT

Gold Standard has cross-referenced the content in this chapter to examples from ACER's official GAMSAT practice materials. It is for you to decide when you want to explore these questions since you may want to preserve some of ACER's materials for timed mock-exam practice.

Examples – Loose bowel movements: Q10 of 1; bilirubin unit with no assumed knowledge: Q62-63 of 3 (not counted in the % Importance for this chapter); regulation of stomach acid, flow chart: Q1-5 of 4; ternary graph unit Q14-17 of 5 (no assumed knowledge; not counted). Note that "Q" is followed by the question number, and, for example, "of 1" refers to booklet number 1 which is referenced in the Spoiler Alert table at the end of Chapter 1. The 15 full-length GAMSAT practice tests by Gold Standard, HEAPS-1 through HEAPS-15, contain specific cross-references to this chapter within the worked solutions. Note that two questions from the ternary graph unit come from HEAPS-5 while the other 4 questions in that unit are novel; the cimetidine flow chart unit contains part of a unit from HEAPS-1. Regarding the ternary graph: Aside from the description with examples in GAMSAT Maths Chapter 3 (GM 3.9), we also have a free explanatory video which you can find in the Gold Standard GAMSAT YouTube channel in the worked solution for ACER's Q14-17 of 5 (this video is also in the Video section of your gamsat-prep.com account).

Chapter Checklist

- ☐ Access your online account to view answers, worked solutions and discussion boards.
- ☐ Reassess your 'learning objectives' for this chapter: Go back to the first page of this chapter and re-evaluate the top 3 boxes and the Introduction.
- ☐ Complete a maximum of 1 page of notes using symbols/abbreviations to represent the entire chapter based on your learning objectives. These are your Gold Notes.
- ☐ Consider your multimedia options based on your optimal way of learning:
    - ☐ Download the free Gold Standard GAMSAT app for your Android device or iPhone.
    - ☐ Create your own, tangible study cards or try the free app: Anki.
    - ☐ Record your voice reading your Gold Notes onto your smartphone (audio files, e.g., *memo* or MP3s) and listen during exercise, transportation, etc.
    - ☐ Try out the Gold Standard GAMSAT online videos at gamsat-prep.com, or you can try other options on YouTube like Khan Academy or Crash Course Biology.
- ☐ Reassess your schedule for your full-length GAMSAT practice tests: ACER and/or HEAPS exams. Ensure that you have scheduled one full day to complete a practice test and 1-2 days for a thorough assessment of worked solutions while adding to your abbreviated Gold Notes.
- ☐ Reassess your progress in scheduling and/or evaluating stress reduction techniques such as regular exercise (sports), yoga, meditation and/or mindfulness exercises (*see* YouTube for suggestions).

THE EXCRETORY SYSTEM
Chapter 10

Memorise	Understand	Importance
* Nothing	* Roles of the excretory system in homeostasis * Blood pressure, osmoregulation, acid-base balance, N waste removal * Formation of urine: glomerular <u>filtration</u>, <u>secretion</u> and <u>reabsorption</u> of solutes * Concentration of urine; counter-current multiplier mechanism	**Low level: 2% of GAMSAT Biology** questions released by ACER are related to content in this chapter (in our estimation). * Note that approximately 75% of the questions in GAMSAT Biology are related to just 7 chapters: 1, 2, 3, 4, 7, 12, and 15.

GAMSAT-Prep.com

Introduction

The excretory system excretes waste. The focus of this chapter is to examine the kidney's role in excretion. This includes eliminating nitrogen waste products of metabolism such as urea. There is no rote learning for this chapter that would be of any significant value for the GAMSAT. Get familiar with the basics and then the practice questions will have you exercising your reasoning and graph-analysis skills which you can apply to many other GAMSAT-question types and topics.

Multimedia Resources at GAMSAT-Prep.com

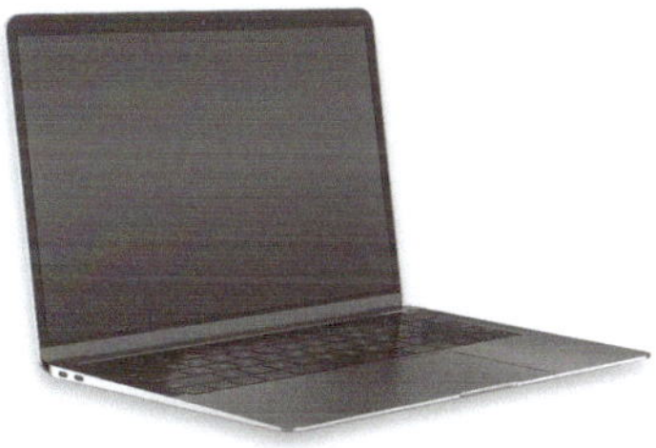

Open Discussion Boards
(gamsat-prep.com/forum)

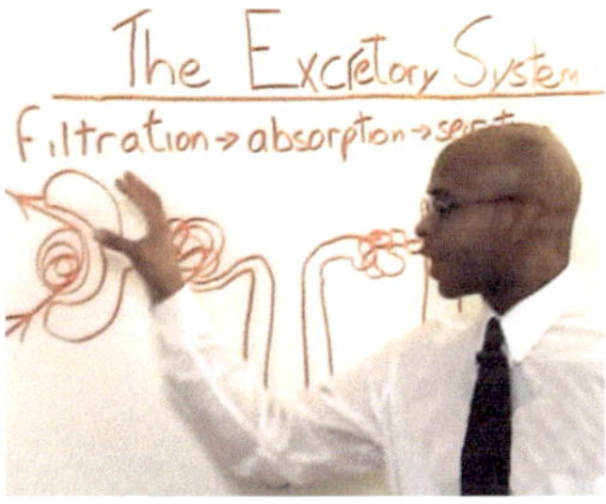

Foundational Videos

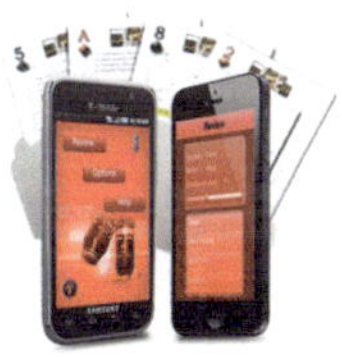

Flashcards

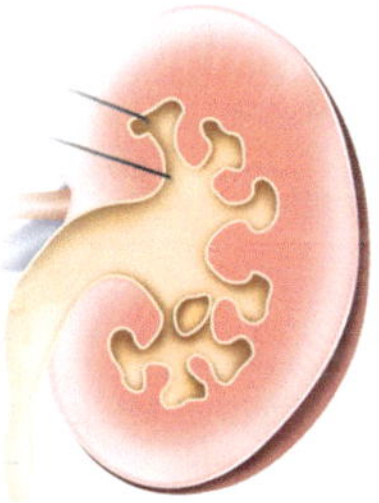

Special Guest

* The real GAMSAT may have advanced-level information presented (i.e. in a passage) but previous knowledge of said information is not required to answer the questions that would follow. Practice questions at the end of this chapter, as well as ACER and GS (HEAPS) practice GAMSATs can help you clarify this point.

10.1 Overview

Excretion is the elimination of substances (usu. wastes) from the body. It begins at the level of the cell. Broken down red blood cells are excreted as bile pigments into the GI tract; CO_2, an end product of cellular aerobic respiration, is blown away in the lungs; urea and ammonia (NH_3), breakdown products of amino acid metabolism, creatinine, a product of muscle metabolism, and H_2O, a breakdown product of aerobic metabolism, are eliminated by the urinary system. In fact, the urinary system eliminates such a great quantity of waste it is often called the excretory system. It is composed of a pair of kidneys, a pair of ureters, one bladder, and one urethra (*see* BIO 10.4).

The composition of body fluids remains within a fairly narrow range. The urinary system is the dominant organ system involved in electrolyte and water homeostasis (*osmoregulation*). It is also responsible for the excretion of toxic nitrogenous compounds (i.e. urea, uric acid, creatinine) and many drugs into the urine. The urine is produced in the kidneys (mostly by the filtration of blood) and is transported, with the help of peristaltic waves, down the tubular ureters to the muscular sack which can store urine, the bladder. Through the process of urination (= *micturition*), urine is expelled from the bladder to the outside via a tubular urethra.

The amount of volume within blood vessels (= *intravascular* or blood volume) and blood pressure are proportional to the rate the kidneys filter blood. Hormones act on the kidney to affect urine formation (*see Endocrine Systems*, BIO 6.3).

10.2 Kidney Structure

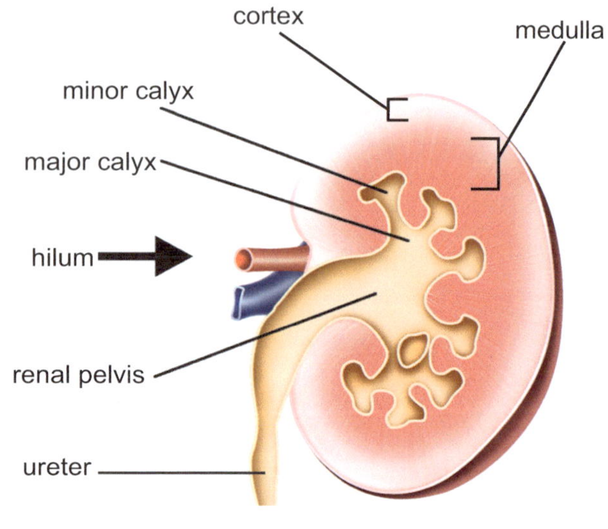

Figure IV.A.10.1: Kidney structure.

The kidney regulates the electrolyte levels in the extracellular fluid and maintains water homeostasis through the production and excretion of urine. The kidney resembles a bean with a concave border (= *the hilum*) where the ureter, nerves, and vessels (blood and lymph) attach. The kidney can be grossly divided into an outer granular-looking **cortex** and an inner dark striated **medulla**. The upper end of the ureter expands into the *renal pelvis* which can be divided into two or three *major calyces*. Each major calyx can be divided into several small branched *minor calyces*. The renal medulla lies deep to the cortex. It

Low-level Importance

is composed of 10-18 medullary pyramids which consist mainly of loop of Henle and collecting tubules. The renal cortex is the superficial layer of the kidney right underneath the capsule. It is composed mainly of renal corpuscles and convoluted tubules.

The kidney is a *filtration-reabsorption-secretion* (excretion) organ. These events are clearly demonstrated at the level of the nephron.

10.3 The Nephron: Filter, Reabsorb, Secrete, Excrete

The nephron is the functional unit of the kidney and consists of the **renal corpuscle** and the **renal tubule**. A renal corpuscle is responsible for the filtration of blood and is composed of a tangled ball of blood capillaries (= *the glomerulus*) and a sac-like structure which surrounds the glomerulus (= *Bowman's capsule*). *Afferent* and *efferent* arterioles lead towards and away from the glomerulus, respectively. The renal tubule is divided into *proximal* and *distal convoluted tubules* with a *loop of Henle* in between. The tube ends in a *collecting duct*.

Blood plasma is **filtered** by the glomerulus through three layers before entering Bowman's capsule. The first layer is formed by the *endothelial cells* of the capillary that possess small holes (= *fenestrae*); the second layer is the *glomerular basement membrane* (BIO 5.3); and the third layer is formed by the negatively charged cells (= *podocytes*) in Bowman's capsule which help repel proteins (most proteins are negatively charged).

The filtration barrier permits passage of water, ions, and small particles from the capillary into Bowman's capsule but prevents pas-

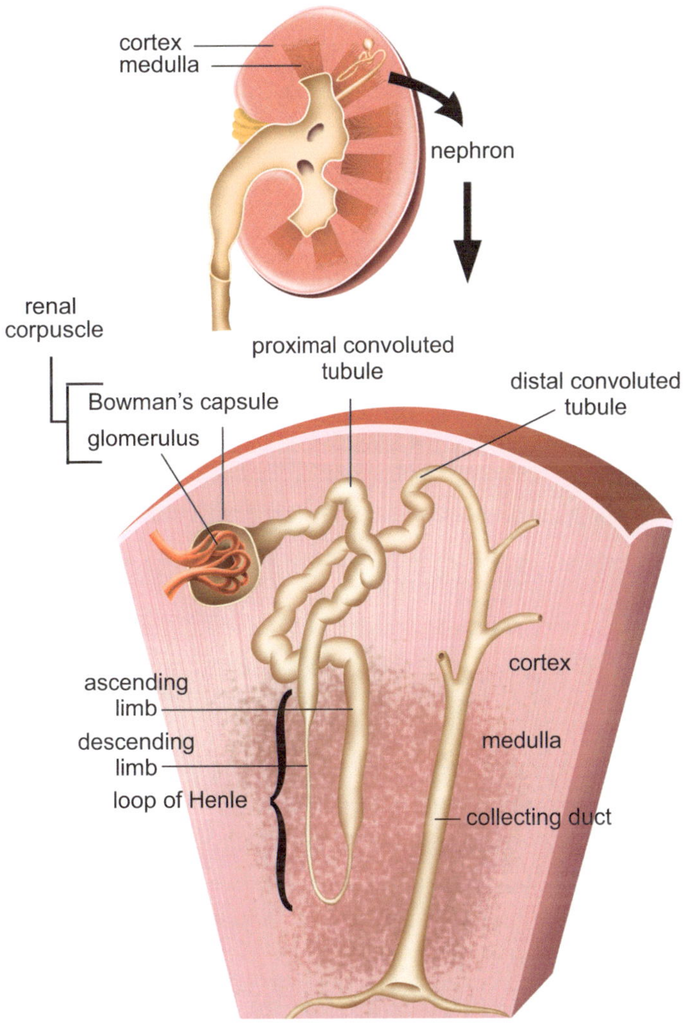

Figure IV.A.10.2: The kidney and its functional unit, the nephron.

Low-level Importance

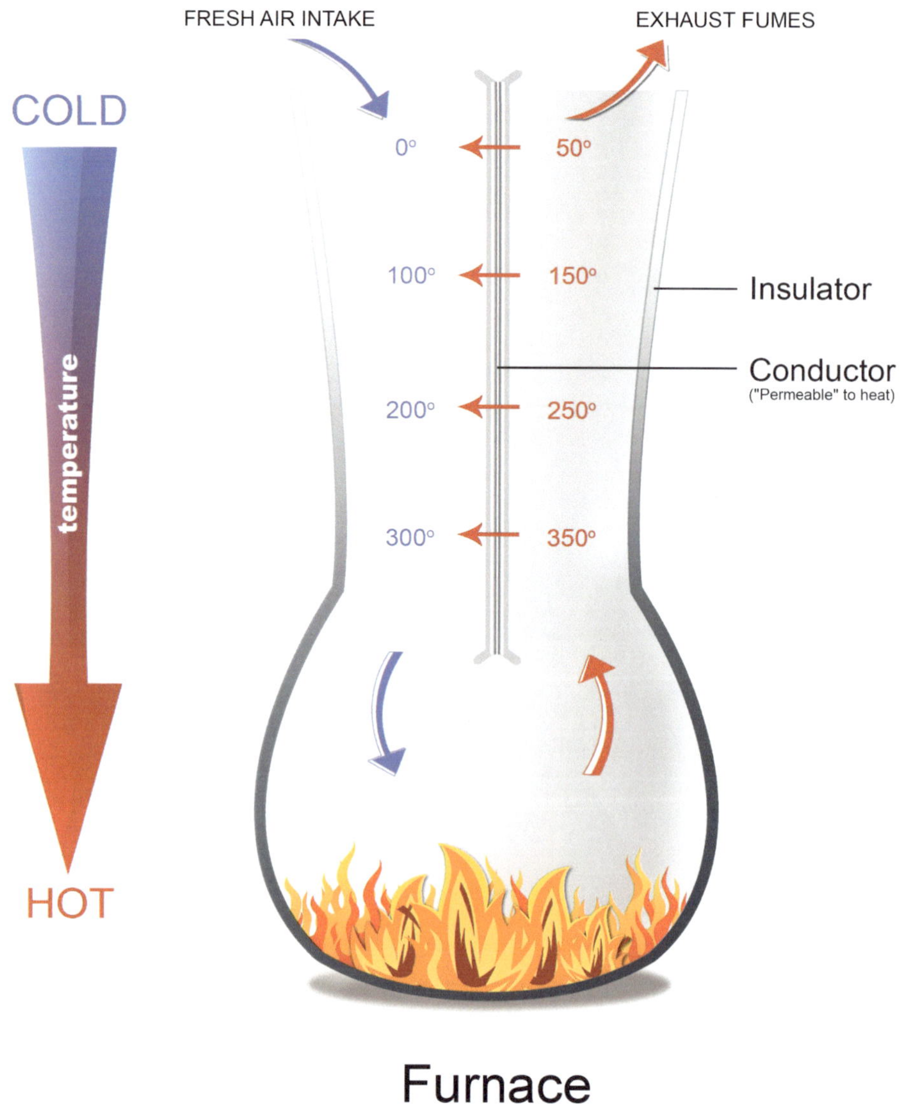

The countercurrent principle depends on a parallel flow arrangement moving in 2 different directions (countercurrent) in close proximity to each other. Our example is that of the air intake and exhaust pipe in this simplified schematic of a furnace.

Heat is transferred from the exhaust fumes to the incoming air.

The small horizontal temperature gradient of only 50° is multiplied longitudinally to a gradient of 300°. This conserves heath that would otherwise be lost.

Figure IV.A.10.3: The countercurrent principle (= counter-current mechanism) using a simplified furnace as an example.

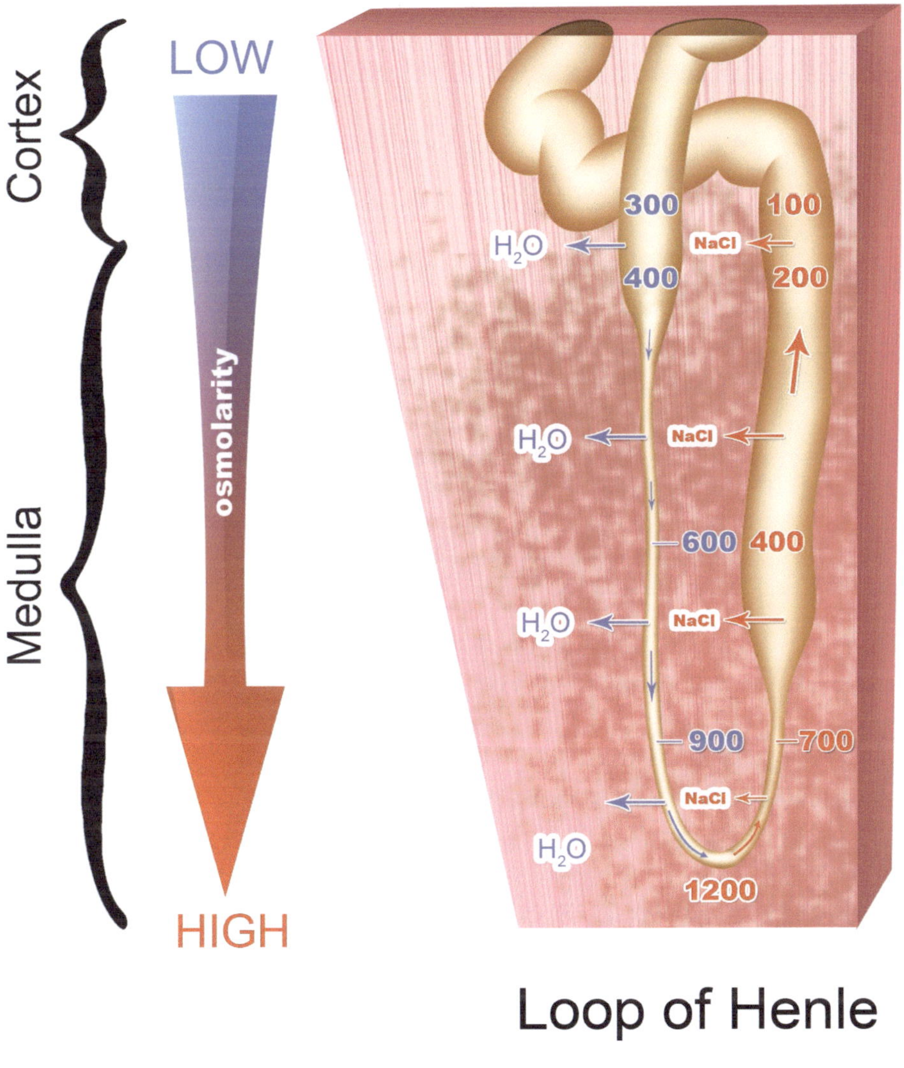

The countercurrent system involving the loop of Henle results in an osmotic gradient increasing from cortex to inner medulla (*juxtamedullary* nephrons). Solutes enter and exit at different segments of the nephron. The descending limb of the loop of Henle is highly permeable to water and relatively impermeable to NaCl (thus the filtrate becomes increasingly hypertonic). The ascending limb is impermeable to water but relatively (through active transport) permeable to NaCl.

Due to the increased osmolarity of the interstitial fluid, water moves out of the descending limb into the interstitial fluid by osmosis. Volume of the filtrate decreases as water leaves. Osmotic concentration of the filtrate increases (1200) as it rounds the hairpin turn of the loop of Henle.

Some of the NaCl leaving the ascending limb moves by diffusion into the descending limb from the interstitial fluid thus increasing the solute concentration in the descending limb. Also, new NaCl in the filtrate continuously enters the tubule inflow to be transported out of the ascending limb into the interstitial fluid. Thus this recycling multiplies NaCl concentration.

Figure IV.A.10.4: The countercurrent principle (= counter-current mechanism) in the loop of Henle.

10.3 The Nephron (cont'd)

sage of large/negatively charged particles (= *ultrafiltration*) and forms a filtrate in the Bowman's space. The rate of filtration is proportional to the net ultrafiltration pressure across the glomerular capillaries. This net pressure, which is usually positive and favors fluid filtration out of the capillary, can be derived from the difference between glomerular capillary hydrostatic pressure, which favors fluid out of the capillary, and the combined effect of glomerular capillary oncotic pressure and Bowman's space *hydrostatic* pressure, which favor fluid back into the capillary. {The oncotic pressure of Bowman's space is typically zero, so it is ignored here; keep in mind that 'oncotic pressure' is simply the osmotic pressure caused by proteins; *see* BIO 7.5.2}

The filtrate, which is similar to plasma but with minimal proteins, now passes into the proximal convoluted tubule (PCT). It is here that the body actively **reabsorbs** compounds that it needs (i.e. proteins, amino acids, and especially glucose); and over 75% of all ions and water are reabsorbed by *obligate* (= required) reabsorption from the PCT. To increase the surface area for absorption, the cells of the PCT have a lot of microvilli (= *brush border*, cf. BIO 1.2). Some substances like H^+, urea and penicillin are **secreted** into the PCT.

From the PCT the filtrate goes through the descending and ascending limbs of the loop of Henle which extend into the renal medulla. The purpose of the loop of Henle is to concentrate the filtrate by the transport of ions (Na^+ and Cl^-) into the medulla which produces an osmotic gradient (= *a countercurrent mechanism*). As a consequence of this system, the medulla of the kidney becomes concentrated with ions and tends to "pull" water out of the renal tubule by osmosis.

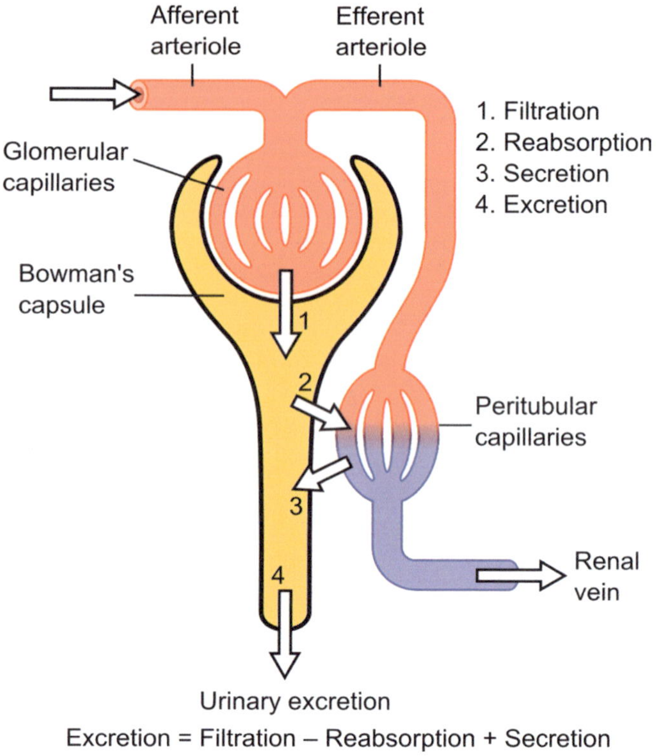

Figure IV.A.10.5: Schematic diagram of the nephron showing 4 key functions. (ref: Madhero88, Wikimedia Commons)

The filtrate now passes on to the distal convoluted tubule (DCT) which reabsorbs ions actively and water passively and secretes various ions (i.e. H^+). Hormones can modulate the reabsorption of substances from the DCT (= *facultative* reabsorption). Aldosterone acts at the DCT to absorb Na^+ which is coupled to the secretion of K^+ and the passive retention of H_2O.

Low-level Importance

Finally the filtrate, now called urine, passes into the collecting duct which drains into larger and larger ducts which lead to renal papillae, calyces, the renal pelvis, and then the ureter. ADH concentrates urine by increasing the permeability of the DCT and the collecting ducts allowing the medulla to draw water out by osmosis. Water returns to the circulation via a system of vessels called the *vasa recta*.

Renin is a hormone (BIO 6.3.5) which is secreted by cells that are "near the glomerulus" (= *juxtaglomerular cells*). At the beginning of the DCT is a region of modified tubular cells which can influence the secretion of renin (= *macula densa*). The juxtaglomerular cells and the macula densa are collectively known as the juxtaglomerular apparatus.

10.4 The Bladder

Urine flow through the ureters to the bladder is propelled by muscular contractions of the ureter wall - peristalsis. The urine is stored in the bladder and intermittently ejected during urination, termed micturition.

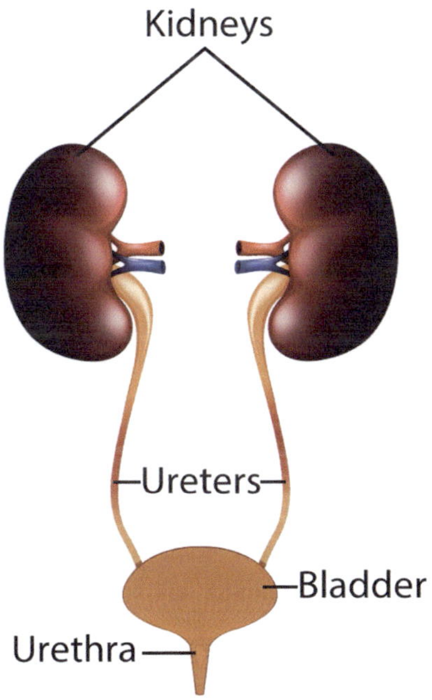

Figure IV.A.10.6: The urinary system.

The bladder is a balloon-like chamber with walls of muscle collectively termed the detrusor muscle. The contraction of this muscle squeezes the urine into the lumen (= *space inside*) of the bladder to produce urination. That part of the detrusor muscle at the base of the bladder, where the urethra begins, functions as a sphincter - the internal urethral sphincter. Beyond the outlet of the urethra is the external urethral sphincter, the contraction of which can prevent urination even when the detrusor muscle contracts strongly.

The basic micturition reflex is a spinal reflex (BIO 6.1.3), which can be influenced by descending pathways from the brain. The bladder wall contains stretch receptors whose afferent fibers enter the spinal cord and stimulate the parasympathetic nerves that supply and stimulate the detrusor muscle. As the bladder fills with urine, the pressure within it increases and the stretch receptors are stimulated, thereby reflexively eliciting stimulation

Low-level Importance

of the parasympathetic neurons and contractions of the detrusor muscle. When the bladder reaches a certain volume, the induced contraction of the detrusor muscle becomes strong enough to open the internal urethral sphincter. Simultaneously, the afferent input from the stretch receptors inhibits, within the spinal cord, the motor neurons that tonically stimulate the external urethral sphincter to contract. Both sphincters are now open and the contraction of the detrusor muscle is able to produce urination.

In summary:

- The internal sphincter is a continuation of the detrusor muscle and is thus composed of smooth muscle under involuntary or autonomic control. This is the primary muscle for preventing the release of urine.
- The external sphincter is made of skeletal muscle is thus under voluntary control of the somatic nervous system (BIO 6.1.4, 6.1.5, 11.2).

CHAPTER 10: The Excretory System

Note: There are no foundational questions for this chapter, and there are no topics to commit to memory. For the excretory system, it is expected that you understand the concepts of diffusion and osmosis which have been explored elsewhere (BIO 1.1.1 and BIO 7.5.2; CHM 5.1.3).

GOLD STANDARD GAMSAT-LEVEL PRACTICE QUESTIONS

1) The nephron is the structural and functional unit of the kidney. The nephron filters via the glomerulus, reabsorbs from the tubules, secretes into the tubules, and excretes the filtrate which becomes urine. Glucose is the most important source of energy for all organisms and so it is not secreted. Para-aminohippuric acid (PAH) is a diagnostic agent useful in medical tests (renal plasma flow) and so it is not reabsorbed by the nephron. Which of the following equations accurately describes the activity of the nephron under normal conditions?

A. Substances in general: *excretion = (filtration + secretion) - reabsorption*
B. Glucose: *excretion = filtration - reabsorption*
C. PAH: *excretion = filtration + secretion*
D. All of the above

Questions 2–6

The nephron, the functional unit of the kidney, is a filtration-resorption-secretion-excretion unit. The nephron contributes to glucose homeostasis by filtering and reabsorbing glucose.

Note that:

- TmG is the maximum reabsorption rate for glucose;
- glucosuria is the excretion of glucose into the urine.

Consider Figure 1.

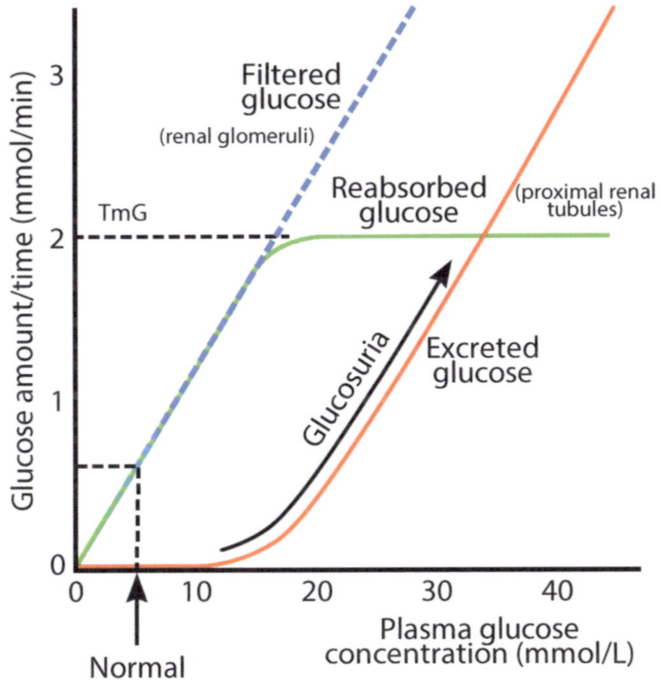

Figure 1

2) Glomerular filtration rate (GFR) is the volume of fluid filtered from the renal (kidney) glomerular capillaries into the Bowman's capsule per unit time. Determine the GFR based on the data from Figure 1.

A. Less than 1 mL/min
B. 5 mL/min
C. 100 mL/min
D. 120 mL/min

3) Based on Figure 1, at 50 mmol/L of plasma glucose concentration, what would be the projected filtered glucose concentration?

A. 2 mmol/L
B. 4 mmol/L
C. 5 mmol/L
D. 6 mmol/L

4) According to Figure 1, which of the following would be expected if 3 mmol/min of glucose is filtered?

A. 33% of the filtered glucose would be excreted
B. 5 mmol/L of plasma glucose concentration
C. Nearly 100% of the filtered glucose would be excreted
D. Under normal conditions, no glucose is excreted from the nephron

5) Some nephrons become glucosuric at lower concentrations than others. Only after the transport maximum of all individual nephrons is exceeded does the urinary excretion become directly proportional to the filtered load. The small amounts excreted before that point have been called "splay". According to Figure 1, splay occurs between which values of plasma glucose concentration?

A. Below 10 mmol/L
B. Between 10-20 mmol/L
C. Between 20-30 mmol/L
D. Above 30 mmol/L

6) According to Figure 1, is it normal to have a relatively small amount of glucose in urine?

A. No, because under normal conditions, filtered and reabsorbed glucose are equal.
B. No, because glucose is vital for metabolism and is thus never excreted.
C. Yes, because 'normal' for everyone varies significantly.
D. Yes, it is not possible to reabsorb unlimited amounts of glucose.

Questions 7–10

The functional unit of the kidney is the urine-producing nephron (*see* Figure 1). Fluid and solutes pass from the capillary [or glomerulus, fed by a small artery labelled (1) in the diagram] which is surrounded by the first part of the nephron called Bowman's capsule. The nephron is capable of concentrating or diluting urine marking a change in the normal solute concentration of urine for humans which ranges from 500-800 mOsm/kg of water. The fluid within the nephron [which includes Bowman's capsule, through to (2) then the descending and ascending limbs of the renal tubule followed by (3) in the diagram, the collecting duct] is often referred to as the filtrate. The Loop of Henle - the long U-shaped portion of the renal tubule - conducts and concentrates the filtrate as it becomes urine.

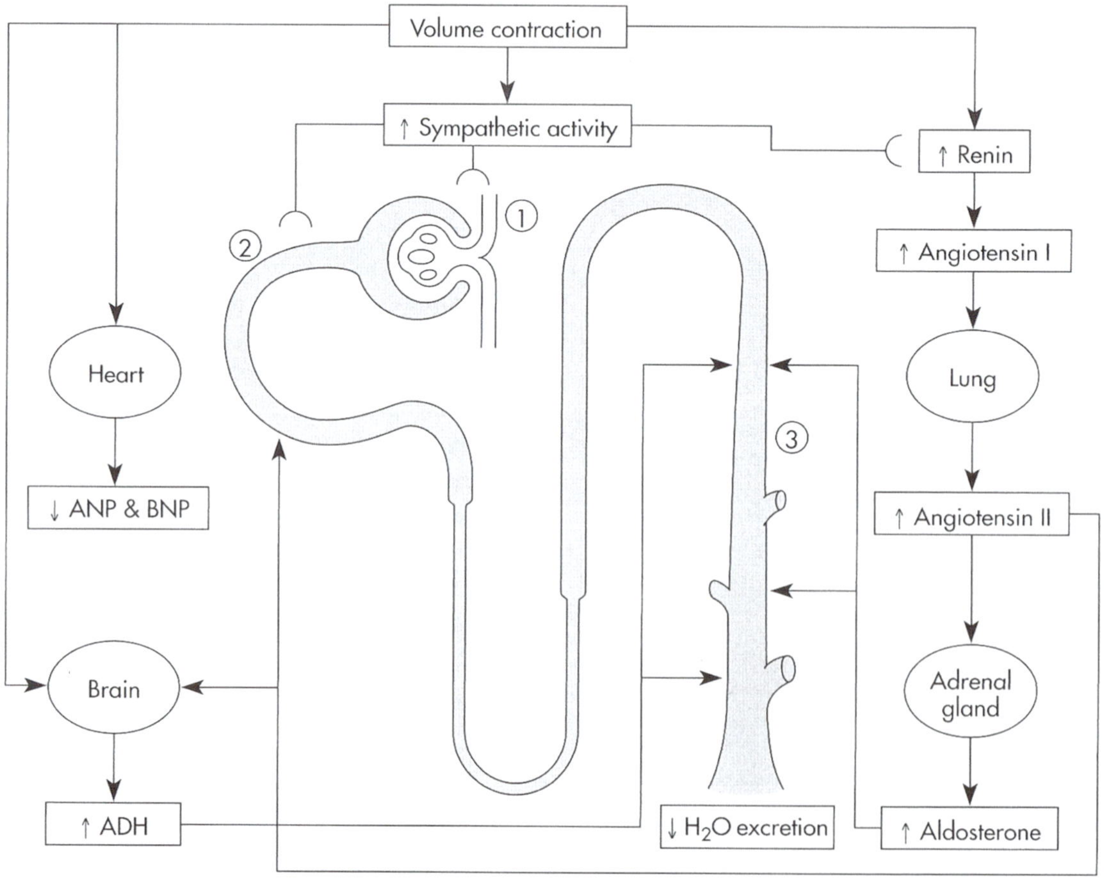

Figure 1: Normal Regulatory responses to extracellular fluid (ECF) volume contraction (reduction of fluid around cells and in blood vessels). The integrated response of the nephron to ECF volume contraction results in the following: decreased glomerular filtration rate (1), increased NaCl and water reabsorption by the proximal tubule and loop of Henle (2), and increased NaCl and water reabsorption by the distal tubule and collecting duct (3). ANP, atrial natriuretic peptide; BNP, brain natriuretic peptide; ADH, antidiuretic hormone. (Lisa M. Harrison-Bernard Advances in Physiology Education Published 1 December 2009 Vol. 33 no. 4, 270-274 DOI: 10.1152/advan.00049.2009)

7) The ascending limb of the renal tubule has a thick (wider) portion which is impermeable to water and solutes. The cells in this part of the nephron use ATP to actively pump sodium and chloride out of the filtrate. Which of the following would be the likely consequence of this active transport on the concentration of the filtrate and the volume of the filtrate, respectively?

A. Increases, decreases
B. Decreases, increases
C. Increases, no change
D. Decreases, no change

8) Which of the following would be most consistent with the urine osmolality if the activity of the enzyme producing ADH in the brain was blocked?

A. 300 mOsm/kg
B. 500 mOsm/kg
C. 800 mOsm/kg
D. 1000 mOsm/kg

9) Figure 1 does not illustrate the action of ANP. Which of the following would NOT be consistent with the pathways illustrated in Figure 1?

A. ANP is secreted in response to an expanded blood volume.
B. ANP decreases aldosterone production.
C. ANP blocks renin and increases blood pressure.
D. **A**, **B** and **C** are consistent with Figure 1.

10) Camels, kangaroo rats and desert rats evolved in hot, arid conditions. Such mammals, as compared to a normal human's nephron, would be expected to have, relatively:

A. longer glomeruli.
B. longer loops of Henle.
C. larger Bowman's capsules.
D. smaller nephrons.

11) The human kidney can be damaged from a number of causes resulting in a patient's inability to filter toxins (e.g. urea) from the body which could result in death. Complete kidney failure is usually first treated with dialysis which "cleans" the blood.

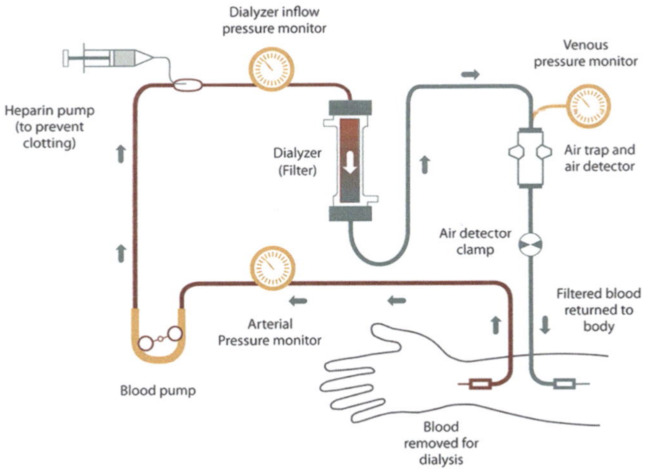

Figure 1: The "dialyzer" is a glass container that has 3 main components: (1) blood percolating through to be cleaned; (2) a dividing membrane; and (3) the dialysate. The latter is liquid containing chemicals used to draw fluids and toxins out of the bloodstream and supply electrolytes and other chemicals to the bloodstream.
(image: kidney.niddk.nih.gov)

All of the following are consistent with the process of dialysis EXCEPT:

A. The membrane in the dialyzer separating the dialysate and the blood must be semi-permeable.
B. The concentration of toxins in the dialysate must increase during dialysis.
C. The concentration of glucose and vital minerals in the dialysate must be similar to that of the patient's blood.
D. Excessive minerals and toxins cross the membrane in the dialyzer by osmosis.

High-level Importance

Questions 12–15

Urine flow through the ureters to the bladder is propelled by muscular contractions of the wall of the ureter - peristalsis. The urine is stored in the bladder and intermittently ejected during urination, termed micturition.

The bladder is a balloon-like chamber with walls of muscle collectively termed the detrusor muscle. The contraction of this muscle squeezes the urine into the lumen of the bladder to produce urination. That part of the detrusor muscle at the base of the bladder, where the urethra begins, functions as a sphincter - the internal urethral sphincter. Beyond the outlet of the urethra is the external urethral sphincter, the contraction of which can prevent urination even when the detrusor muscle contracts strongly.

The basic micturition reflex is a spinal reflex, which can be influenced by descending pathways from the brain. The bladder wall contains stretch receptors whose afferent fibers enter the spinal cord and stimulate the parasympathetic nerves that supply and stimulate the detrusor muscle. As the bladder fills with urine, the pressure within it increases and the stretch receptors are stimulated, thereby reflexively eliciting stimulation of the parasympathetic neurons and contractions of the detrusor muscle. When the bladder reaches a certain volume, the induced contraction of the detrusor muscle becomes strong enough to open the internal urethral sphincter. Simultaneously, the afferent input from the stretch receptors inhibits, within the spinal cord, the motor neurons that tonically stimulate the external urethral sphincter to contract. Both sphincters are now open and the contraction of the detrusor muscle is able to produce urination.

12) The passage infers that the internal and external urethral sphincters consist of:

A. skeletal and smooth muscle, respectively.
B. skeletal muscle and connective tissue, respectively.
C. smooth muscle and skeletal muscle, respectively.
D. smooth muscle and connective tissue, respectively.

13) Through the process of micturition, urine is expelled from the bladder into the:

A. urethra.
B. ureter.
C. major calyx.
D. minor calyx.

14) On a very hot day, the bladder would likely contain:

A. a large amount of urine hypertonic to blood plasma.
B. a large amount of urine hypotonic to blood plasma.
C. a small amount of urine hypertonic to blood plasma.
D. a small amount of urine hypotonic to blood plasma.

15) The passage indicates that the internal urethral sphincter is:

A. closed when the detrusor muscle is relaxed.
B. open when the detrusor muscle is relaxed.
C. not under the direct control of the detrusor muscle.
D. innervated directly by motor neurons extending from the descending pathways.

SPOILER ALERT

Gold Standard has cross-referenced the content in this chapter to examples from ACER's official GAMSAT practice materials. It is for you to decide when you want to explore these questions since you may want to preserve some of ACER's materials for timed mock-exam practice.

Examples – Straight dimensional analysis, Q3 of 1; trap set if you study health/biomed/med-related and tried rote learning: Q5 of 1; extrapolate a line: Q63 of 4. Note that "Q" is followed by the question number, and, for example, "of 1" refers to booklet number 1 which is referenced in the Spoiler Alert table at the end of Chapter 1. The 15 full-length GAMSAT practice tests by Gold Standard, HEAPS-1 through HEAPS-15, contain specific cross-references to this chapter within the worked solutions. Note that for another unit practicing linear extrapolation, you can try the Breast/Infant Milk Lead graph in Chapter 14 of this book.

Chapter Checklist

- ☐ Access your online account to view answers, worked solutions and discussion boards.
- ☐ Reassess your 'learning objectives' for this chapter: Go back to the first page of this chapter and re-evaluate the top 3 boxes and the Introduction.
- ☐ Complete a maximum of 1 page of notes using symbols/abbreviations to represent the entire chapter based on your learning objectives. These are your Gold Notes.
- ☐ Consider your multimedia options based on your optimal way of learning:
  - ☐ Download the free Gold Standard GAMSAT app for your Android device or iPhone.
  - ☐ Create your own, tangible study cards or try the free app: Anki.
  - ☐ Record your voice reading your Gold Notes onto your smartphone (audio files, e.g., *memo* or MP3s) and listen during exercise, transportation, etc.
  - ☐ Try out the Gold Standard GAMSAT online videos at gamsat-prep.com, or you can try other options on YouTube like Khan Academy or Crash Course Biology.
- ☐ Reassess your schedule for your full-length GAMSAT practice tests: ACER and/or HEAPS exams. Ensure that you have scheduled one full day to complete a practice test and 1-2 days for a thorough assessment of worked solutions while adding to your abbreviated Gold Notes.
- ☐ Reassess your progress in scheduling and/or evaluating stress reduction techniques such as regular exercise (sports), yoga, meditation and/or mindfulness exercises (*see* YouTube for suggestions).

THE MUSCULOSKELETAL SYSTEM
Chapter 11

Memorise	Understand	Importance
* Nothing	* Basic categories of muscles * Support, mobility, peripheral circulatory assistance, thermoregulation (shivering reflex) * Skeletal system: structural rigidity/support, calcium storage, physical protection * Skeletal structure: specialisation of bone types, basic joint, endo/exoskeleton	**Medium level: 6% of GAMSAT Biology** questions released by ACER are related to content in this chapter (in our estimation). * Note that approximately 75% of the questions in GAMSAT Biology are related to just 7 chapters: 1, 2, 3, 4, 7, 12, and 15.

GAMSAT-Prep.com

Introduction

The musculoskeletal system (= locomotor system) permits the movement of organisms with the use of muscle and bone. Other uses include providing form and stability for the organism; protection of vital organs (i.e. skull, rib cage); storage for calcium and phosphorous as well as containing a critical component to the production of blood cells (skeletal system).

Multimedia Resources at GAMSAT-Prep.com

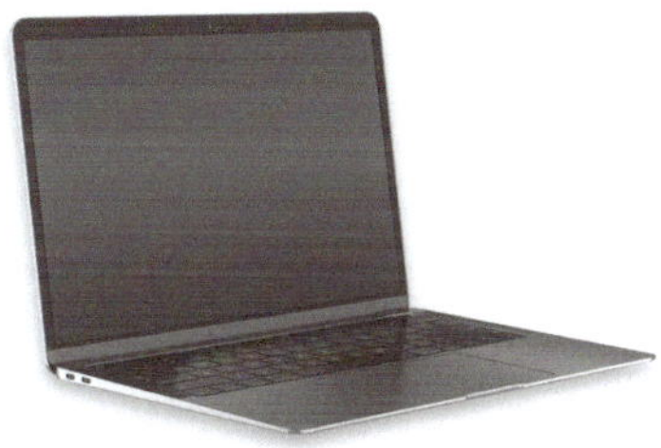

Open Discussion Boards
(*gamsat-prep.com/forum*)

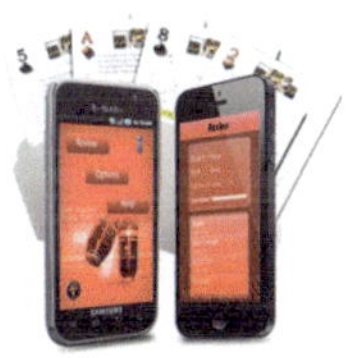

Flashcards

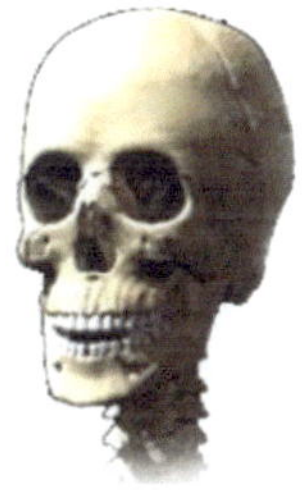

Special Guest

* The real GAMSAT may have advanced-level information presented (i.e. in a passage) but previous knowledge of said information is not required to answer the questions that would follow. Practice questions at the end of this chapter, as well as ACER and GS (HEAPS) practice GAMSATs can help you clarify this point.

11.1 Overview

The musculoskeletal system supports, protects and enables body parts to move. Muscles convert chemical energy (i.e. ATP, creatine phosphate) into mechanical energy (→ contraction). Thus body heat is produced, body fluids are moved (i.e. lymph), and body parts can move in accordance with lever systems of muscle and bone.

11.2 Muscle

Medium-level Importance

There are many general features of muscle. A latent period is the lag between the stimulation of a muscle and its response. A twitch is a single contraction in response to a brief stimulus which lasts for a fraction of a second. Muscles can either *contract* or *relax* but they cannot actively expand. When muscles are stimulated frequently, they cannot fully relax - this is known as *summation*. Tetany is a sustained contraction (a summation of multiple contractions) that lacks even partial relaxation. If tetany is maintained, the muscle will eventually fatigue or tire. Muscle tone (*tonus*) occurs because even when a muscle appears to be at rest, some degree of sustained contraction is occurring.

The cellular characteristics of muscle have already been described (*see Contractile Cells and Tissues,* BIO 5.2). We will now examine the gross features of the three basic muscle types.

Cardiac muscle forms the walls of the heart and is responsible for the pumping action. Its contractions are continuous and are initiated by inherent mechanisms (i.e., they are myogenic) and modulated by the autonomic nervous system. Its activity is decreased by the parasympathetic nervous system and increased by the sympathetic nervous system. The sinoatrial node (SA node) or *pacemaker* contains specialised cardiac muscle cells in the right atrium which initiate the contraction of the heart (BIO 7.2). The electrical signal then progresses to the atrioventricular node (AV node) in the cardiac muscle (myocardium) - between the atria and ventricles - then through the bundle of His which splits and branches out to Purkinje fibers which can then stimulate the contraction of the ventricles (systole; BIO 7.2).

Smooth Muscle has two forms. One type occurs as separate fibers and can contract in response to motor nerve stimuli. These are found in the iris (*pupillary dilation or constriction*) and the walls of blood vessels (*vasodilation or constriction)*. The second and more dominant form occurs as sheets of muscle fibers and is sometimes called *visceral muscle*. It forms the walls of many hollow visceral organs like the stomach, intestines, uterus, and the urinary bladder. Like cardiac muscle, its contractions are inherent, involuntary, and rhythmic. Visceral muscle is responsible for peristalsis. Its contractility is usually slow and can be modulated by the autonomic nervous system, hormones, and local metabolites. The activity of visceral muscle is increased by the parasympathetic nervous system and decreased by the sympathetic nervous system.

Skeletal muscle is responsible for voluntary movements. This includes the skeleton and organs such as the tongue and the globe of the eye. Its cells can form a syncytium which is a mass of cells which merge and can function together. Thus skeletal muscle can contract and relax relatively rapidly (*see the Reflex Arc,* BIO 6.1.3).

It should be noted that there are 2 meanings of the word "syncytium" when describing muscle cells. A classic example is the formation of large multinucleated skeletal muscle cells produced from the fusion of thousands of individual muscle cells (= *myocytes*) as alluded to in the previous paragraph ("true syncytium"). However, "syncytium" can also refer to cells that are interconnected by gap junctions (BIO 1.4), as seen in cardiac muscle cells and certain smooth muscle cells, and are thus synchronised electrically during an action potential ("functional syncytium").

Most skeletal muscles act across joints. Each muscle has a movable end (= *the insertion*) and an immovable end (= *the origin*). When a muscle contracts its insertion is moved towards its origin. When the angle of the joint decreases it is called flexion, when it increases it is called extension. Abduction is movement away from the midline of the body and adduction is movement toward the midline. {A**dd**uction is a**dd**icted to the mi**dd**le (= midline)}

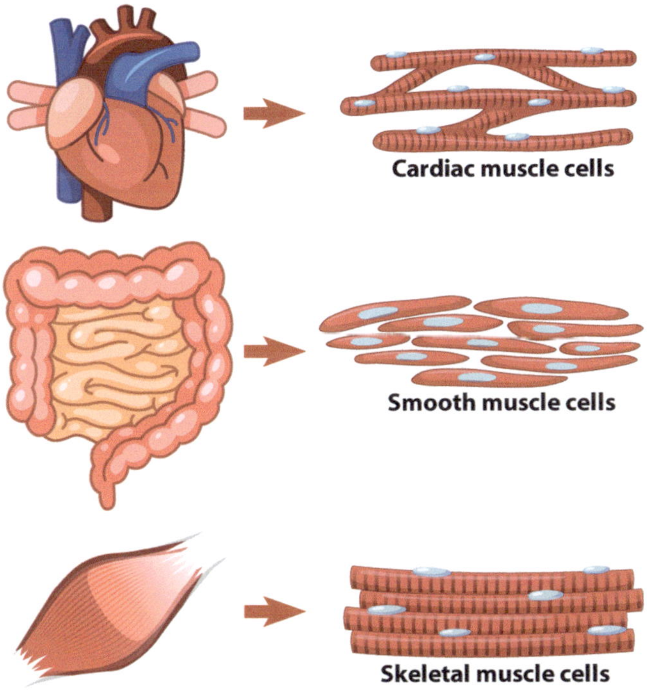

Figure IV.A.11.0: Types of muscle tissue. Notice that both cardiac and skeletal muscle have striated cells (dark lines; BIO 5.2) due to the presence of sarcomeres.

Muscles which assist each other are synergistic (for example: while the deltoid muscle abducts the arm, other muscles hold the shoulder steady). Muscles that can move a joint in opposite directions are antagonistic (for example: at the elbow the biceps can flex while the triceps can extend).

Control of skeletal muscle originates in the cerebral cortex. Skeletal muscle is innervated by the somatic nervous system. Motor (*efferent*) neurons carry nerve impulses from the CNS to synapse with muscle fibers at the *neuromuscular junction.* The terminal end of the motor neuron (motor end plate) can secrete acetylcholine which can depolarise the muscle fiber (BIO 5.1, 5.2). One motor neuron can depolarise many muscle fibers (= *a motor unit*).

The autonomic nervous system can supply skeletal muscle with more oxygenated blood in emergencies (sympathetic response) or redirect the blood to the viscera during relaxed states (parasympathetic response).

Skeletal muscle can be categorised as Type I or Type II. Type I fibers (= *cells*) appear red because of the oxygen-binding protein myoglobin (BIO 7.5.1). These fibers are suited for endurance and are slow to fatigue since they use oxidative metabolism to generate ATP (BIO 4.7-4.10). Type II fibers are white due to the absence of myoglobin and a reliance on glycolytic enzymes (BIO 4.5, 4.6). These fibers are efficient for short bursts of speed and power and use both oxidative metabolism and anaerobic metabolism depending on the particular sub-type. Type II myocytes are quicker to fatigue.

Medium-level Importance

11.3 The Skeletal System

The microscopic features of bone and cartilage have already been described (*see Connective Cells and Tissues*, BIO 5.4.3/4). We will now examine the relevant gross features of the skeletal system.

The bones of the skeleton have many functions: **i)** acting like levers that aid in **body movement**; **ii)** the **storage** of inorganic salts like calcium and phosphorus (and to a lesser extent sodium and magnesium); **iii)** the production of blood cells (= **hematopoiesis**) in the metabolically active red marrow of the spongy parts of many bones. Bone also has a yellow marrow which contains fat storage cells.

11.3.1 Bone Structure and Development

Bone structure can be classified as follows: **i)** long bones which have a long shaft, the diaphysis, that is made up mostly of compact bone and expanded ends, like arm and leg bones; **ii)** short bones which are shaped like long bones but are smaller and have only a thin layer of compact bone surrounding a spongy bone interior; **iii)** flat bones which have broad surfaces like the skull, ribs, and the scapula and have two layers of compact bones with a layer of spongy bone in the middle; **iv)** irregular bones like the vertebrae and many facial bones and consist of a thin layer of compact bone covering a spongy bone

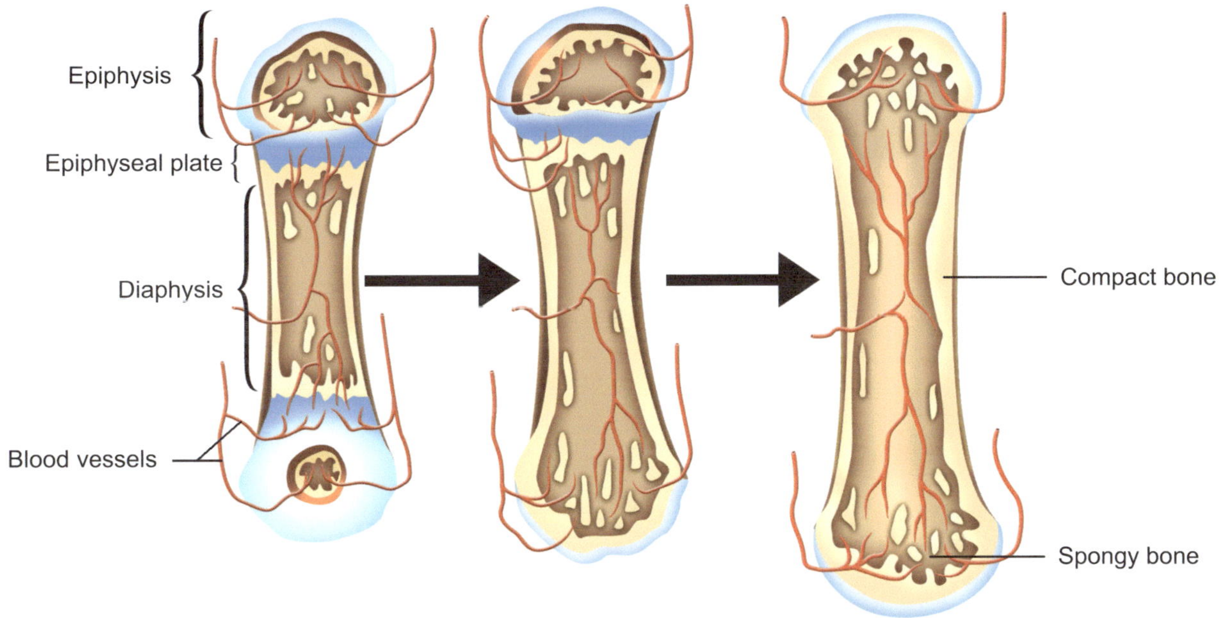

Figure IV.A.11.1: Bone structure and development.

interior. Bone structure can also be classified as: **i)** <u>primary bone</u>, also known as immature or woven bone, which contains many cells and has a low mineral content; **ii)** <u>secondary bone</u>, also known as mature or lamellar bone, which has a calcified matrix arranged in regular layers, or lamella.

The rounded expanded end of a long bone is called the *epiphysis* which contains <u>spongy bone</u>. The epiphysis is covered by fibrous tissue (*the periosteum*) and it forms a joint with another bone. Spongy bone contains bony plates called *trabeculae* (= *spicules)*. The shaft of the bone which connects the expanded ends is called the *diaphysis.* It is predominately composed of <u>compact bone</u>. This kind of bone is very strong and resistant to bending and has no trabeculae or bone marrow cavities.

Animals that fly have less dense, more light bones (spongy bone) in order to facilitate flying. Animals that swim do not need to have as strong bones as land animals as the buoyant force of the water takes away from the everyday stress on the bones. In the adult, yellow marrow is likely to be found in the diaphysis while red marrow is likely to be found in the epiphysis.

Bone growth occurs in two ways, intramembranous and endochondral bone formation. Both formations produce bones that are histologically identical. Intramembranous bone formation begins as layers of membranous connective tissue, which are later calcified by osteoblasts. Most of the flat bones are formed by this process. Endochondral bone formation is the process by which most of long bones are formed. It begins with hyaline cartilage that functions as a template for the bone to grow on.

Vascularisaton of the cartilage causes the transformation of cartilage cells to bone cells (osteoblasts), which later form a cartilage-calcified bone matrix. The osteoblasts continue to replace cartilage with bone and the osteoclasts create perforations to form bone marrow cavities. In children one can detect an **epiphyseal growth plate** on X-ray. This plate is a disk of cartilage between the epiphysis and diaphysis where bone is being actively deposited (= *ossification*).

11.3.2 Joint Structure

Medium-level Importance

Articulations or joints are junctions between bones. They can be **immovable** like the dense connective tissue sutures which hold the flat bones of the skull together; **partly movable** like the hyaline and fibrocartilage joints on disks of the vertebrae; or **freely movable** like the synovial joints which are the most prominent joints in the skeletal system. Synovial joints contain a joint capsule composed of outer ligaments and an inner layer (= *the synovial membrane*) which secretes a lubricant (= *synovial fluid*).

Freely movable joints can be of many types. For example, ball and socket joints have a wide range of motion, like the shoulder and hip joints. On the other hand, hinge joints allow motion in only one plane like a hinged door (i.e. the knee, elbow, and interphalangeal joints).

11.3.3 Cartilage

The microscopic aspects of cartilage have already been discussed (*see Dense Connective Tissue*, BIO 5.4.2/3). Opposing and mobile surfaces of bone are covered by various forms of cartilage. As already mentioned, joints with hyaline or fibrocartilage allow little movement.

Ligaments attach bone to bone. They are formed by dense bands of fibrous connective tissue which reinforce the joint capsule and help to maintain bones in the proper anatomical arrangement.

Tendons connect muscle to bone. They are formed by the densest kind of fibrous connective tissue. Tendons allow muscular forces to be exerted even when the body (*or belly*) of the muscle is at some distance from the action.

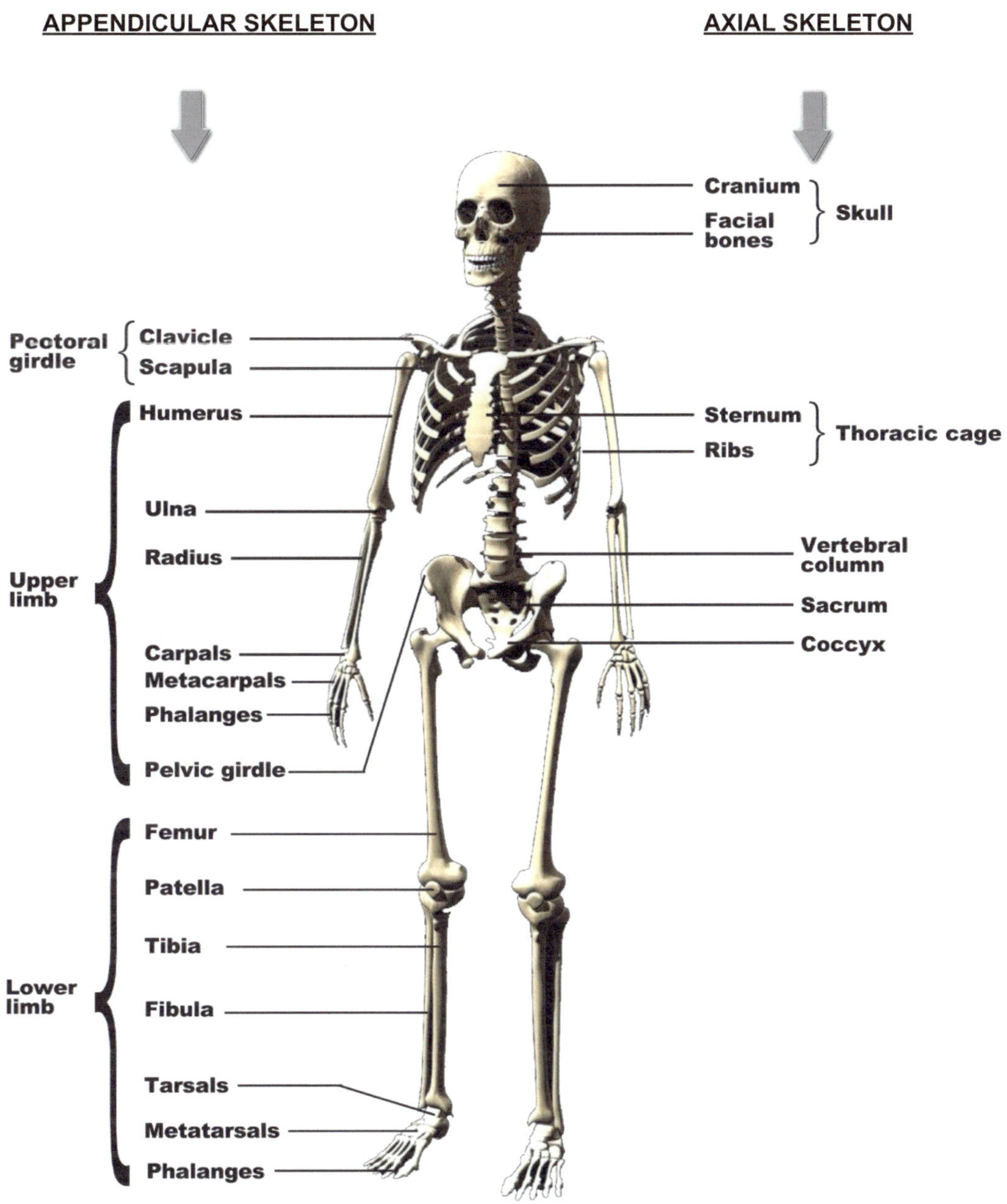

Figure IV.A.11.2: Skeletal structure. Note: in brackets some common relations - scapula (shoulder blade), clavicle (collarbone), carpals (wrist), metacarpals (palm), phalanges (fingers), tibia (shin), patella (kneecap), tarsals (ankle), metatarsals (foot), phalanges (toes), vertebral column (backbone). Note that the appendicular skeleton includes the bones of the appendages, the pectoral girdle, and the pelvic girdle. The axial skeleton consists of the skull, vertebral column, and the rib cage.

CHAPTER 11: The Musculoskeletal System

High-level Importance

GOLD STANDARD FOUNDATIONAL GAMSAT PRACTICE QUESTIONS

1) As red muscle fibers go from a resting state to a rapidly contracting state, which of the following occurs?

A. Increased rate of consumption of oxygen
B. Decreased rate of production of carbon dioxide
C. Decreased rate of hydrolysis of ATP
D. Decreased rate of degradation of glucose

2) Suppose that the oxygen supply to continuously contracting red muscles fibers is abruptly cut off. Which of the following processes would occur in the muscles?

A. Increased rate of synthesis of muscle glycogen
B. Increased rate of production of ATP
C. Increased rate of production of carbon dioxide
D. Increased rate of production of lactic acid

3) Which of the following metabolic processes predominates in rapidly contracting white muscle fibers?

A. Oxidative phosphorylation
B. Alcoholic fermentation
C. Glycolysis
D. Krebs Citric Acid Cycle reaction

GOLD STANDARD GAMSAT-LEVEL PRACTICE QUESTIONS

4) Consider the following diagram that demonstrates the growth of the canine femur (leg bone).

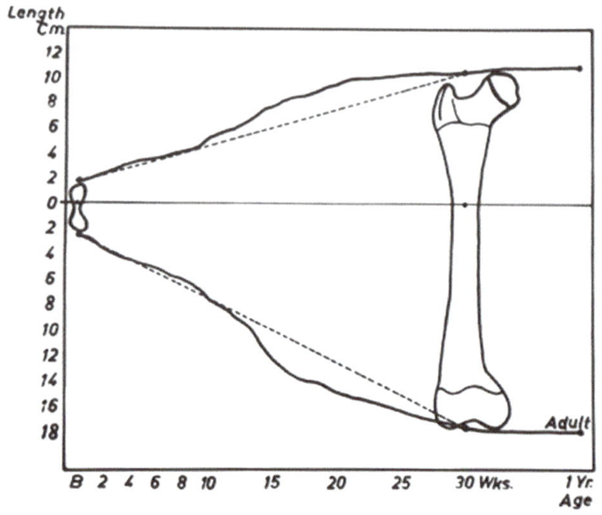

Figure 1: Chart drawn from radiographic overlay tracings of the canine femur at intervals from birth to one year of age. The 0 point on the vertical axis is the level of the nutrient foramen (opening for blood vessels). Riser WH: Growth and development of the normal canine pelvis. JAVRS 14:24, 1973.

Using Figure 1, determine the rate of growth of the femur from birth until 6 months of age.

A. 1.3×10^{-6} m/s
B. 1.3×10^{-8} m/s
C. 1.3×10^{-10} m/s
D. 1.3×10^{-12} m/s

5) The patella (i.e. kneecap) is a thick, mostly circular bone which articulates with the femur (thigh bone) and covers and protects the front (anterior) part of the knee joint. Approximate the rate of growth of the anterior surface area of the human patella from birth to age 20 years old.

A. 1.1×10^{-4} cm^2 per hour
B. 1.1×10^{-4} nm^2 per hour
C. 1.1×10^{-2} cm^2 per second
D. 1.1×10^{-2} nm^2 per second

Note that there are fewer questions as compared to other chapters because of overlap: ideas related to muscle and bone have been tested intermittently from chapters 5 to 10.

SPOILER ALERT

Gold Standard has cross-referenced the content in this chapter to examples from ACER's official GAMSAT practice materials. It is for you to decide when you want to explore these questions since you may want to preserve some of ACER's materials for timed mock-exam practice.

Examples – Muscle extensors and flexors in a flow chart: Q87-91 of 3; using dimensional analysis to determine the rate of growth of a body part in m/s: Q105 of 5. Note that "Q" is followed by the question number, and, for example, "of 1" refers to booklet number 1 which is referenced in the Spoiler Alert table at the end of Chapter 1. The 15 full-length GAMSAT practice tests by Gold Standard, HEAPS-1 through HEAPS-15, contain specific cross-references to this chapter within the worked solutions. Note that the patella calculation in this chapter comes from HEAPS-6.

Chapter Checklist

- ☐ Access your online account to view answers, worked solutions and discussion boards.
- ☐ Reassess your 'learning objectives' for this chapter: Go back to the first page of this chapter and re-evaluate the top 3 boxes and the Introduction.
- ☐ Complete a maximum of 1 page of notes using symbols/abbreviations to represent the entire chapter based on your learning objectives. These are your Gold Notes.
- ☐ Consider your multimedia options based on your optimal way of learning:
    - ☐ Download the free Gold Standard GAMSAT app for your Android device or iPhone.
    - ☐ Create your own, tangible study cards or try the free app: Anki.
    - ☐ Record your voice reading your Gold Notes onto your smartphone (audio files, e.g., *memo* or MP3s) and listen during exercise, transportation, etc.
    - ☐ Try out the Gold Standard GAMSAT online videos at gamsat-prep.com, or you can try other options on YouTube like Khan Academy or Crash Course Biology.
- ☐ Reassess your schedule for your full-length GAMSAT practice tests: ACER and/or HEAPS exams. Ensure that you have scheduled one full day to complete a practice test and 1-2 days for a thorough assessment of worked solutions while adding to your abbreviated Gold Notes.
- ☐ Reassess your progress in scheduling and/or evaluating stress reduction techniques such as regular exercise (sports), yoga, meditation and/or mindfulness exercises (*see* YouTube for suggestions).

THE RESPIRATORY SYSTEM
Chapter 12

Memorise

* Basic structures and function

Understand

* Basic functions: thermoregulation, gas exchange, etc.
* Protection against disease, particulate matter
* Breathing mechanisms: diaphragm, rib cage, differential pressure; Henry's Law
* Resiliency and surface tension effects
* The carbonic acid-bicarbonate buffer

Importance

Medium level: 8% of GAMSAT Biology questions released by ACER are related to content in this chapter (in our estimation).
* Note that approximately 75% of the questions in GAMSAT Biology are related to just 7 chapters: 1, 2, 3, 4, 7, 12, and 15.

Introduction

The respiratory system permits the exchange of gases with the organism's environment. This critical process occurs in the microscopic space between alveoli and capillaries. It is here where molecules of oxygen and carbon dioxide passively diffuse between the gaseous external environment and the blood. As you have done before, get familiar with the basics and then the practice questions will have you exercising your reasoning and graph-analysis skills which you can apply to many other GAMSAT-question types and topics.

Multimedia Resources at GAMSAT-Prep.com

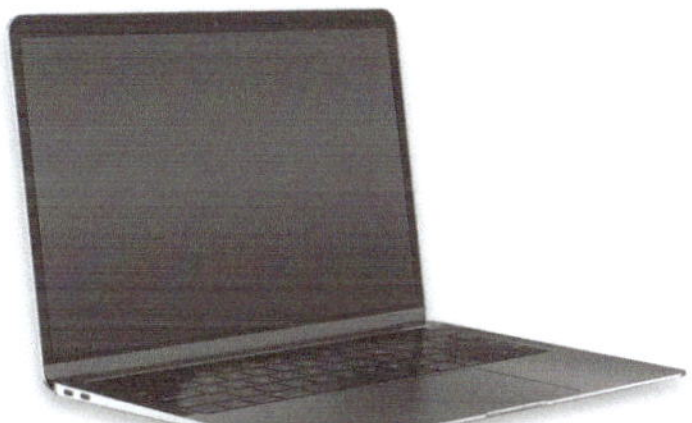

Open Discussion Boards
(*gamsat-prep.com/forum*)

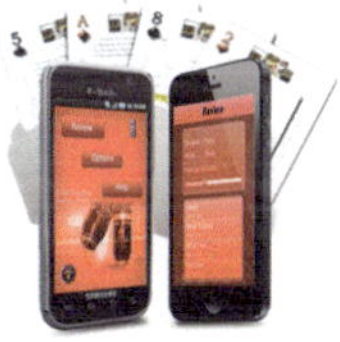

Flashcards

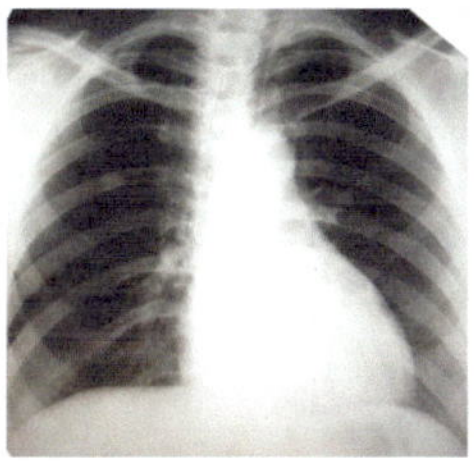

Special Guest

* The real GAMSAT may have advanced-level information presented (i.e. in a passage) but previous knowledge of said information is not required to answer the questions that would follow. Practice questions at the end of this chapter, as well as ACER and GS (HEAPS) practice GAMSATs can help you clarify this point.

12.1 Overview

There are two forms of respiration: cellular respiration which refers to the oxidation of organic molecules (*see* BIO 4.4 - 4.10) and mechanical respiration where the gases related to cellular respiration are exchanged between the atmosphere and the circulatory system (O_2 in and CO_2 out).

The respiratory system, which is concerned with mechanical respiration, has the following principal functions:

- providing a conducting system for the exchange of gases
- the filtration of incoming particles
- to help control the water content and temperature (= *thermoregulation*) of the incoming air
- to assist in speech production, the sense of smell, and the regulation of pH.

The respiratory system is composed of the lungs and a series of airways that connect the lungs to the external environment, deliver air to the lungs and perform gas exchange.

Medium-level Importance

12.2 The Upper Respiratory Tract

The respiratory system can be divided into an *upper* and *lower respiratory tract* which are separated by the pharynx. The **upper respiratory tract** is composed of the nose, the nasal cavity, the sinuses, and the nasopharynx. This portion of the respiratory system warms, moistens and filters the air before it reaches the lower respiratory system. The nose (*nares*) has receptors for the sense of smell. It is guarded by hair to entrap coarse particles. The nasal cavity, the hollow space behind the nose, contains a ciliated mucous membrane (= a form of *respiratory epithelium*) to entrap smaller particles and prevent infection (this arrangement is common throughout the respiratory tract; for cilia *see the Generalised Eukaryotic Cell*, BIO 1.2). The nasal cavity adjusts the humidity and temperature of incoming air. The nasopharynx helps to equilibrate pressure between the environment and the middle ear via the eustachian tube (BIO 6.2.3).

12.3 The Lower Respiratory Tract

The **lower respiratory tract** is composed of the larynx which contains the vocal cords, the trachea which divides into left and right main bronchi which continue to divide into smaller airways (→ 2° bronchi → 3° bronchi → bronchioles → terminal bronchioles). The terminal bronchioles are the most distal part of the conducting portion of the respira-

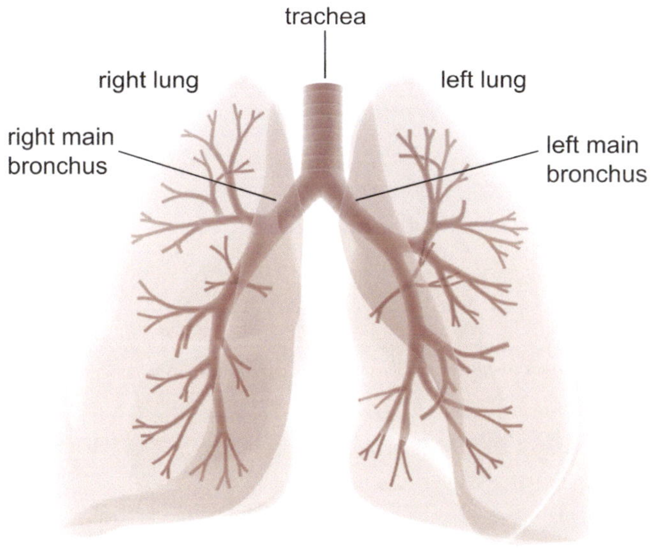

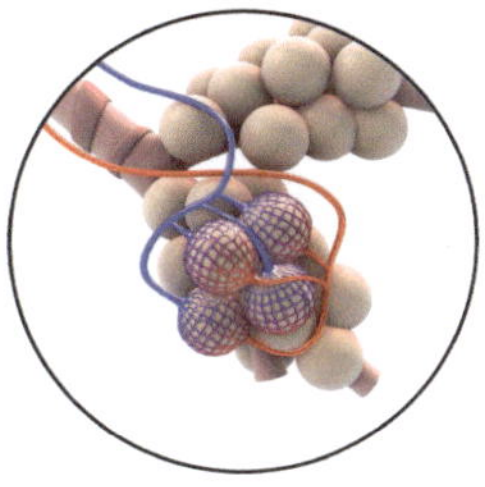

Figure IV.A.12.1: Illustration representing the lower respiratory tract including the dividing bronchial tree and grape-shaped alveoli with blood supply. Note that "right" refers to the patient's perspective which means the left side from your perspective.

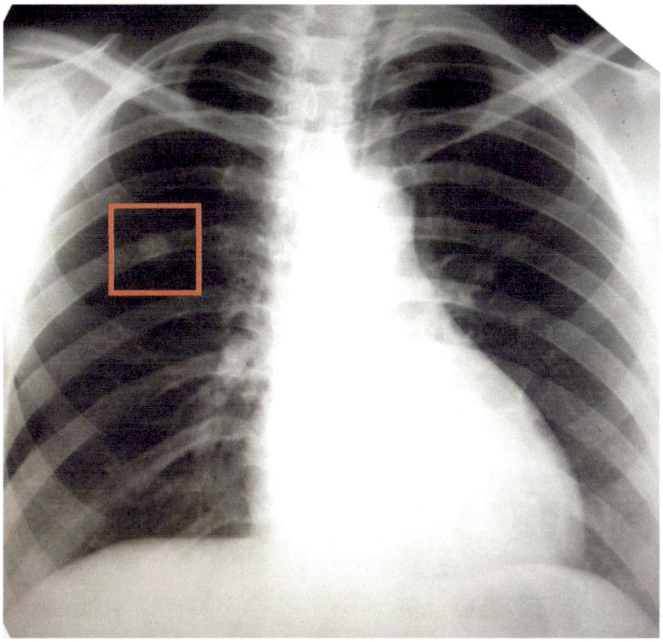

Figure IV.A.12.2: Chest x-ray of an adult male smoker. Notice the coin-shaped shadow in the right lung which presented with coughing blood. Further tests confirmed the presence of a right lung cancer. Cancer-causing chemicals (carcinogens) can irritate any of the cells lining the lower respiratory tract.

tory system. Starting from respiratory bronchioles → alveolar ducts → alveolar sacs until the level of <u>the alveolus</u>, these are considered the respiratory portion of respiratory system, where gas exchange takes place.

It is in these microscopic air sacs called *alveoli* that O_2 diffuses through the alveolar walls and enters the blood in nearby capillaries (where the concentration or *partial pressure* of O_2 - pO_2 - is lowest and pCO_2 is highest), and CO_2 diffuses from the blood through the walls to enter the alveoli (where pCO_2 is lowest and pO_2 is highest). Gas exchange occurs by diffusion (BIO 1.1.1) across the blood-gas barrier between the alveolar airspace and the capillary lumen. The blood-gas barrier is composed of three layers: type I pneumocyte cells, fused basal laminae and the endothelium of capillaries. *Alveolar macrophages* are phagocytes which help to engulf particles which reach the alveolus. A *surfactant* is secreted into alveoli by special lung cells (*pneumocytes type II*). The surfactant reduces surface tension and prevents the fragile alveoli from collapsing.

Sneezing and coughing, which are reflexes mediated by the medulla, can expel particles from the upper and lower respiratory tract, respectively.

The **lungs** are separated into left and right and are enclosed by the diaphragm and the thoracic cage. It is covered by a membrane (= *pleura*) which secretes a lubricant to reduce friction while breathing. The lungs contain the air passages, nerves, alveoli, blood and lymphatic vessels of the lower respiratory tract.

12.4 Breathing: Structures and Mechanisms

Inspiration is active and occurs according to the following main events: **i)** nerve impulses from the phrenic nerve cause the muscular diaphragm to contract; as the dome shaped diaphragm moves downward, the thoracic cavity increases; **ii)** simultaneously, the intercostal (= *between ribs*) muscles and/or certain neck muscles may contract further increasing the thoracic cavity (the muscles mentioned here are called *accessory respiratory muscles* and under normal circumstances the action of the diaphragm is much more important); **iii)** as the size of the thoracic cavity increases, its internal pressure decreases leaving it relatively negative; **iv)** the relatively positive atmospheric pressure forces air into the respiratory tract thus inflating the lungs.

Expiration is passive and occurs according to the following main events: **i)** the diaphragm and the accessory respiratory muscles relax and the chest wall pushed inward; **ii)** the elastic tissues of the lung, thoracic cage, and the abdominal organs recoil to their original position; **iii)** this recoil increases the pressure within the lungs (making the pressure relatively positive) thus forcing air out of the lungs and passageways.

Medium-level Importance

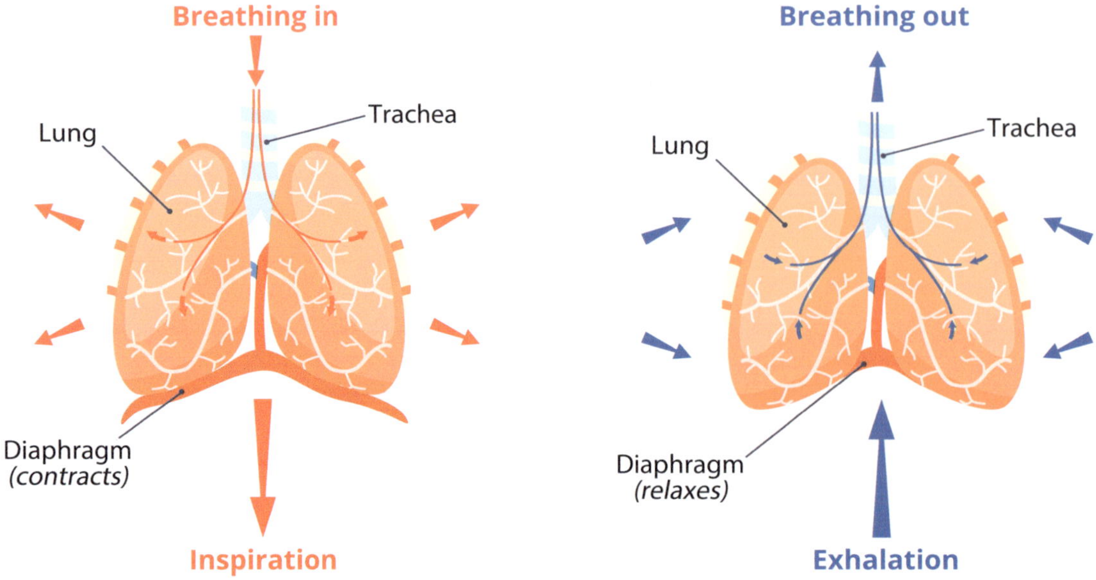

Figure IV.A.12.3: Breathing.

12.4.1 Control of Breathing

Though voluntary breathing is possible (!), normally breathing is involuntary, rhythmic, and controlled by the *respiratory centre* in the medulla of the brain stem. The respiratory centre is sensitive to pH of the cerebrospinal fluid (CSF). An increase in blood CO_2 or consequently, decrease in pH of the CSF, acts on the respiratory centre and stimulates breathing, returning the arterial pCO_2 (partial pressure of carbon dioxide) back to normal. The increase in blood CO_2 and the decrease in pH are two interrelated events since CO_2 can be picked up by hemoglobin forming carbaminohemoglobin (about 20%, BIO 7.5.1), but it can also be converted into carbonic acid by dissolving in blood plasma (about 5%) or by conversion in red blood cells by the enzyme *carbonic anhydrase* (about 75%). The reaction is summarised as follows:

$$CO_2 + H_2O \leftrightarrow \underset{\text{carbonic acid}}{H_2CO_3} \leftrightarrow \underset{\text{bicarbonate}}{HCO_3^-} + H^+$$

According to Henry's Law, the concentration of a gas dissolved in solution is directly proportional to its partial pressure. From the preceding you can see why the respiratory system, through the regulation of the partial pressure of CO_2 in blood, also helps in maintaining pH homeostasis (= a buffer). More generally, the carbonic acid-bicarbonate buffer is the most important buffer for maintaining acid-base balance in the blood and helps to maintain pH around 7.4.

12.4.2 Henry's Law, Pop and The Bends

Higher gas pressure and lower temperature cause more gas to dissolve in a liquid. When a carbonated drink (soda/pop) is manufactured, water is chilled, optimally to just above freezing, in order to permit the maximum amount of carbon dioxide to dissolve. Then CO_2 is pumped in at high pressure, the pressure is maintained by closing the container (can or bottle), which forces the carbon dioxide to dissolve into the liquid, creating carbonic acid (Le Chatelier's principle; CHM 9.9) and giving 'pop' its tang. Flat soda tastes strange, or at least less pleasant, because of the loss of carbonic acid due to the release of carbon dioxide bubbles/fizz.

So pop is stored in a way to seal pressure, preventing gas escape and maintaining the supersaturation of CO_2 in the solvent. It is pressure and temperature that drive the outgassing process.

Diving underwater exposes the body to increasing pressure (PHY 6.1). A diving cylinder (scuba tank) is used to store and trans-

Medium-level Importance

port high pressure breathing gas. As the dive becomes deeper, inhaled gas is absorbed into body tissue in higher concentrations than normal (Henry's Law). Surfacing from a deep dive underwater, unused gases (inert) like nitrogen try to do the same thing in your bloodstream that happens when you open a container of pop. The release of these bubbles (outgassing) produces the symptoms of decompression sickness (= 'the bends') that can be painful or even fatal. {We have placed GAMSAT-level practice questions based on Henry's Law in General Chemistry Chapter 4.}

CHAPTER 12: The Respiratory System

GOLD STANDARD FOUNDATIONAL GAMSAT PRACTICE QUESTIONS

1) Which of the following does NOT occur during inspiration?

A. Increased pressure within the chest cavity
B. Contraction of the rib cage muscles
C. Downward displacement of the diaphragm
D. Increased diameter of the chest

2) Active transport assumes particular importance in all but which of the following structures?

A. Cells of the large intestine
B. Alveoli
C. Nerve and muscle cells
D. Loop of Henle

GOLD STANDARD GAMSAT-LEVEL PRACTICE QUESTIONS

3) Figure 1 demonstrates the basic aspects of lung function. Note that the bell jar is sealed except for the inlet/outlet of the rubber tube. The 'thoracic' space represents the area between the balloon and the bell jar/diaphragm.

Of the following events, which one occurs first in the sequence preceding the inflation of the balloon?

A. The volume of air inside the balloon increases.
B. The volume of 'thoracic' air increases.
C. Pressure decreases in the 'thoracic' space.
D. Pressure decreases inside of the balloon.

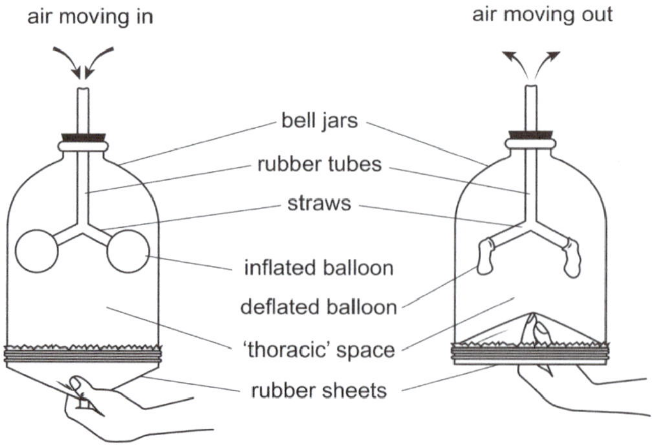

Figure 1

Questions 4–6

Consider the pneumotachogram in Figure 1.

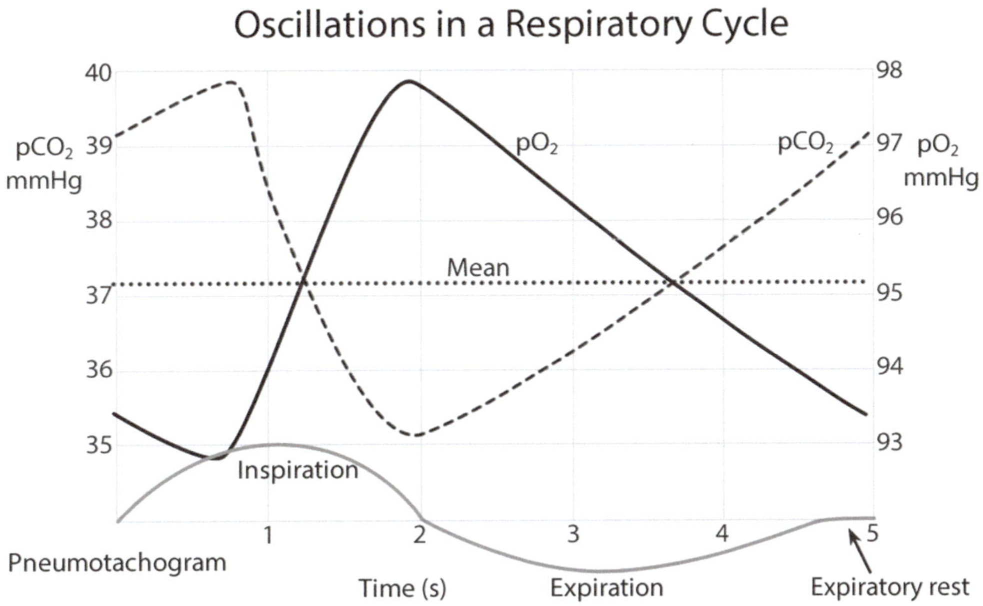

Figure 1: Pneumotachogram showing the rate of airflow during tidal breathing as well as changes in the partial pressures of oxygen (pO_2, solid line) and carbon dioxide (pCO_2, dashed line) in the alveoli during a complete respiratory cycle.

4) According to Figure 1, which of the following best approximates the minimum difference in the oxygen and carbon dioxide partial pressures during a respiratory cycle?

A. 0 mmHg
B. Between 50 and 55 mmHg
C. Between 55 and 60 mmHg
D. More than 60 mmHg

5) Which of the following statements is consistent with Figure 1?

A. The oxygen and carbon dioxide partial pressures are equal at approximately 3.7 seconds in the respiratory cycle.
B. Carbon dioxide partial pressure exceeds oxygen partial pressure during 2 phases of the respiratory cycle.
C. Carbon dioxide partial pressure rises throughout the period of expiration.
D. The mean oxygen and carbon dioxide partial pressures are the same.

6) The tidal volume is the amount of air inspired (or expired) during normal tidal breathing. In a healthy adult, tidal volume is approximately 7 mL/kg of body mass. Minute ventilation is the total volume of air entering the lungs in a minute. Using the information in Figure 1, and considering a 60-kg healthy female, which of the following best approximates her minute ventilation?

A. 4 L
B. 5 L
C. 6 L
D. 7 L

Questions 7–11

The volume of air that flows into or out of an alveolus per unit time is directly proportional to the pressure difference between the atmosphere and alveolus and inversely proportional to the resistance to flow caused by the airways. During normal relaxed breathing, about 500 mL of air flows in and out of the lungs. This is the tidal volume. After expiration, approximately 2.5 litres of air remains in the lungs which is referred to as the functional residual capacity. A spirometer is an instrument for measuring air inhaled and exhaled; it provides a simple way of determining most of the lung volumes and capacities that are measured in pulmonary function tests. The minute ventilation can be calculated as follows:

$$\text{Minute ventilation} = \text{Tidal volume} \times \text{Respiratory rate}$$

Airway resistance is: i) directly proportional to the magnitude of the viscosity between the flowing gas molecules; ii) directly proportional to the length of the airway; and iii) inversely proportional to the fourth power of the radius of the airway.

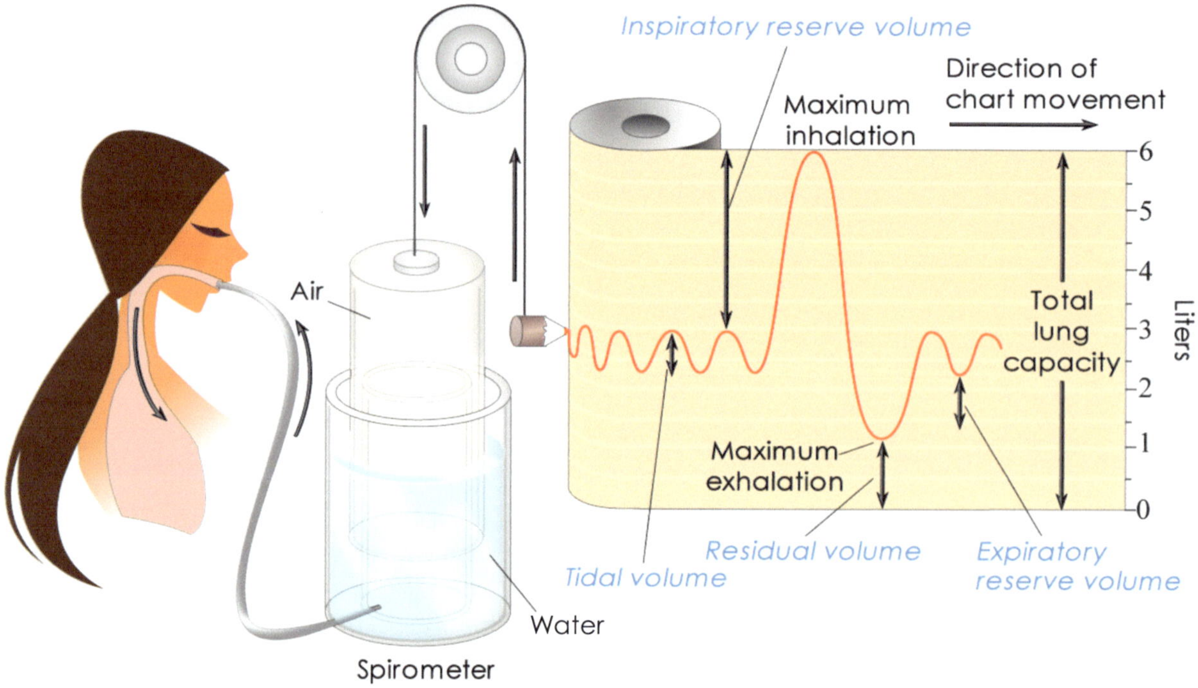

Figure 1: The four lung volumes measured by spirometer. Note that there are 4 key lung capacities: (1) the functional residual capacity which is the sum of the residual volume and the expiratory reserve volume (= ERV which is the maximum volume that can be exhaled following a normal quiet exhalation); (2) the vital capacity (VC) is the maximum volume that can be exhaled following a maximal inhalation; VC = inspiratory reserve volume (IRV) + tidal volume (VT) + ERV; (3) the inspiratory capacity (IC) is the maximum volume that can be inhaled following a normal quiet exhalation; IC = IRV + VT; (4) total lung capacity is the amount of air in the lung after maximal inhalation.

Resistance to air flow in the lung is normally small thus small pressure differences allow large volumes of air to flow. Physical, neural and chemical factors affect airway radii and therefore resistance. Transpulmonary pressure is a physical factor which exerts a distending force on the airways and alveoli. Such a force is critical to prevent small airways from collapsing.

The rate of respiration is primarily dependent on the concentration of carbon dioxide in the blood. As carbon dioxide levels rise, chemoreceptors in blood vessels are stimulated to discharge neuronal impulses to the respiratory centre in the medulla oblongata in the brain stem. The respiratory centre would then send impulses to the diaphragm causing an increase in the rate of contraction thus increasing the respiratory rate.

7) Given a resting respiratory rate of 12 breaths per minute, give an approximation of the minute ventilation.

A. 2.5 L/min
B. 5.0 L/min
C. 6.0 L/min
D. 30 L/min

8) Which of the following is consistent with the total lung capacity?

A. The amount of air inhaled and exhaled normally at rest
B. The sum of the residual volume and the expiratory reserve volume
C. The maximum volume that can be exhaled following a maximal inhalation
D. The maximum volume of air present in the lungs

9) During inspiration, transpulmonary pressure should:

A. increase, increasing airway radius and decreasing airway resistance.
B. increase, increasing airway radius and increasing airway resistance.
C. decrease, decreasing airway radius and decreasing airway resistance.
D. decrease, decreasing airway radius and increasing airway resistance.

10) Lateral traction refers to the process by which connective tissue fibers maintain airway patency by continuously pulling outward on the sides of the airways. As the lungs expand these fibers become stretched. Thus during inspiration lateral traction acts:

A. in the same direction as transpulmonary pressure, by increasing the viscosity of air.
B. in the opposite direction to transpulmonary pressure, by decreasing the viscosity of air.
C. in the same direction as transpulmonary pressure, by increasing the airway radius.
D. in the opposite direction to transpulmonary pressure, by increasing the airway radius.

11) The Heimlich Maneuver is used to aid individuals who are choking on matter caught in the upper respiratory tract through the application of a sudden abdominal pressure with an upward thrust. The procedure includes:

A. forcing the diaphragm downward, increasing thoracic size and causing a passive expiration.
B. forcing the diaphragm upward, increasing thoracic size and causing a forced expiration.
C. forcing the diaphragm upward, reducing thoracic size and causing a forced expiration.
D. forcing the diaphragm upward, increasing thoracic size and causing a passive expiration.

Questions 12–15

At 29 029 feet, Mount Everest is the world's highest mountain and one of the most dangerous. As of 2020, about 6.5% of the roughly 4000 climbers who have attempted a summit died, most in an area called the Death Zone where the percentage of oxygen in the air is too low and tissues receive an insufficient amount of oxygen. Figure 1 shows the percentage of hemoglobin in the blood that is saturated with oxygen to form oxyhemoglobin as a function of the partial pressure of oxygen in the air. A saturation percentage below 90 is considered low.

As the oxygen partial pressure decreases, climbers become susceptible to hypoxia, a condition that occurs when the body is deprived of an adequate supply of oxygen. Hypoxia can lead to fatigue, nausea and potentially unconsciousness. Past a certain point there is not enough oxygen to sustain the body. Figure 2 shows the relationship between the total pressure for different altitudes and the volume percentage of oxygen.

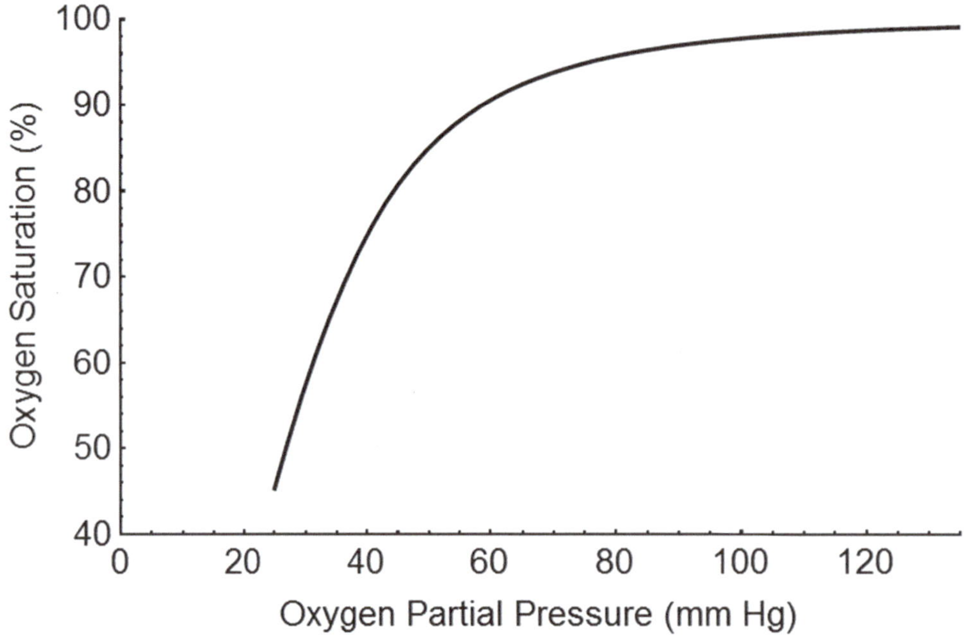

Figure 1: Percentage of oxygen saturation in hemoglobin versus the oxygen partial pressure.
(adapted from Julie-Ann Collins, Aram Rudenski, John Gibson, Luke Howard and Ronan O'Driscoll, Breathe, 2015)

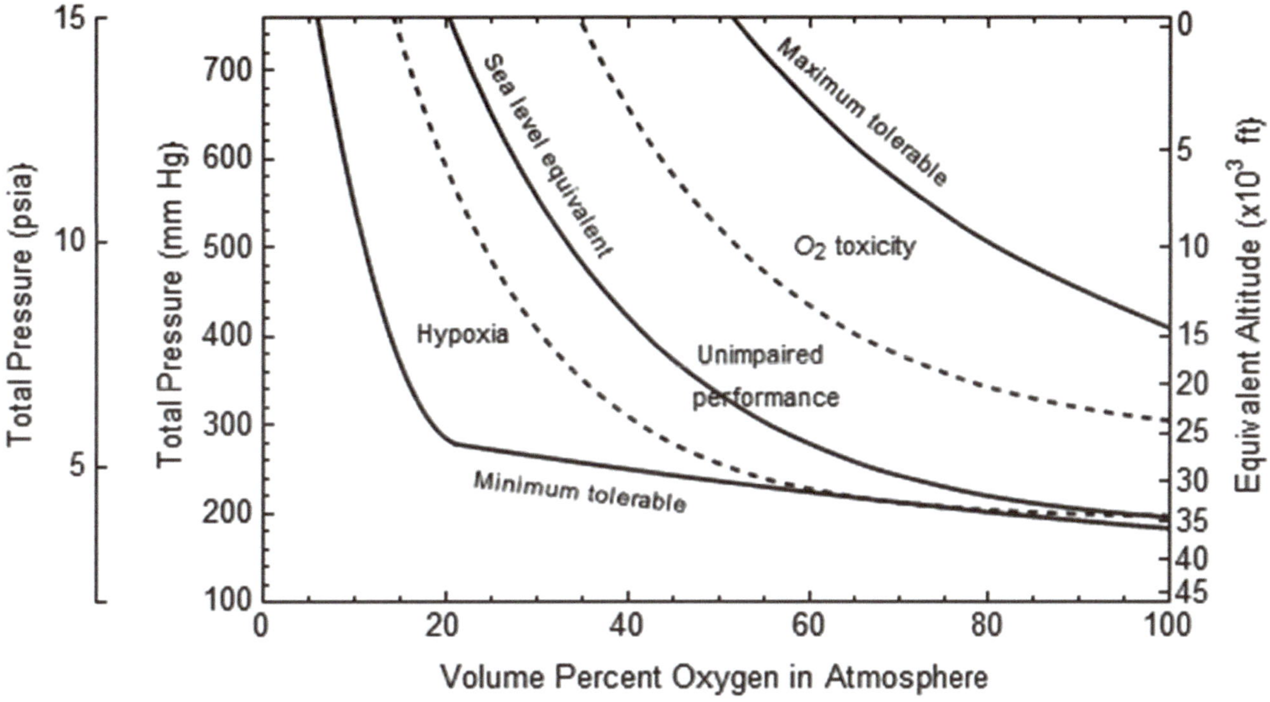

Figure 2: Pressure and oxygen percentage as a function of altitude above sea level.
(adapted from Man-System Integration Standards Volume 1, National Aeronautics and Space Administration, 1995)

12) Climbers have a higher chance of surviving the Death Zone if they take supplemental oxygen delivered through a face mask. How does the supplemental oxygen affect the body?

A. Increases activity under normal conditions
B. Increases percent oxygen saturation
C. Decreases oxygen partial pressure
D. Decreases chance of oxygen toxicity

13) Based on Figure 2, at sea level, which of the following is the best approximation of the optimal oxygen partial pressure?

A. 1-3 psia
B. 2-6 psia
C. 6-8 psia
D. 8-10 psia

14) Based on Figure 1 and Figure 2, at 5 psia of total pressure, what is the best approximation of the minimum percentage of oxygen-saturated hemoglobin a climber needs?

A. 20%
B. 45%
C. 60%
D. More than 80%

15) At 20 000 feet above sea level, approximate the volume percent oxygen at which hypoxia begins.

A. 15%
B. 35%
C. 45%
D. 60%

High-level Importance

SPOILER ALERT

Gold Standard has cross-referenced the content in this chapter to examples from ACER's official GAMSAT practice materials. It is for you to decide when you want to explore these questions since you may want to preserve some of ACER's materials for timed mock-exam practice.

Examples – Two bell-jar model questions but ACER moved the location: Depending on the edition that you have, it is either Q24-25 of 1, or Q16-17 of 3. As an example of examiners' convergent evolution, the questions offer some similarity to ours. Note that "Q" is followed by the question number, and, for example, "of 1" refers to booklet number 1 which is referenced in the Spoiler Alert table at the end of Chapter 1. The 15 full-length GAMSAT practice tests by Gold Standard, HEAPS-1 through HEAPS-15, contain specific cross-references to this chapter within the worked solutions. Note that the double y-axis pneumotachogram unit in GAMSAT-level practice questions in this chapter comes from HEAPS-7.

Chapter Checklist

- ☐ Access your online account to view answers, worked solutions and discussion boards.
- ☐ Reassess your 'learning objectives' for this chapter: Go back to the first page of this chapter and re-evaluate the top 3 boxes and the Introduction.
- ☐ Complete a maximum of 1 page of notes using symbols/abbreviations to represent the entire chapter based on your learning objectives. These are your Gold Notes.
- ☐ Consider your multimedia options based on your optimal way of learning:
  - ☐ Download the free Gold Standard GAMSAT app for your Android device or iPhone.
  - ☐ Create your own, tangible study cards or try the free app: Anki.
  - ☐ Record your voice reading your Gold Notes onto your smartphone (audio files, e.g., *memo* or MP3s) and listen during exercise, transportation, etc.
  - ☐ Try out the Gold Standard GAMSAT online videos at gamsat-prep.com, or you can try other options on YouTube like Khan Academy or Crash Course Biology.
- ☐ Reassess your schedule for your full-length GAMSAT practice tests: ACER and/or HEAPS exams. Ensure that you have scheduled one full day to complete a practice test and 1-2 days for a thorough assessment of worked solutions while adding to your abbreviated Gold Notes.
- ☐ Reassess your progress in scheduling and/or evaluating stress reduction techniques such as regular exercise (sports), yoga, meditation and/or mindfulness exercises (*see* YouTube for suggestions).

THE SKIN AS AN ORGAN SYSTEM
Chapter 13

Memorise	Understand	Importance
* Nothing	* Skin system: homeostasis and osmoregulation * Functions in thermoregulation: hair, erectile musculature, fat layer for insulation * Vasoconstriction and vasodilation in surface capillaries * Physical protection: nails, calluses, hair; protection against abrasion, disease organisms * Relative impermeability to water	**Low level: 0% of GAMSAT Biology** questions released by ACER are related to content in this chapter (in our estimation). * Note that approximately 75% of the questions in GAMSAT Biology are related to just 7 chapters: 1, 2, 3, 4, 7, 12, and 15.

GAMSAT-Prep.com

Introduction

Skin is composed of layers of epithelial tissues which protect underlying muscle, bone, ligaments and internal organs. Thus skin has many roles including protecting the body from microbes, insulation, temperature regulation, sensation and synthesis of vitamin D.

The topic of this chapter is a conventional introductory-level subject and thus within the scope of possible - though very unlikely - GAMSAT-assumed knowledge in a future exam. Despite the 'low level of importance', the GAMSAT-level practice questions at the end of this chapter include dimensional analysis and graph analysis which both apply to many other question types.

Multimedia Resources at GAMSAT-Prep.com

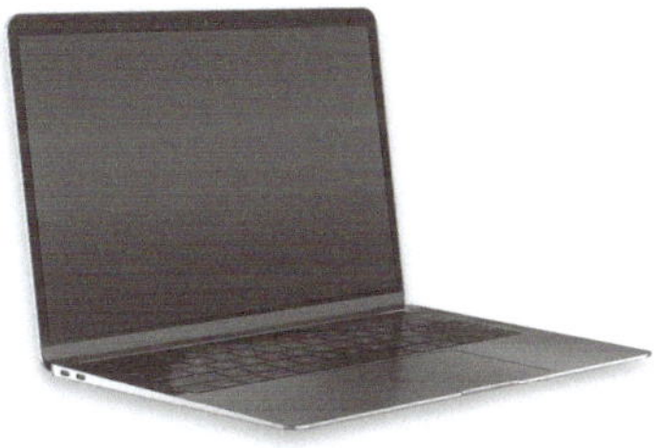

Open Discussion Boards
(*gamsat-prep.com/forum*)

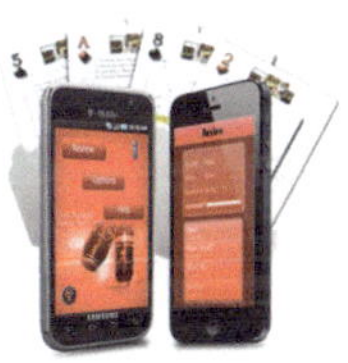

Flashcards

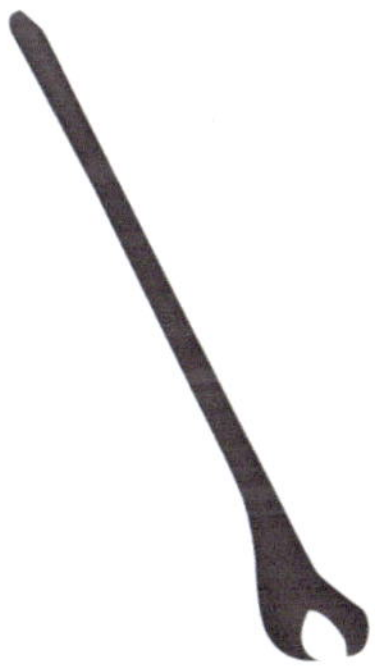

Special Guest

* The real GAMSAT may have advanced-level information presented (i.e. in a passage) but previous knowledge of said information is not required to answer the questions that would follow. Practice questions at the end of this chapter, as well as ACER and GS (HEAPS) practice GAMSATs can help you clarify this point.

13.1 Overview

The skin, or *integument*, is the body's largest organ. The following represents its major functions:

* **Physical protection:** The skin protects against the onslaught of the environment including UV light, chemical, thermal or even mechanical agents. It also serves as a barrier to the invasion of microorganisms.

* **Sensation:** The skin, being the body's largest sensory organ, contains a wide range of sensory receptors including those for pain, temperature, light touch, and pressure.

* **Metabolism:** Vitamin D synthesis can occur in the epidermis of skin (*see Endocrine Systems*, BIO 6.3). Also, energy is stored as fat in subcutaneous adipose tissue.

* **Thermoregulation and osmoregulation:** Skin is vital for the homeostatic mechanism of thermoregulation and to a lesser degree osmoregulation. Hair (*piloerection*, which can trap a layer of warm air against the skin's surface) and especially subcutaneous fat (*adipose tissue*) insulate the body against heat loss. Shivering, which allows muscle to generate heat, and decreasing blood flow to the skin (= *vasoconstriction*) are important in emergencies.

On the other hand, heat and water loss can be increased by increasing blood flow to the multitude of blood vessels (= *vasodilation*) in the dermis (cooling by radiation), the production of sweat (which forms spheres to minimise surface tension; PHY 6.1.5), and the evaporation of sweat due to the heat at the surface of the skin; thus the skin cools. {Remember: the **hypothalamus** also regulates body temperature (*see The Nervous System*, BIO 6.1); it is like a thermostat which uses other organs as tools to maintain our body temperatures at about 37 °C (98.6 °F)}.

13.2 The Structure of Skin

Low-level Importance

Skin is divided into three layers: **i)** the outer **epidermis** which contains a stratified squamous keratinised epithelium; **ii)** the inner **dermis** which contains vessels, nerves, muscle, and connective tissues; **iii)** the innermost **subcutaneous layer**, known as hypodermis, which contains adipose and a loose connective tissue; this layer binds to any underlying organs.

The epidermis is divided into several different layers or *strata*. The deepest layer, *stratum basale*, contains actively dividing cells (keratinocytes) which are nourished by the vessels in the dermis. The mitotic activity of keratinocytes can keep regenerating epidermis approximately every 30 days. As these cells continue to divide, older epidermal cells are pushed towards the surface of the skin - *away from the nutrient providing dermal layer*; thus in time they die. Simultaneously, these cells are actively producing strands of a tough, fibrous, waterproof protein called keratin. This process is called *keratinisation*. The two preceding events lead to the formation of an outermost layer (= *stratum corneum*) of keratin-filled dead cells which are devoid of organelles and are continuously shed by a process called *desquamation*.

Melanin is a dark pigment produced by cells (= *melanocytes*) whose cell bodies are usually found in the stratum basale. Melanin absorbs light thus protects against UV light induced cell damage (i.e. sunburns, skin cancer). Individuals have about the same number of melanocytes - regardless of race. Melanin production depends on genetic factors (i.e. race) and it can be stimulated by exposure to sunlight (i.e. tanning).

Langerhans cells have long processes and contain characteristic tennis-racket-shaped Birbeck granules. They function as antigen presenting cells in the immune response (BIO 8.2, 8.3).

Merkel cells are present in the richly innervated areas of stratum basale. They are responsible for receiving afferent nerve impulses and function as sensory mechanoreceptors (BIO 6.1.1).

The dermis is composed of dense irregular connective tissue including type I collagen fibers and a network of elastic fibers. It contains the blood vessels which nourish the various cells in the skin. It also contains motor fibers and many types of sensory nerve fibers such as fine touch receptors, pressure receptors and cold receptors.

13.3 Skin Appendages

The **appendages** of the skin include hair, sebaceous glands and sweat glands. Hair is a modified keratinised structure produced by a cylindrical downgrowth of epithelium *(= hair follicle)*. The follicle extends into the dermis (sometimes the subcutaneous tissue as well). The arrector pili muscle attaches to the connective tissue surrounding a hair follicle. When this bundle of smooth muscle contracts (= *piloerection*), it elevates the hair and "goose bumps" are produced.

The sebaceous glands are lobular acinar glands that empty their ducts into the hair follicles. They are most abundant on the face, forehead and scalp. They release an oily/waxy secretion called sebum to lubricate and waterproof the skin.

Sweat glands can be classified as either eccrine sweat glands, which are simple tubular glands present in the skin throughout the body or apocrine sweat glands, which are large specialised glands located only in certain areas of the body (i.e. areola of the nipple, perianal area, axilla which is the "armpit") and will not function until puberty.

We have previously explored endocrine glands and saw how they secrete their products - without the use of a duct - directly into the bloodstream (BIO 6.3). Alternatively, endo-

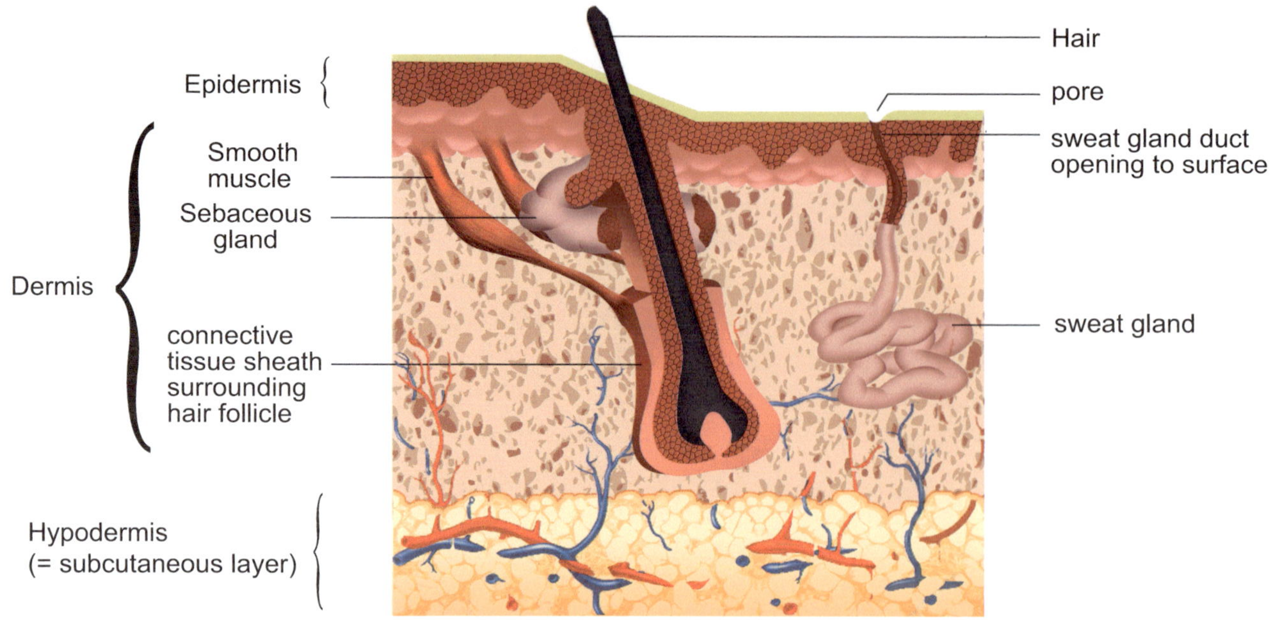

Figure IV.A.13.1: Skin structure with appendages.

crine products may diffuse into surrounding tissue (*paracrine signaling*) where they often affect only target cells near the release site.

An exocrine gland is distinguished by the fact that it excretes its product via a duct to some environment external to itself, either inside the body (BIO 9.3, 9.4) or on a surface of the body. Examples of exocrine glands include the sebaceous glands, sweat glands, salivary glands, mammary glands, pancreas and liver.

Holocrine (= *wholly secretory*) is a type of glandular secretion in which the entire secreting cell, along with its accumulated secretion, forms the secreted matter of the gland; for example, the sebaceous glands. Apocrine concentrates products at the free end of the secreting cell and are thrown off along with a portion of the cytoplasm (i.e. mammary gland, axilla). Eccrine, apocrine and holocrine are subdivisions of exocrine.

13.3.1 Nails, Calluses

Nails are flat, translucent, keratinised coverings near the tip of fingers and toes. In humans, nails grow at an average rate of 3 mm (0.12 in) per month.

A callus is a toughened, thickened area of skin. It is usually created in response to repeated friction or pressure thus they are normally found on the hands or feet.

Low-level Importance

CHAPTER 13: The Skin as an Organ System

GOLD STANDARD FOUNDATIONAL GAMSAT PRACTICE QUESTIONS

1) Which of the following best describes why perspiring causes a reduction in body temperature?

A. Perspiration causes vasoconstriction.
B. Perspiration carries heated water to the surface.
C. Perspiration removes excess Na^+ and Cl^- ions from cells.
D. Perspiration evaporates and cools skin.

2) Which of the following is the best way to reduce body temperature?

A. Constrict skeletal muscle.
B. Reduce insulin levels.
C. Increase kidney function.
D. Relax smooth muscle of blood vessels.

3) Water droplets on skin tend to resemble spheres as opposed to other shapes so as to:

A. minimise surface tension.
B. maximise the area to volume ratio.
C. minimise cohesive forces.
D. maximise adhesive forces.

4) Which of the following functions is NOT associated with the skin?

A. Detection of sensory information
B. Synthesis of C vitamins
C. Protection of underlying structures
D. Maintenance of normal body temperatures

GOLD STANDARD GAMSAT-LEVEL PRACTICE QUESTIONS

5) Estimate the average rate of growth for head hair of an average person.

A. 5×10^{-7} m/s
B. 5×10^{-9} m/s
C. 5×10^{-11} m/s
D. 5×10^{-13} m/s

Questions 6–10

Sweat is a watery fluid containing between 0.1 and 0.4% sodium chloride, sodium lactate and urea. It is less concentrated than blood plasma and is secreted by the activity of sweat glands under the control of pseudomotor neurons. These neurons are part of the sympathetic nervous system and they relay impulses from the hypothalamus.

When sweat evaporates from the skin surface, energy as latent heat of evaporation is lost from the body and this reduces body temperature. Experiments have now confirmed that sweating only occurs as a result of a rise in core body temperature. Blood from the carotid vessels flows to the hypothalamus and these experiments have indicated its role in thermoregulation. Inserting a thermistor against the eardrum gives an acceptable estimate of hypothalamic temperature.

6) The transport of electrolytes in sweat from blood plasma to the sweat glands is best accounted for by which of the following processes?

A. Osmosis
B. Diffusion
C. Active transport
D. All of the above

7) Drinking iced water results in a lowering of core body temperature. Thus, a trial exposing the skin to heat while drinking iced water would result in which of the following according to the passage?

A. If the person had been sweating prior to exposure to the trial then there would be an increase in sweating.
B. If the person had been sweating prior to exposure to the trial then there would be a decrease in sweating.
C. Irrespective of whether the person had been sweating prior to the trial, there would be an increase in sweating followed by a decrease in sweating.
D. Irrespective of whether the person had been sweating prior to the trial, there would be no change in sweat production.

Questions 8–10 refer to Figure 1.

8) During the first 20 minutes, the temperature and evaporation rate remain relatively constant because during this time:

A. evaporation was at a minimum.
B. the energy loss was not constant.
C. the subject was allowed to equilibrate with his surroundings.
D. 45 °C was considerably higher than the mean body temperature.

9) The relationship between hypothalamic temperature and rate of sweating could be best described as:

A. direct, suggesting that the rate of sweating is controlled by hypothalamic activity.
B. direct, suggesting that hypothalamic activity is controlled by the rate of sweating.
C. inverse, suggesting that changes in the rate of sweating occur in the opposite direction to changes in hypothalamic temperature.
D. independent, suggesting that the rate of sweating and hypothalamic activity change independently of each other.

10) Shortly after ingestion of the iced water, skin temperature rises. This can best be explained by which of the following?

A. As the evaporation rate falls, latent heat is no longer being lost from the skin, causing a rise in skin temperature.

B. The unusually high temperature of the chamber over the 30 minute period caused the rise in temperature.

C. The skin temperature rose to counteract the disturbance in body temperature caused by ingestion of the iced water.

D. Change in skin temperature always occurs in the opposite direction to change in hypothalamic temperature.

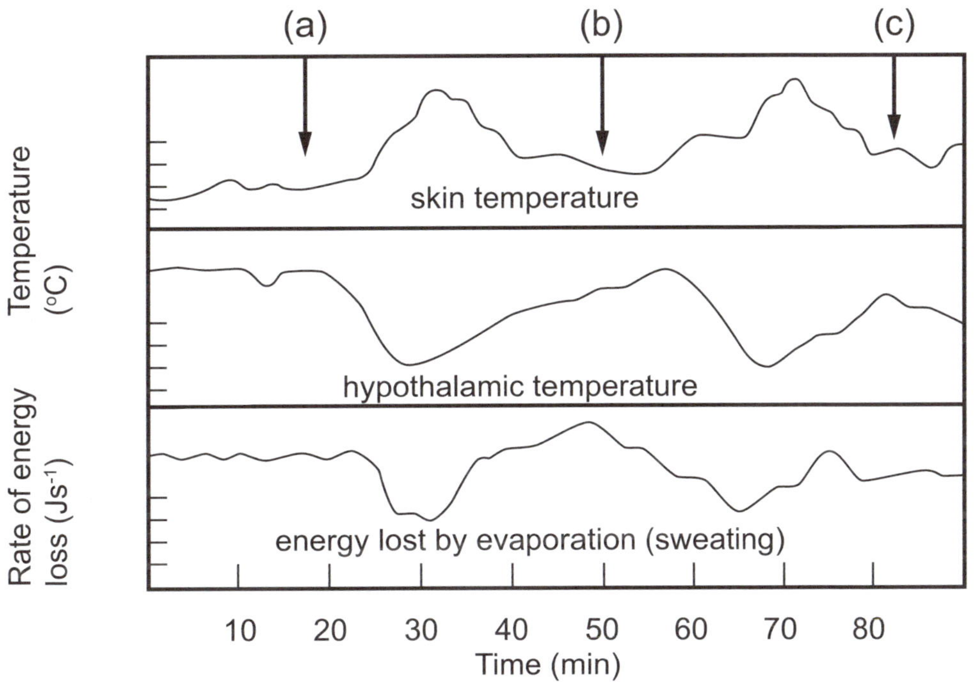

Figure 1: The relation between skin temperature, hypothalamic temperature and rate of evaporation for a human in a warm chamber (45 °C). Iced water is swallowed at points labeled (a), (b) and (c).

High-level Importance

SPOILER ALERT

Gold Standard has cross-referenced the content in this chapter to examples from ACER's official GAMSAT practice materials. It is for you to decide when you want to explore these questions since you may want to preserve some of ACER's materials for timed mock-exam practice.

Example – Using dimensional analysis to determine the rate of growth of your fingernails in m/s: Q105 of 5. Note that "Q" is followed by the question number, and, for example, "of 1" refers to booklet number 1 which is referenced in the Spoiler Alert table at the end of Chapter 1. The 15 full-length GAMSAT practice tests by Gold Standard, HEAPS-1 through HEAPS-15, contain specific cross-references to this chapter within the worked solutions. Note that the sweat/graph unit is from HEAPS-6; femur, patella, height, heart rate and other areas of growth are also among the HEAPS exams.

Chapter Checklist

- ☐ Access your online account to view answers, worked solutions and discussion boards.
- ☐ Reassess your 'learning objectives' for this chapter: Go back to the first page of this chapter and re-evaluate the top 3 boxes and the Introduction.
- ☐ Complete a maximum of 1 page of notes using symbols/abbreviations to represent the entire chapter based on your learning objectives. These are your Gold Notes.
- ☐ Consider your multimedia options based on your optimal way of learning:
  - ☐ Download the free Gold Standard GAMSAT app for your Android device or iPhone.
  - ☐ Create your own, tangible study cards or try the free app: Anki.
  - ☐ Record your voice reading your Gold Notes onto your smartphone (audio files, e.g., *memo* or MP3s) and listen during exercise, transportation, etc.
  - ☐ Try out the Gold Standard GAMSAT online videos at gamsat-prep.com, or you can try other options on YouTube like Khan Academy or Crash Course Biology.
- ☐ Reassess your schedule for your full-length GAMSAT practice tests: ACER and/or HEAPS exams. Ensure that you have scheduled one full day to complete a practice test and 1-2 days for a thorough assessment of worked solutions while adding to your abbreviated Gold Notes.
- ☐ Reassess your progress in scheduling and/or evaluating stress reduction techniques such as regular exercise (sports), yoga, meditation and/or mindfulness exercises (*see* YouTube for suggestions).

REPRODUCTION AND DEVELOPMENT
Chapter 14

Memorise

* Male and female reproductive structures, functions
* Ovum, sperm: differences in formation, relative contribution to next generation

Understand

* Gametogenesis by meiosis
* Embryogenesis: stages of early development
* Cell specialisation, communication in development, gene regulation in development
* Programmed cell death; basics: the menstrual cycle

Importance

Medium level: 5% of GAMSAT Biology questions released by ACER are related to content in this chapter (in our estimation).
* Note that approximately 75% of the questions in GAMSAT Biology are related to just 7 chapters: 1, 2, 3, 4, 7, 12, and 15.

GAMSAT-Prep.com

Introduction

Reproduction refers to the process by which new organisms are produced. The process of development follows as the single-celled zygote grows into a fully-formed adult. These two processes are fundamental to life as we know it.

The most important chapter in this book, Chapter 7, makes a return in Chapter 14's GAMSAT-level practice questions: Dimensional analysis and the fetus, the oxygen dissociation curve for the fetus, and a flow chart (number puzzle) for fetal circulation. These all represent classic GAMSAT fare.

Multimedia Resources at GAMSAT-Prep.com

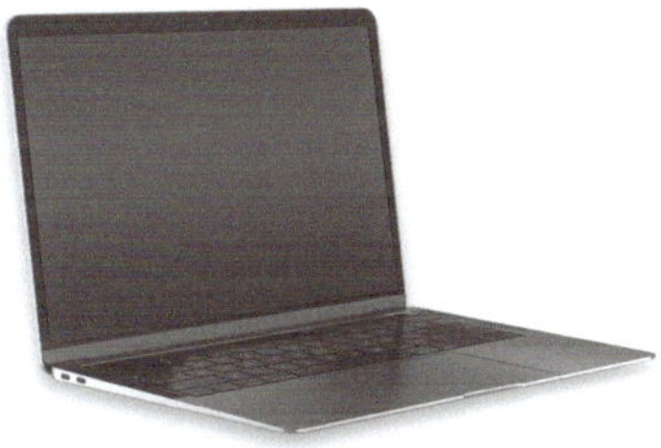

Open Discussion Boards
(gamsat-prep.com/forum)

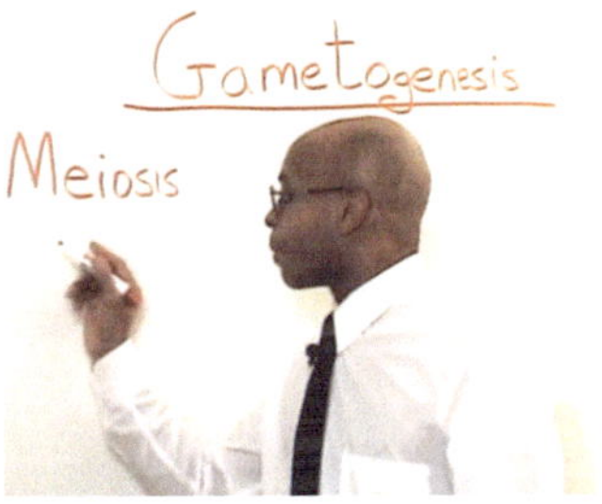

Foundational Videos

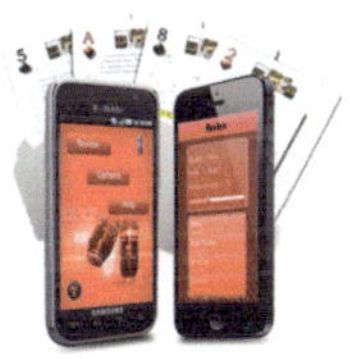

Flashcards

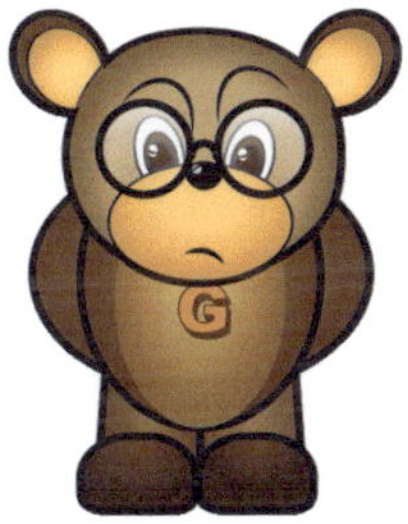

Special Guest

* The real GAMSAT may have advanced-level information presented (i.e. in a passage) but previous knowledge of said information is not required to answer the questions that would follow. Practice questions at the end of this chapter, as well as ACER and GS (HEAPS) practice GAMSATs can help you clarify this point.

14.1 Organs of the Reproductive System

Gonads are the organs which produce gametes (= germ cells = reproductive cells). The female gonads are the two ovaries which lie in the pelvic cavity. Opening around the ovaries and connecting to the uterus are the Fallopian tubes (= *oviducts*) which conduct the egg (= *ovum*) from the ovary to the uterus. The uterus is a muscular organ. Part of the uterus (= the cervix) protrudes into the vagina or *birth canal*. The vagina leads to the external genitalia. The vulva includes the openings of the vagina, various glands, and folds of skin which are large (= labia majora) and small (= labia minora). The clitoris is found between the labia minora at the anterior end of the vulva. Like the glans penis, it is very sensitive as it is richly innervated. However, the clitoris is unique in being the only organ in the human body devoted solely to sensory pleasure.

The male gonads are the two testicles (= *testes*) which are suspended by spermatic cords in a sac-like scrotum outside the body cavity (this is because the optimal temperature for spermatogenesis is less than body temperature). Sperm (= *spermatozoa*) are produced in the seminiferous tubules in the testes and then continue along a system of ducts including: the epididymis where sperm complete their maturation and are collected and stored; the vas deferens which leads to the ejaculatory duct which in turn leads to the penile urethra which conducts to the exterior. The accessory organs include the seminal vesicles, the bulbourethral and prostate glands. They are exocrine glands whose secretions contribute greatly to the volume of the *ejaculate* (= semen = seminal fluid). The penis is composed of a body or shaft, which contains an erectile tissue which can be engorged by blood; a penile urethra which can conduct either urine or sperm; and a very sensitive head or glans penis which may be covered by foreskin (= *prepuce*, which is removed by circumcision).

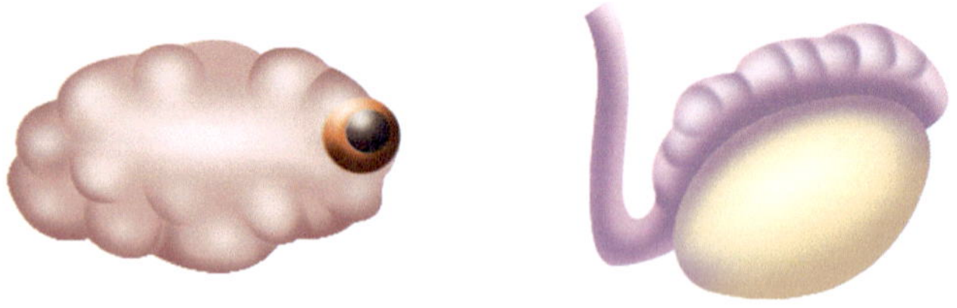

Figure IV.A.14.0: An ovulating ovary and a testicle with spermatic cord.

Medium-level Importance

14.2 Gametogenesis

Gametogenesis refers to the production of gametes (eggs and sperm) which occurs by meiosis (*see Mitosis*, BIO 1.3, *for comparison*). Meiosis involves two successive divisions which can produce four cells from one parent cell. The first division, the reduction division, reduces the number of chromosomes from $2n$ (= *diploid*) to n (= *haploid*) where n = 23 for humans. This reduction division occurs as follows: i) in **prophase I** the chromosomes appear (= *condensed chromatin*), the nuclear membrane and nucleoli disappear and the spindle fibers become organised. Homologous paternal and maternal chromosomes pair[1] (= *synapsis*) forming a tetrad as each pair of homologous chromosomes consists of four chromatids. The exchange of genetic information (DNA) may occur by crossing over between homologous chromosomes at sites called *chiasmata*, therefore redistributing maternal and paternal genetic information ensuring variability; **ii)** in **metaphase I** the synaptic pairs of chromosomes line up midway between the poles of the developing spindle (= *the equatorial plate*). Thus each pair consists of 2 chromosomes (= 4 chromatids), each attached to a spindle fiber; **iii)** in **anaphase I** the homologous chromosomes migrate to opposite poles of the spindle, separating its paternal chromosomes from maternal ones. Thus, each daughter cell will have a unique mixture of paternal and maternal origin of chromosomes. In contrast to anaphase in mitosis, the two chromatids remain held together. Consequently, the centromeres do *not* divide; **iv)** in **telophase I** the parent cell divides into two daughter cells (= *cytokinesis*), the nuclear membranes and nucleoli reappear, and the spindle fibers are no longer visible. Each daughter cell now contains 23 chromosomes (1*n*).

The first meiotic division is followed by a short interphase I and then the second meiotic division which proceeds essentially the same as mitosis. Thus prophase II, metaphase II, anaphase II, and telophase II proceed like the corresponding mitotic phases.

Gametogenesis in males (= *spermatogenesis*) proceeds as follows: before the age of sexual maturity only a small number of primordial germ cells (= *spermatogonia*) are present in the testes. There are two types of spermatogonia, type A and type B. Type A spermatogonia (2*n*) are mitotically active and continuously provide a supply of type A or type B spermatogonia. Type B spermatogonia (2*n*) undergo meiosis and will give rise to primary spermatocytes. After sexual maturation these cells prolifically multiply throughout a male's life.

In the seminiferous tubules, the type B spermatogonia (2*n*) enter meiosis I and undergo chromosome replication forming primary spermatocytes with 2*n* chromosomes. Primary spermatocytes complete meiosis I producing two secondary spermatocytes with 1*n* chromosomes. Secondary spermatocytes quickly enter meiosis II without an intervening S phase to form four spermatids. Spermatids are haploid (1*n*) cells (*see* Fig. IV.A.14.0a *au verso*).

In summary, each primary spermatocyte results in the production of four spermatids. Spermatids undergo a post-meiotic cytodifferentiation whereby spermatids are transformed into **four** motile sperm (1*n*) through a process called *spermiogenesis*.

Sperm can be divided into: **i)** a *head* which is oval and contains the nucleus with its 23 chromosomes {since the nucleus carries either an X or Y sex chromosome, sperm determine the sex of the offspring}. The head is partly surrounded by the acrosome which contains enzymes (esp. hyaluronidase) which

Medium-level Importance

[1]synapsing homologous chromosomes are often called tetrads or bivalents.

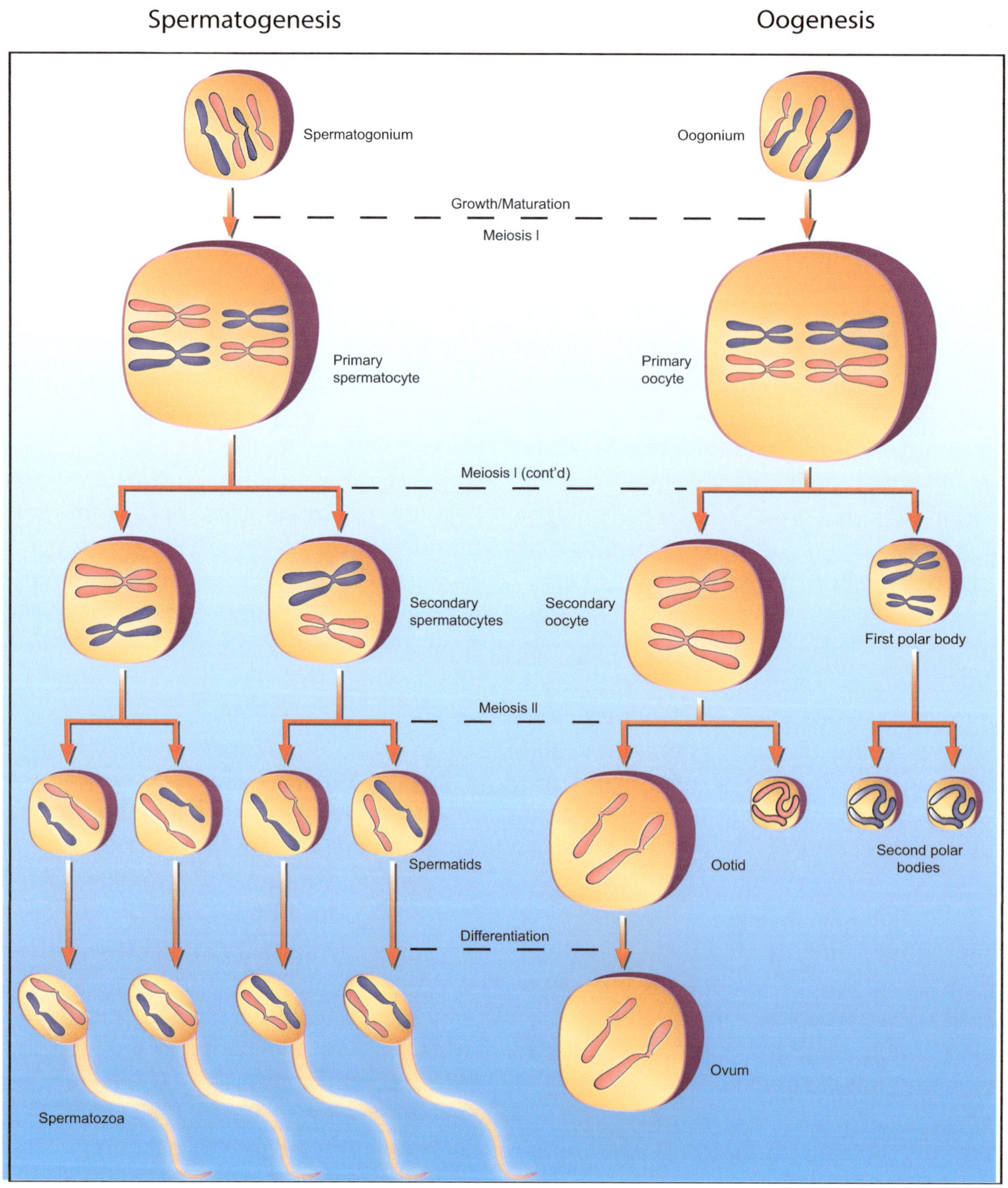

Figure IV.A.14.0a: Gametogenesis.

help the sperm penetrate the egg. The release of these enzymes is known as the acrosome reaction; **ii)** the *body* of the sperm contains a central core surrounded by a large number of mitochondria for power; and **iii)** the *tail* constitutes a flagellum which is critical for the cell's locomotion. Newly formed sperm are incapable of fertilisation until they undergo a process called capacitation, which happens in the female reproductive duct. After removal of its protein coating, the sperm becomes capable of fertilisation. Also in the seminiferous tubules are Sertoli cells which support and nourish developing sperm and Leydig cells which produce and secrete testosterone. While LH stimulates the latter, FSH stimulates primary spermatocytes to undergo meiosis. {Remember: LH = Leydig, FSH = spermatogenesis}

Gametogenesis in females (= *oogenesis*) proceeds as follows: in fetal development, groups of cells (= *ovarian or primordial follicles*) develop from the germinal epithelium of the ovary and differentiate into oogonia (2*n*). Oogonia (2*n*) enter meiosis I and undergo DNA replication producing primary oocytes (2*n*) which are surrounded by epithelia (= *follicular cells*) in the primordial follicle. The oocytes remain arrested in prophase I of meiosis until ovulation which occurs between the ages of about 13 (sexual maturity) and 50 (menopause). Thus, unlike males, all female germ cells are present at birth. Some follicles degenerate and are called *atretic*. During puberty, when the ovarian cycle begins, up to 20 primordial follicles may begin to differentiate to *Graafian follicles*. During this development, meiosis continues. In response to an LH surge from the pituitary gland, the primary oocyte (2*n*) completes meiosis I just prior to ovulation to form the secondary oocyte (1*n*) and the first polar body, which will probably degenerate. The secondary oocyte is surrounded by (from the inside out): a thick, tough membrane (= *the zona pellucida*), follicular cells (= *the corona radiata*), and estrogen-secreting thecal cells. It then enters meiosis II and remains arrested in metaphase of meiosis II until fertilisation occurs.

Of the twenty or so maturing follicles, all the remaining secondary follicles will degenerate (= *atresia*) except for one which becomes the Graafian (mature) follicle. In response to the LH surge, the secondary oocyte leaves the ruptured Graafian follicle in the process called ovulation. This ovum, along with its zona pellucida and corona radiata, migrate to and through the Fallopian tube (oviduct) where a sperm may penetrate the secondary oocyte (= *fertilisation*). If fertilisation occurs then the second meiotic division proceeds, forming a mature oocyte, known as ovum, (1*n*) and a second polar body; if fertilisation does not occur, then the ovum degenerates. Unlike in males, each primary germ cell (oocyte) produces one gamete and not four. This is a consequence of the production of *polar bodies* which are degenerated nuclear material. Up to three polar bodies can be formed: one from the division of the primary oocyte, one from the division of the secondary oocyte, and sometimes the first polar body divides.

Both animals and land plants produce ova ('eggs'; singular: ovum). The ovum is one of the largest cells in the human body. Ooplasm is the *yolk* of the ovum which includes cytoplasm and nutrition.

Medium-level Importance

14.3 The Menstrual Cycle

The "period" or menstrual cycle occurs in about 28 days and can be divided as follows: i) **Menses:** the first four days (days 1-4) of the cycle are notable for the menstrual blood flow. This occurs as a result of an estrogen and progesterone withdrawal which leads to vasoconstriction in the uterus causing the uterine lining (= *endometrium*) to disintegrate and slough away; ii) **Follicular** (ovary) or **Proliferative Phase** (days 5-14): FSH stimulates follicles to mature, and all but one of these follicles will stop growing, and the one dominant follicle in the ovary will continue to mature into a Graafian follicle, which in turn produces and secretes estrogen. Estrogen causes the uterine lining to thicken (= proliferate); iii) **Ovulation**: a very high concentration of estrogen is followed by an LH surge (estrogen-induced LH surge) at about day 15 (midcycle) which stimulates ovulation; iv) **Luteal** or **Secretory Phase** (days 15-28): the follicular cells degenerate into the corpus luteum which secretes estrogen *and* progesterone. Progesterone is responsible for a transient body temperature rise immediately after ovulation and it stimulates the uterine lining to become more vascular and glandular. Estrogen continues to stimulate uterine wall development and, along with progesterone, inhibits the secretion of LH and FSH (= negative feedback).

If the ovum is fertilised, the implanted embryo would produce the hormone *human chorionic gonadotropin* (= hCG) which would stimulate the corpus luteum to continue the secretion of estrogen and progesterone {hCG is the basis for most pregnancy tests}. If there is no fertilisation, the corpus luteum degenerates causing a withdrawal of estrogen and progesterone thus the cycle continues [*see* i) *in the preceding paragraph*].

Estrous vs. menstrual cycles: Mammals with estrous cycles reabsorb the endometrium if conception does not occur during that cycle. Also, they are generally only sexually active during a specific phase of their cycle ("in heat"). In contrast, females of species with menstrual cycles (i.e. humans) can of course be sexually active at any time in their cycle, and the endometrium is shed monthly.

Medium-level Importance

14.4 The Reproductive Sequence

During sexual stimulation parasympathetic impulses in the male lead to the dilatation of penile arteries combined with restricted flow in the veins resulting in the engorgement of the penis with blood (= *an erection*). In the female, the preceding occurs in a similar manner to the clitoris, along with the expansion and increase in secretions in the vagina. Intercourse or copulation may lead to orgasm which includes many responses from the sympathetic nervous system. In the male, the ejaculation of semen accompanies orgasm. In the female, orgasm is accompanied by many reflexes including an increase in muscular activity of the uterus and the Fallopian tubes. The latter may help in the transport of the already motile sperm to reach the tubes where the egg might be.

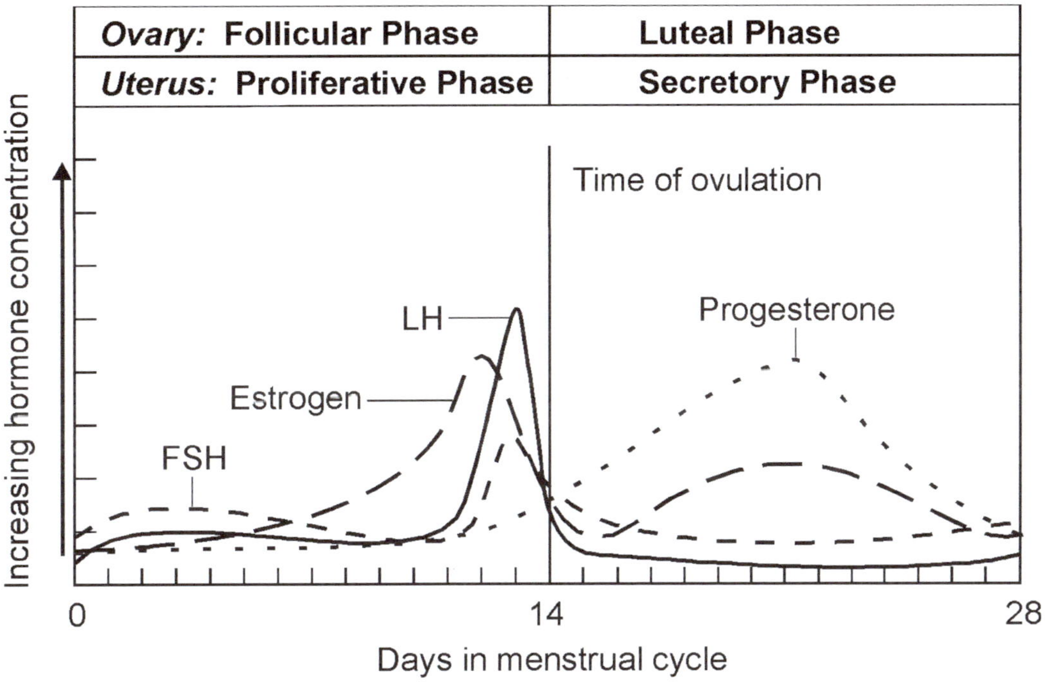

Figure IV.A.14.1: Changing hormone concentration during the menstrual cycle.

14.5 Embryogenesis

The formation of the embryo or *embryogenesis* occurs in a number of steps within two weeks of fertilisation. Many parts of the developing embryo take shape during this period (= *morphogenesis*).

Penetration of the zona pellucida leads to the *cortical reaction*, in which the secondary oocyte is no longer permeable to other sperm.

Fertilisation is a sequence of events which include: the sperm penetrating the corona radiata and the zona pellucidum due to the release of lytic enzymes from the acrosome known as the acrosome reaction; the fusion of the plasma membranes of the sperm and egg; the egg, which is really a secondary oocyte, becomes a mature ovum by completing the second meiotic division; the nuclei of the ovum and sperm are now called *pronuclei*; the male and female pronuclei fuse forming a zygote (2*n*). Fertilisation, which normally occurs in the Fallopian tubes, is completed within 24 hours of ovulation.

Cleavage consists of rapid, repeated mitotic divisions beginning with the zygote. Because the resultant daughter cells or

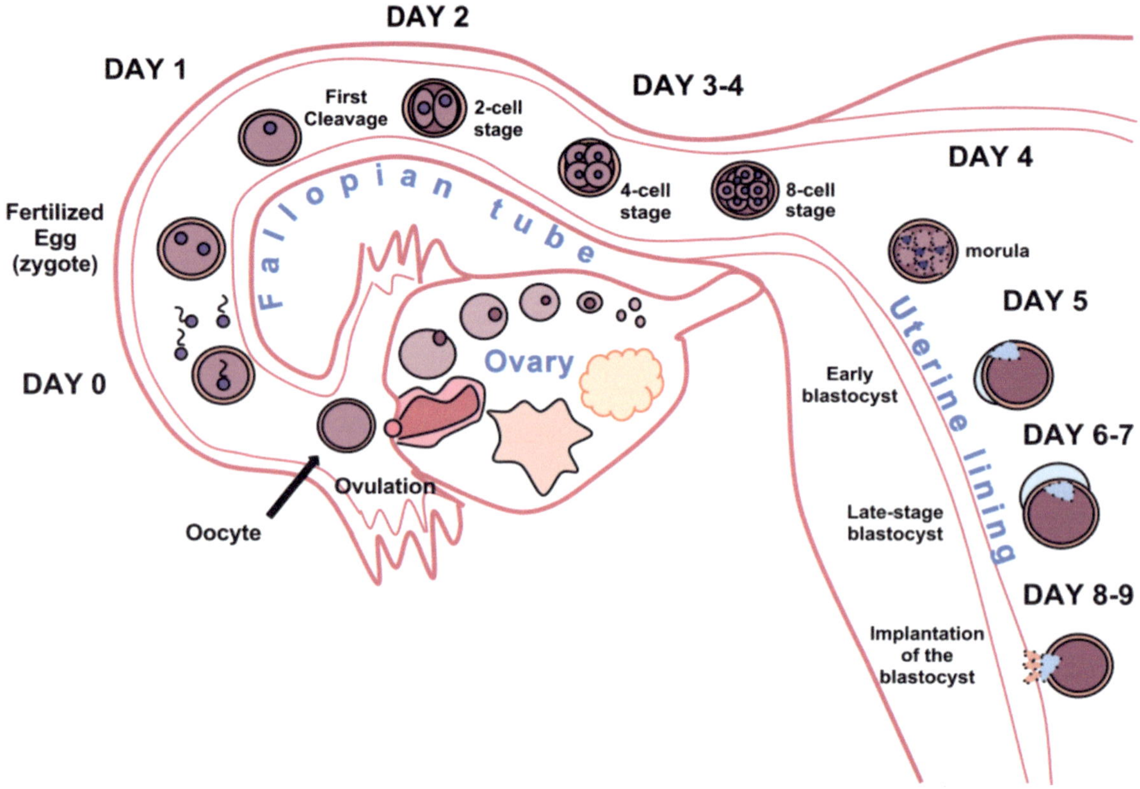

Figure IV.A.14.2: Human fertilisation. The sperm and ovum unite through fertilisation, creating a zygote that will evolve into a blastocyst which implants in the uterine wall via the uterine lining (*endometrium*) where it will continue to develop over the course of 9 months. (ref: α)

blastomeres are still contained within the zona pellucidum, the cytoplasmic mass remains constant. Thus the increasing number of cells requires that each daughter cell be smaller than its parent cell. A morula is a solid ball of about 16 blastomeres which enters the uterus.

Blastulation is the process by which the morula develops a fluid filled cavity (= *blastocoel*) thus converting it to a blastocyst. Since the zona pellucidum degenerates at this point, the blastocyst is free to implant in the uterine lining or endometrium. The blastocyst contains some centrally located cells (= *the inner cell mass*) called the embryoblast which develops into the embryo. The outer cell mass called the trophoblast becomes part of the placenta.

Implantation is the process by which the zona pellucida must degenerate before the blastocyst can implant into the endometrium of the uterus. Once implantation

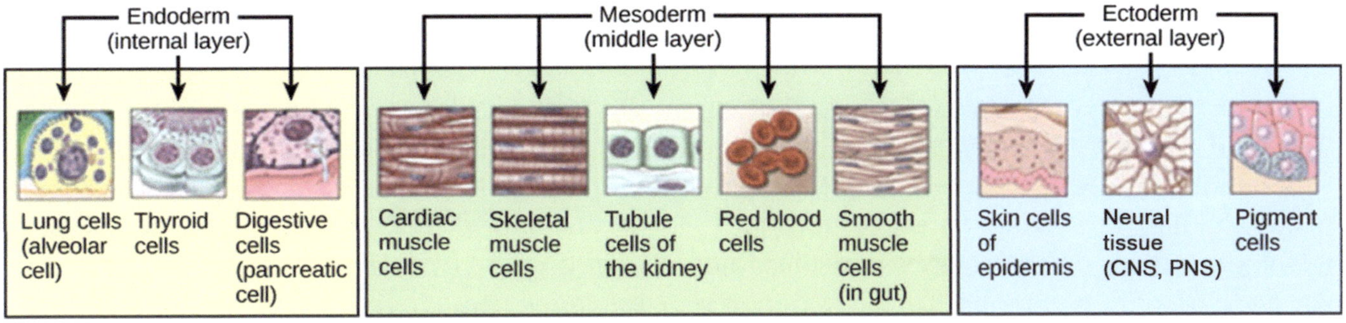

Figure IV.A.14.3: Germ layers differentiate. (ref: β)

is completed, the blastocyst becomes surrounded by layers of cells that further invade the endometrium.

Gastrulation is the process by which the blastula invaginates, and the inner cell mass is converted into a three layered (= *trilaminar*) disk. The trilaminar disk includes the **three primary germ layers**: an outer ectoderm, a middle mesoderm, and an inner endoderm. The ectoderm will develop into the epidermis and the nervous system; the mesoderm will become muscle, connective tissue (incl. blood, bone), and circulatory, reproductive and excretory organs; the endoderm will become the epithelial linings of the respiratory tract, and digestive tract, including the glands of the accessory organs (i.e. the liver and pancreas). During this stage the embryo may be called a gastrula.

Neurulation is the process by which the neural plate and neural folds form and close to produce the neural tube. The neural plate is formed by the thickening of ectoderm which is induced by the developing *notochord*. The notochord is a cellular rod that defines the axis of the embryo and provides some rigidity. Days later, the neural plate invaginates along its central axis producing a central neural groove with neural folds on each side. The neural folds come together and fuse thus converting the neural plate into a neural tube which separates from the surface ectoderm. Special cells on the crest of the neural folds (= *neural crest cells*) migrate to either side of the developing neural tube to a region called the neural crest.

As a consequence, we are left with **three** regions: the surface ectoderm which will become the epidermis; the neural tube which will become the central nervous system (CNS); and the neural crest which will become cranial and spinal ganglia and nerves, and the medulla of the adrenal gland. During this stage the embryo may be called a *neurula*.

Medium-level Importance

14.5.1 Mechanisms of Development

Though this is a subject which is still poorly understood, it seems clear that morphogenesis relies on the coordinated interaction of genetic and environmental factors. When the zygote passes through its first few divisions, the blastomeres remain indeterminate or uncommitted to a specific fate. As development proceeds the cells become increasingly committed to a specific outcome (i.e. neural tube cells → CNS). This is called **determination**.

In order for a cell to specialise it must differentiate into a committed or determined cell. Since essentially all cells in a person's body have the same amount of genetic information, differentiation relies on the *difference* in the way these genes are *activated*. For example, though brain cells (neurons) have the same genes as osteoblasts, neurons do not activate such genes (otherwise we would have bone forming in our brains!). The general mechanism by which cells differentiate is called **induction**.

Induction can occur by many means. If two cells divide unevenly, the cell with more yolk (e.g., cytoplasm and nutrients) might have the necessary amount of a substance which could *induce* its chromosomes to activate cell-specific genes. Furthermore, sometimes a cell, through contact (i.e. *contact inhibition*) or the release of a chemical mediator, can influence the development of nearby cells (*recall that the notochord induces the development of the neural plate;* BIO 14.5). The physical environment (pH, temperature, etc.) may also influence the development of certain cells. Irrespective of what form of induction is used, the signal must be translated into an intracellular message which influences the genetic activity of the responding cells.

Programmed cell-death (PCD = apoptosis) is death of a cell in any form, which is controlled by an intracellular program. PCD is carried out in a regulated process directed by DNA which normally confers advantage during an organism's life-cycle. PCD serves fundamental functions during tissue development. For example, the development of the spaces between your fingers requires cells to undergo PCD.

Thus cells specialise and develop into organ systems (*morphogenesis*). The embryo develops from the second to the ninth week, followed by the fetus which develops from the ninth week to birth (*parturition*).

Medium-level Importance

14.6 The Placenta

The **placenta** is a complex vascular structure formed by part of the maternal endometrium (= *the decidua basalis*) and cells of embryonic origin (= *the chorion*). The placenta begins to form when the blastocyst implants in the endometrium. A cell layer from the embryo invades the endometrium with fingerlike bumps (= *chorionic villi*) which project into intervillous spaces which contain maternal blood. Maternal spiral arteries enter the intervillous spaces allowing blood to circulate.

The placenta has three main functions: **i)** the **transfer** of substances necessary for the development of the embryo or fetus from the mother (O_2, H_2O, carbohydrates, amino acids, IgG antibodies - BIO 8.2, vitamins, etc.) and the **transfer** of wastes from the embryo or fetus to the mother (CO_2, urea, uric acid, etc.); **ii)** the placenta can synthesise substances (i.e. glycogen, fatty acids) to use as an energy source for itself and the embryo or fetus; **iii)** the placenta produces and secretes a number of hormones including human chorionic gonadotropin (hCG), estrogen and progesterone. The hCG rescues the corpus luteum from regression and stimulates its production of progesterone.

14.7 Fetal Circulation

Medium-level Importance

Consider the following: the fetus has lungs but does not breathe O_2. In fact, the placenta is, metaphorically, the "fetal lung." Oxygenated and nutrient-rich blood returns to the fetus from the placenta via the left umbilical vein. Most of the blood is directed to the inferior vena cava through the ductus venosus. From there, blood joins the deoxygenated and nutrient-poor blood from the superior vena cava and empties into the right atrium. However, most of the blood is diverted from the pulmonary circulation (bypassing the right ventricle) to the left atrium via a hole in the atrial septum: the patent foramen ovale (for adult circulation and anatomy, *see* chapter 7). Blood then enters the left ventricle and is distributed through the body (systemic circulation) via the aorta (*see* Fig.IV.A.14.4 *au verso*).

Some blood in the right atrium enters into the right ventricle and then proceeds into the pulmonary trunk. However, resistance in the collapsed lung is high and the pulmonary artery pressure is higher than it is in the aorta. Consequently, most of the blood bypasses the lung via the ductus arteriosus back to the aorta.

Blood circulates through the body and is sent back to the placenta via right and left umbilical arteries. The placenta re-oxygenates this deoxygenated and nutrient-poor blood and returns it to the fetus through the umbilical vein and the cardiovascular cycle repeats. Notice that in the fetus, oxygenated and nutrient-rich blood can be carried by veins to the right chambers of the heart which cannot occur in normal adult circulation. Also note that fetal hemoglobin binds to oxygen more strongly (*higher oxygen affinity*) than adult hemoglobin, enabling the transfer of oxygen from mother to fetus.

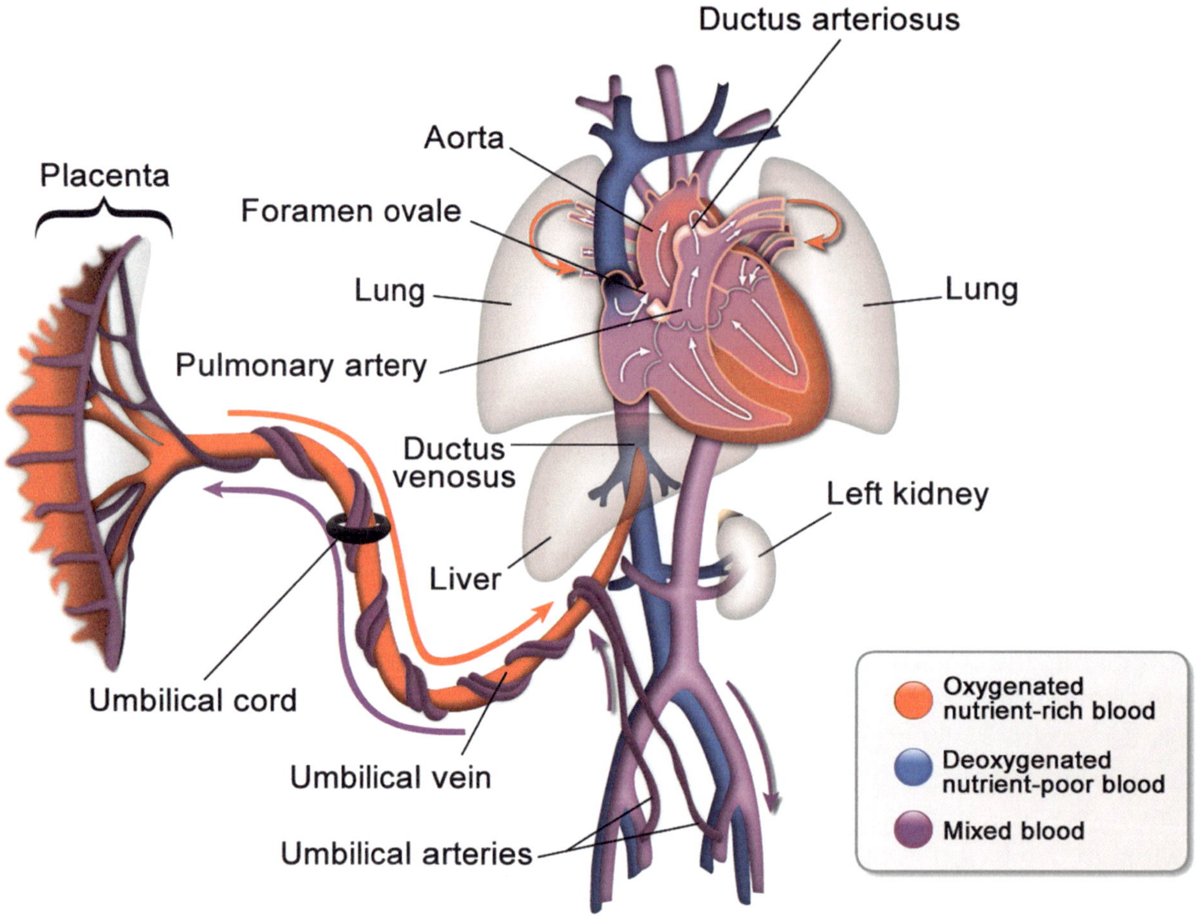

Figure IV.A.14.4: Fetal circulation.

14.8 Fetal Sexual Development

The normal sexual development of the fetus depends on the genotype (XX female, XY male), the morphology of the internal organs and gonads, and the phenotype or external genitalia. Later, these many factors combine to influence the individual's self-perception along with the development of secondary sexual characteristics (i.e. breast development in females, hair growth and lower pitched voice in males).

Every fetus, regardless of genotype, has the capacity to become a normally formed individual of either sex. Development naturally proceeds towards "female" unless there is a Y chromosome factor present. Thus the XX genotype leads to the maturation of the Müllerian ducts into the uterus, Fallopian tubes, and part of the vagina. The primitive gonad will develop into a testis only if the Y chromosome is present and encodes the appropriate factor and eventually the secretion of testosterone. Thus the XY genotype leads to the involution of the Müllerian ducts and the maturation of the Wolffian ducts into the vas deferens, seminiferous tubules and prostate.

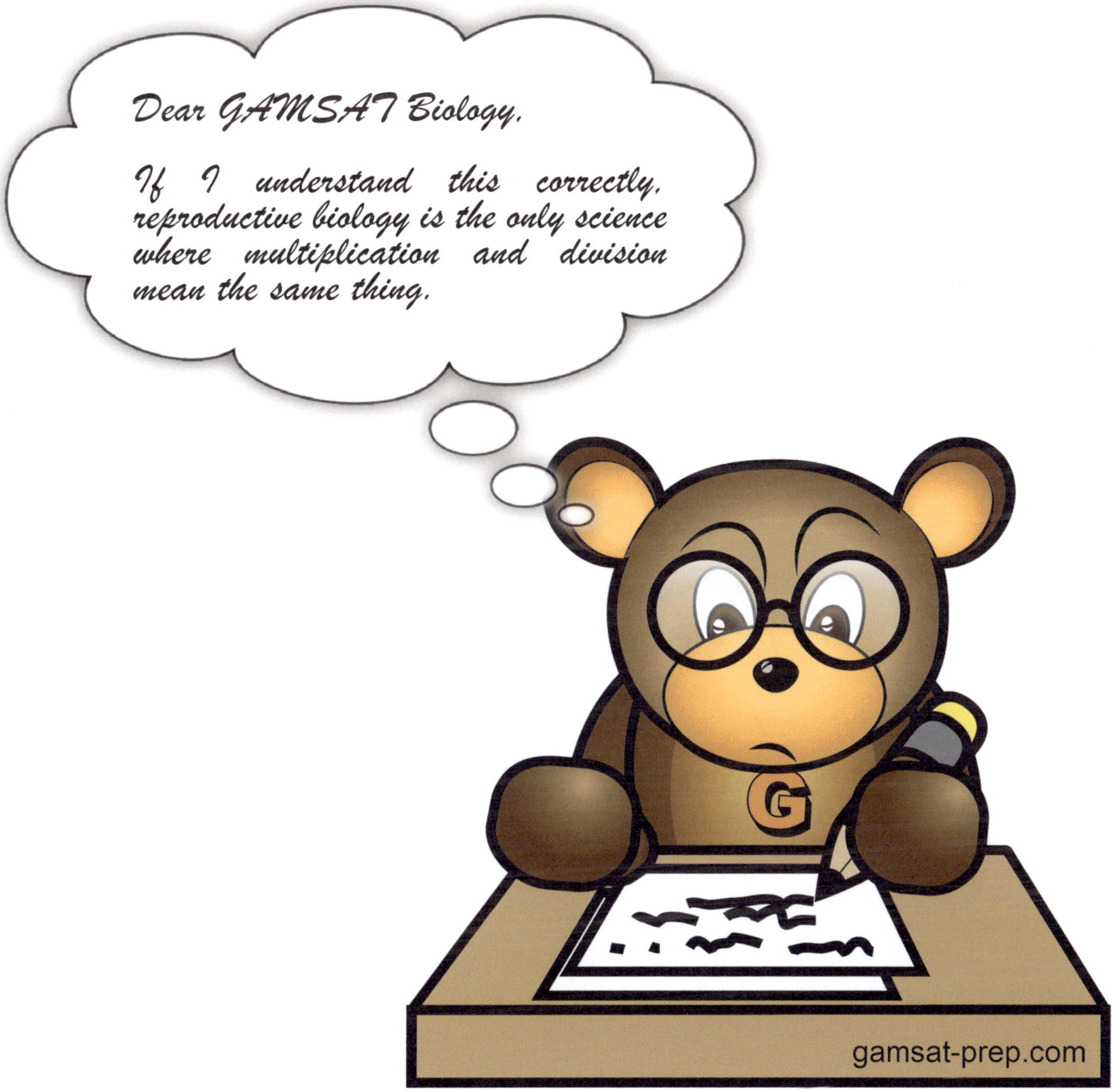

High-level Importance

CHAPTER 14: Reproduction and Development

GOLD STANDARD FOUNDATIONAL GAMSAT PRACTICE QUESTIONS

1) Down's syndrome, in which $2n = 47$, is one of the most common forms of chromosomal abnormalities. This results from the failure of one pair of homologous chromosomes to separate during meiosis. During which of the meiotic phases would this likely occur?

A. Metaphase I
B. Metaphase II
C. Anaphase I
D. Anaphase II

2) In general terms, what is the primary genetic difference between a brain cell and a muscle cell?

A. The amount of DNA
B. The number of chromosomes
C. The number of genes
D. The expression of genes

3) After fertilisation, the zygote will develop into a female if:

A. the zygote possesses an X chromosome.
B. the primary oocyte possesses an X chromosome.
C. the egg possesses an X chromosome.
D. the sperm possesses an X chromosome.

4) Which of the following correctly describes a species that has a chromosome number of $2n = 16$?

A. The species has 16 sets of chromosomes per cell.
B. Each cell has 8 homologous pairs.
C. During anaphase there will be 32 separate chromosomes.
D. The species is diploid with 8 chromosomes per cell.

GOLD STANDARD GAMSAT-LEVEL PRACTICE QUESTIONS

5) A 35-kg child has approximately 2.5 litres of blood which circulates approximately once per minute. For this child:

- 100 cm^3 of blood in the pulmonary artery carries about 55 cm^3 of CO_2.
- 100 cm^3 of the blood in the pulmonary vein carries about 50 cm^3 of CO_2.

What is the approximate volume of CO_2 excreted per minute from this child?

A. 55 cm^3
B. 125 cm^3
C. 250 cm^3
D. 2500 cm^3

Questions 6–7

Consider the following diagram.

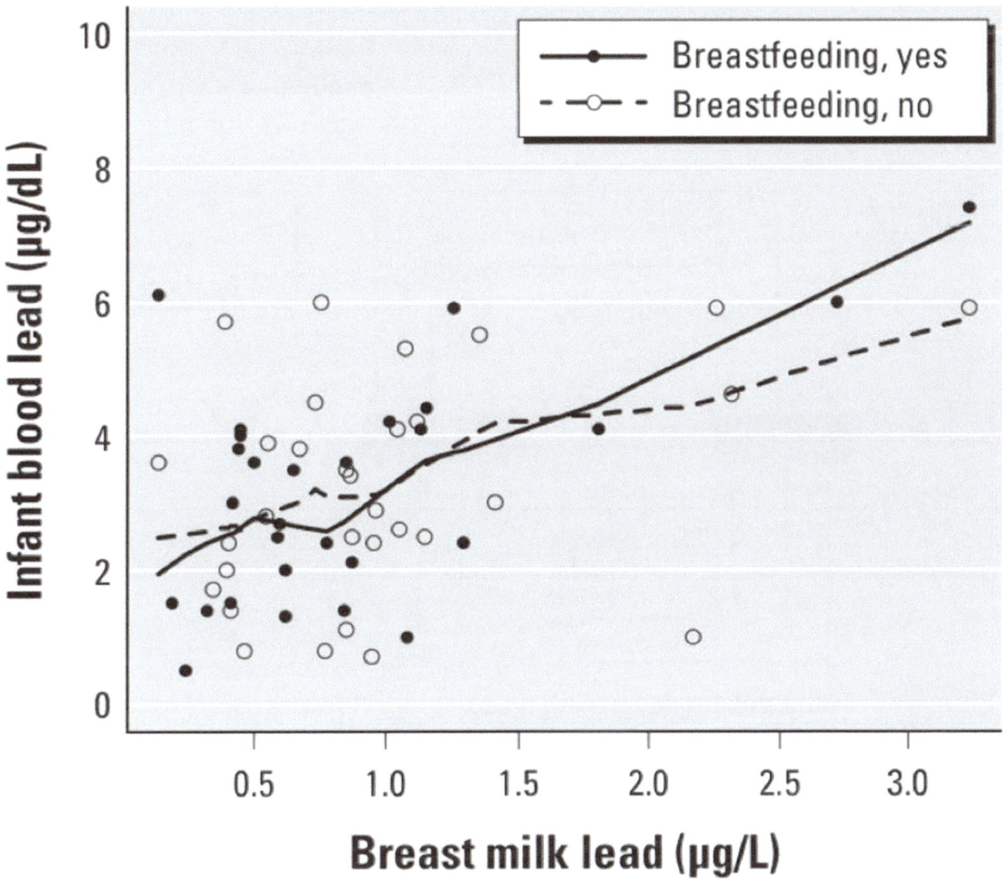

Figure 1: Association between infant blood lead and breast milk lead, separated by infants who were breastfed, and those who were not.
(Ettinger, A. et al. *Environ Health Perspect*. 2014; 122(1): 87)

6) According to Figure 1, when breast milk lead is at 1.0 µg/L, as compared to infant blood lead, breast milk lead is approximately:

A. the same concentration.
B. 2.5 times less.
C. 3 times less.
D. 30 times less.

7) How much milk breast lead would be projected if the difference in infant blood lead between breastfeeding and non-breastfeeding trials is doubled that present at 2.5 µg/L breast milk lead?

A. 3.0 µg/L
B. 4.0 µg/L
C. 4.5 µg/L
D. 5.0 µg/L

8) Apoptosis is the process of programmed cell death that can occur in multicellular organisms. The proteins involved in apoptosis are associated with pathways for cell cycle arrest and DNA repair. These processes are mostly regulated through the interplay of various proteins involved in feedback loops including some of the ones shown in Figure 1.

According to Figure 1, CDK2 activity would most reasonably increase due to all of the following EXCEPT:

A. degradation of p21.
B. high cyclin G concentrations.
C. a mutation in the gene that produces PTEN.
D. high p53 concentrations.

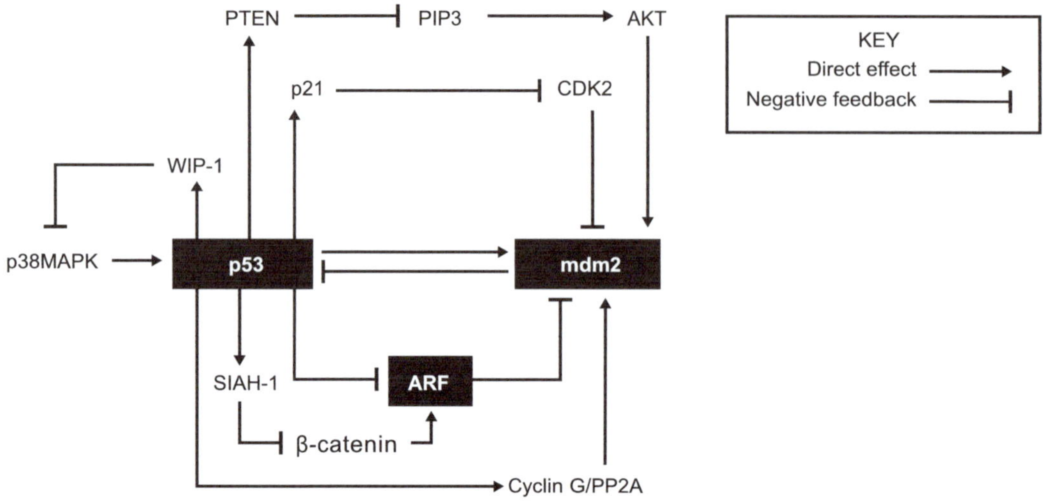

Figure 1: Feedback loops forming a regulatory network affecting apoptosis, cell cycle arrest and DNA repair. (Bioformatics Institute)

9) Figure 1 shows the oxygen dissociation curves for hemoglobin from an adult and a fetus.

Which one of the following statements describes the difference in the behaviour of the two types of hemoglobin?

A. Adult hemoglobin has a higher oxygen affinity than fetal hemoglobin.
B. Adult hemoglobin cannot carry as much oxygen as fetal hemoglobin.
C. Fetal hemoglobin has a higher oxygen affinity than adult hemoglobin.
D. Fetal hemoglobin cannot carry as much oxygen as adult hemoglobin.

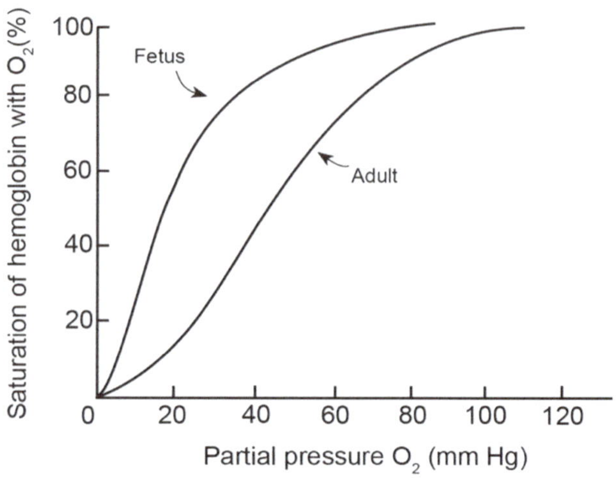

Figure 1

Question 10

The body mass index (BMI) provides a measure of the relative mass based on the weight and height of an individual.

- Metric units: BMI = Weight[kg] / (Height[m] × Height[m])
- Imperial units: BMI = 703 × Weight[lb] / (Height[in] × Height[in])

Consider Figure 1.

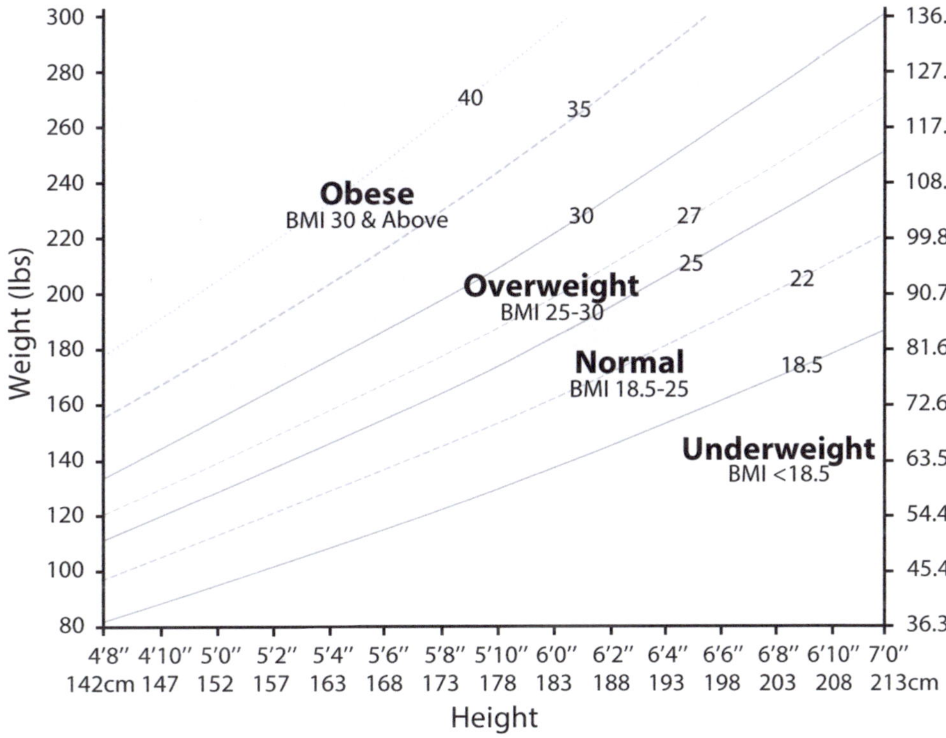

Figure 1: Body Mass Index (BMI) Chart for Adults. Intermittent shading from upper left to bottom right represents Obese, Overweight, Normal, and Underweight, respectively. Note that Height is given in feet (′) and inches (″) as well as centimetres (cm). For example, a 'Normal' BMI of 22 can be seen for a person who 6′0″ or 183 cm, and 160 lbs or 72.6 kg. Adapted from Vertex 42 LLC.

10) Which of the following statements is most accurate?

A. A height of 1.75 m with a weight of 96 kg is categorised as 'overweight'.

B. With an increase in height, the effect of height on the ratio that constitutes BMI is exponential, whereas the change in weight has a linear effect.

C. An increase in weight by 5 kg due to muscle is likely to have a greater impact on the BMI than an increase of 5 kg due to fat.

D. Doubling the weight in kilograms for a person who is 'underweight' is more likely to make that person 'obese' as compared to doubling their weight in lbs.

High-level Importance

Questions 11–12

Cardiac output is the amount of blood the heart pumps through the circulatory system in a minute. This is simple in the adult where there are essentially two equal serial circulations: systemic and pulmonary. However, in the fetus, who has two unequal parallel circulations due to fetal shunts, distribution of blood is given by the percentage of combined ventricular output (CVO), which is the combined output of left and right ventricles.

A human model using catheters in fetal sheep was studied to determine the CVO through the heart and major vessels. The numbers in Figure 1 represent the CVO in various structures, though some values have been replaced by red bold letters.

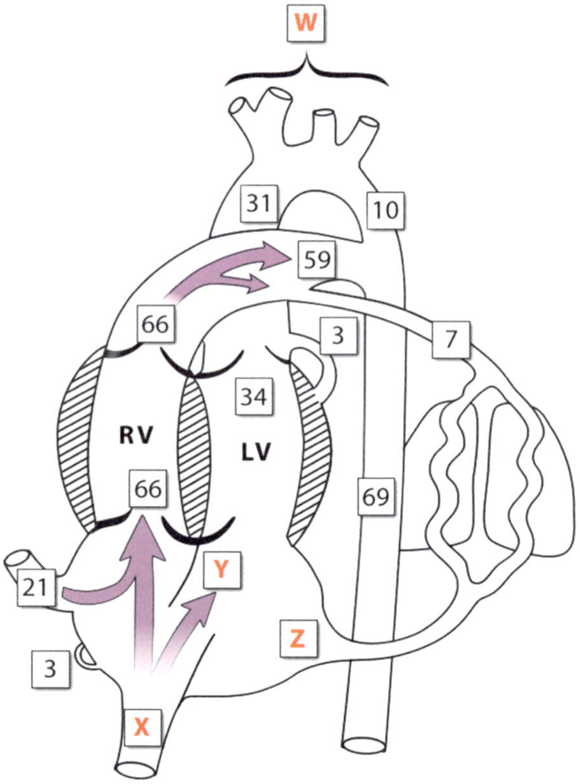

Figure 1: Diagrammatic representation of fetal circulation and CVO. RV: right ventricle; LV: left ventricle. (Modified from: Rudolph AM; Congenital Diseases of the Heart)

11) Which of the following likely represents the CVO at **W**?

A. 10%
B. 21%
C. 41%
D. 100%

12) Which of the following best approximates the CVO at **X**?

A. 70%
B. 100%
C. (**Z** + **Y**)%
D. (**X** – **Y** + 66)%

13) The karyotype represents the number and visual appearance of the chromosomes in the cell nuclei of an organism. The following is an illustration of the karyotype of a particular rat kangaroo found in Western Australia.

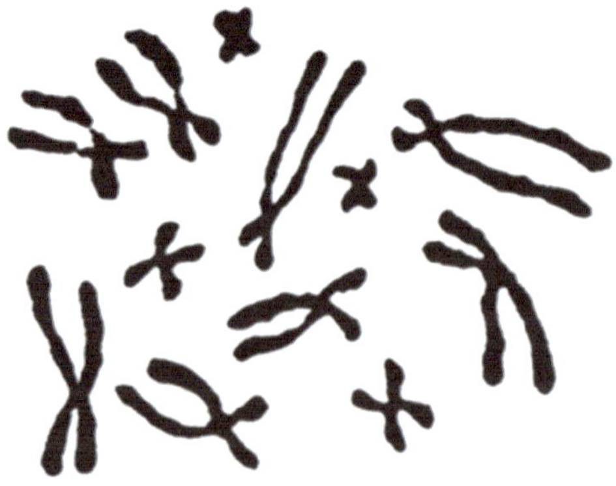

Which of the following is most consistent with the chromosome number indicated by the illustration?

A. Haploid chromosome number = 24
B. Diploid chromosome number = 24
C. Haploid chromosome number = 12
D. Diploid chromosome number = 12

Questions 14–15

Consider Figure 1.

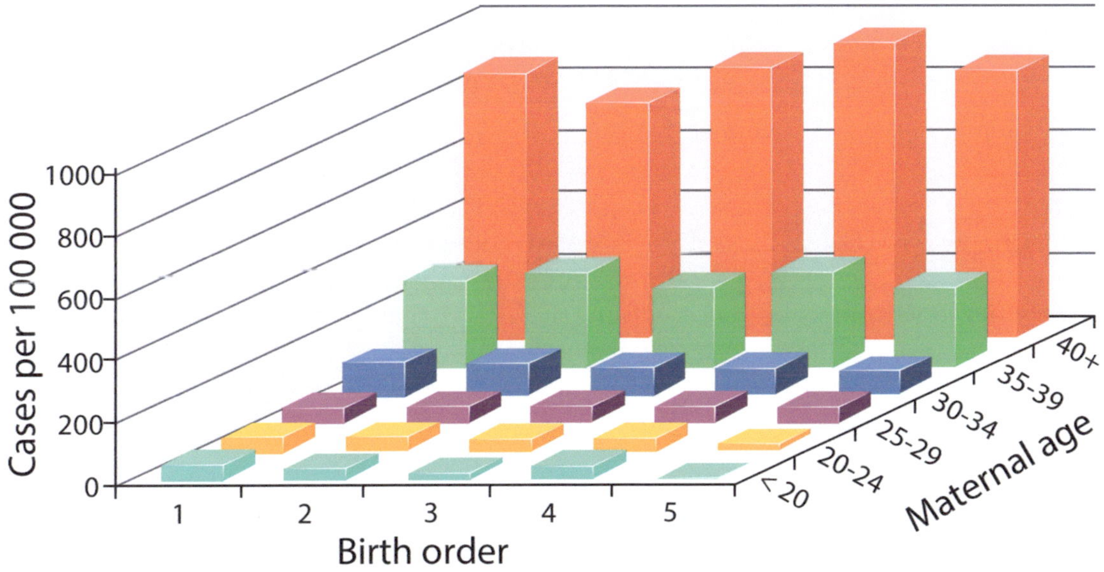

Figure 1: Stratifying the prevalence of Down's syndrome per 100 000 live births by both birth order and maternal age. (Ref: Boston University School of Public Health, LaMorte, MD; 2020)

14) A 42-year-old woman is pregnant with her second child. Given the data in Figure 1, what is the percent chance that she would have a child with Down's syndrome?

- **A.** Greater than 50%
- **B.** Between 10% and 50%
- **C.** Between 5% and 10%
- **D.** Below 1%

15) A patient wonders whether or not the number of live births she has had in the past significantly affects her risk of having a child with Down's syndrome. Based on the data in Figure 1, which of the following would be a rational response?

- **A.** The likelihood depends on the age of the mother.
- **B.** There is little or no correlation with birth order.
- **C.** There is a significant increase in the likelihood with increasing birth order.
- **D.** There is a significant decrease in the likelihood with increasing birth order.

SPOILER ALERT

Gold Standard has cross-referenced the content in this chapter to examples from ACER's official GAMSAT practice materials. It is for you to decide when you want to explore these questions since you may want to preserve some of ACER's materials for timed mock-exam practice.

Examples – What phase of meiosis? Q94 of 3; graph extrapolation: Q63-65 of 4; percent puzzle cardiac output: Q31-34 of 5. Note that "Q" is followed by the question number, and, for example, "of 1" refers to booklet number 1 which is referenced in the Spoiler Alert table at the end of Chapter 1. The 15 full-length GAMSAT practice tests by Gold Standard, HEAPS-1 through HEAPS-15, contain specific cross-references to this chapter within the worked solutions. Note that the apoptosis question is from HEAPS-6; the 3D graph of Down's syndrome risk is from HEAPS-7 (but of course, in black and white!).

Chapter Checklist

- ☐ Access your online account to view answers, worked solutions and discussion boards.
- ☐ Reassess your 'learning objectives' for this chapter: Go back to the first page of this chapter and re-evaluate the top 3 boxes and the Introduction.
- ☐ Complete a maximum of 1 page of notes using symbols/abbreviations to represent the entire chapter based on your learning objectives. These are your Gold Notes.
- ☐ Consider your multimedia options based on your optimal way of learning:
  - ☐ Download the free Gold Standard GAMSAT app for your Android device or iPhone.
  - ☐ Create your own, tangible study cards or try the free app: Anki.
  - ☐ Record your voice reading your Gold Notes onto your smartphone (audio files, e.g., *memo* or MP3s) and listen during exercise, transportation, etc.
  - ☐ Try out the Gold Standard GAMSAT online videos at gamsat-prep.com, or you can try other options on YouTube like Khan Academy or Crash Course Biology.
- ☐ Reassess your schedule for your full-length GAMSAT practice tests: ACER and/or HEAPS exams. Ensure that you have scheduled one full day to complete a practice test and 1-2 days for a thorough assessment of worked solutions while adding to your abbreviated Gold Notes.
- ☐ Reassess your progress in scheduling and/or evaluating stress reduction techniques such as regular exercise (sports), yoga, meditation and/or mindfulness exercises (*see* YouTube for suggestions).

References

α: Figure IV.A.14.2
Human fertilisation, labels modified from Ttrue12 Wikimedia Commons.

β: Figure IV.A.14.3
Germ layers differentiate, label modified from CNX Wikimedia Commons.

GENETICS

Chapter 15

Memorise

* Define: phenotype, genotype, gene, locus, allele (single and multiple)
* Homo/heterozygosity, wild type, recessiveness, complete/co-dominance
* Incomplete dominance, gene pool
* Sex-linked characteristics, sex determination

Understand

* Importance of meiosis; compare/contrast with mitosis
* Segregation of genes, assortment, linkage, recombination
* Single/double crossovers
* Hardy-Weinberg Principle
* Test cross: back cross, concepts of parental, F1 and F2 generations; evaluating a pedigree

Importance

High level: 10% of GAMSAT Biology questions released by ACER are related to content in this chapter (in our estimation).
* Note that approximately 75% of the questions in GAMSAT Biology are related to just 7 chapters: 1, 2, 3, 4, 7, 12, and 15.

GAMSAT-Prep.com

Introduction

Genetics is the study of heredity and variation in organisms. The observations of Gregor Mendel in the mid-nineteenth century gave birth to the science which would reveal the physical basis for his conclusions – DNA – about 100 years later.

This is the last of the 3 'high-level importance' chapters. Approximately 45% of GAMSAT Biology questions among ACER's official practice materials contain content related to 3 chapters: 1, 7 and 15, this chapter. Also, be forewarned: despite the fact that a dihybrid cross (BIO 15.3) is time consuming, it appears in 3 separate ACER GAMSAT practice booklets.

Multimedia Resources at GAMSAT-Prep.com

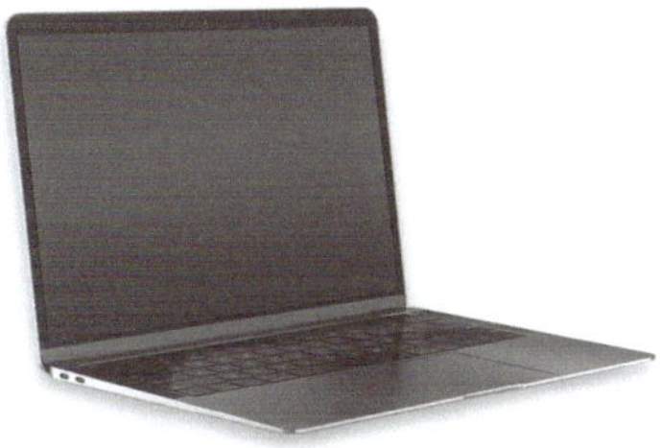

Open Discussion Boards
(*gamsat-prep.com/forum*)

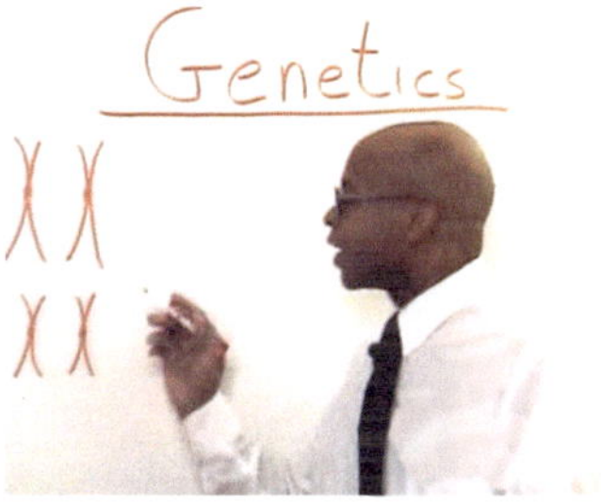

Foundational Videos

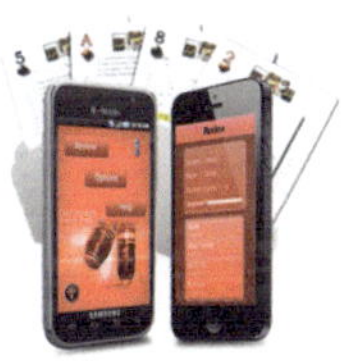

Flashcards

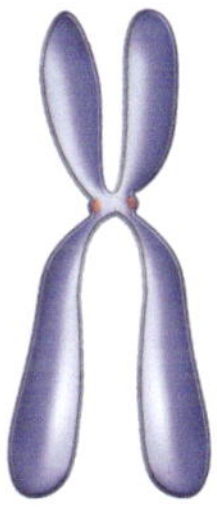

Special Guest

* The real GAMSAT may have advanced-level information presented (i.e. in a passage) but previous knowledge of said information is not required to answer the questions that would follow. Practice questions at the end of this chapter, as well as ACER and GS (HEAPS) practice GAMSATs can help you clarify this point.

15.1 Background Information

Genetics is a branch of biology which deals with the principles and mechanics of heredity; in other words, the *means* by which *traits* are passed from parents to offspring. To begin, we will first examine some relevant definitions - a few of which we have already discussed.

Chromosomes are a complex of DNA and proteins (incl. histones; BIO 1.2.2). A gene is that sequence of DNA that codes for a protein or polypeptide. A locus is the *position* of the gene on the DNA molecule. Recall that humans inherit 46 chromosomes - 23 from maternal origin and 23 from paternal origin (BIO 14.2). A given chromosome from maternal origin has a counterpart from paternal origin which codes for the same products. This is called a **homologous pair** of chromosomes.

Any homologous pair of chromosomes have a pair of genes which codes for the same product (i.e. hair colour). Such pairs of genes are called **alleles**. Thus for one gene product, a nucleus contains one allele from maternal origin and one allele from paternal origin. If both alleles are identical (i.e. they code for the same hair colour), then the individual is called **homozygous** for that trait. If the two alleles differ (i.e. one codes for dark hair while the other codes for light hair), then the individual is called **heterozygous** for that trait.

The set of genes possessed by a particular organism is its genotype. The appearance or phenotype of an individual is expressed as a consequence of the genotype and the environment. Consider a heterozygote that expressed one gene (dark hair) but not the other (light hair). The expressed gene would be called dominant while the other unexpressed allele would be called recessive. The individual would have dark hair as their phenotype, yet their genotype would be heterozygous for that trait. The dominant allele is expressed in the phenotype. This is known as Mendel's Law of Dominance.

It is common to symbolise dominant genes with capital letters (A) and recessive genes with small letters (a). From the preceding paragraphs, we can conclude that with two alleles, three genotypes are possible: homozygous dominant (AA), heterozygous (Aa), and homozygous recessive (aa). Note that this only results in two phenotypes since both AA and Aa express the dominant gene, while only aa expresses the recessive gene.

Each individual carries **two** alleles while populations may have many or **multiple alleles**. Sometimes these genes are not strictly dominant or recessive. There may be degrees of blending (= *incomplete dominance*) or sometimes two alleles may be equally dominant (= *codominance*). ABO blood types are an important example of multiple alleles with codominance.

Incomplete dominance occurs when the phenotype of the heterozygote is an intermediate of the phenotypes of the homozygotes. A classic example is flower colour in snapdragon: the snapdragon flower colour is red for homozygous dominant and white for homozygous recessive. When the red homozygous flower is crossed with the white homozygous flower, the result yields a 100% pink snapdragon flower. The pink snapdragon is the result of the combined effect of both dominant and recessive genes.

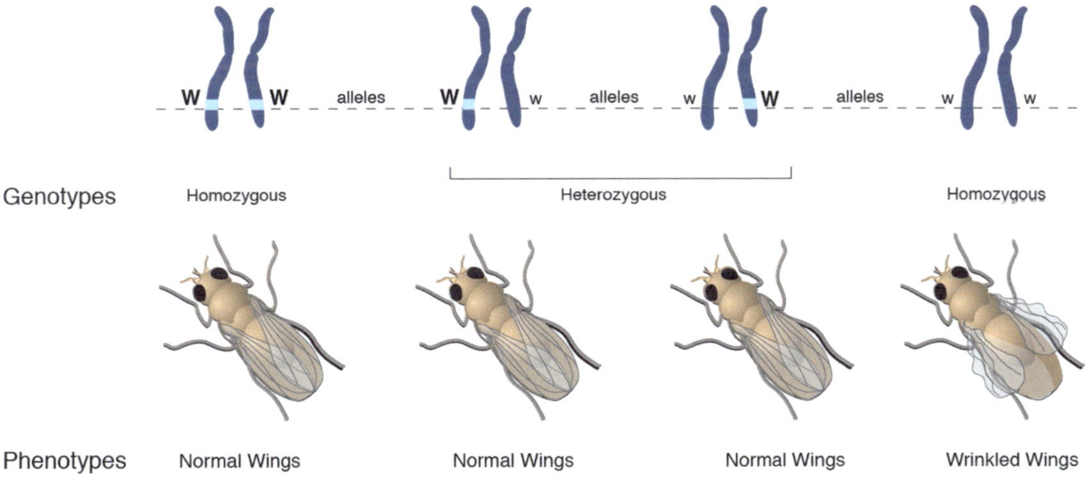

Figure IV.A.15.1: Genotype vs. phenotype; dominant allele W, recessive allele w, in a fly. (Courtesy: National Human Genome Research Institute)

15.2 ABO Blood Types

Codominance occurs when multiple alleles exist for a particular gene and more than one is dominant. When a dominant allele is combined with a recessive allele, the phenotype of the recessive allele is completely masked. But when two dominant alleles are present, the contributions of both alleles do not overpower each other and the phenotype is the result of the expression of both alleles. A classic example of codominance is the ABO blood type in humans.

Red blood cells can have various antigens (BIO 8.1) or *agglutinogens* on their plasma membranes which aid in blood typing. The important two are antigens A and B. If the red blood cells have only antigen A, the blood type is A; if they have only antigen B, then the blood type is B; if they have both antigens, the blood type is AB; if neither antigen is present, the blood type is O. There are three allelic genes in the population (I^A, I^B, i^O). Two are codominant (I^A, I^B) and one is recessive (i^O). Thus in a given population, there are six possible genotypes which result in four possible phenotypes:

Genotype	*Phenotype*
I^AI^A, I^Ai^O	blood type A
I^BI^B, I^Bi^O	blood type B
I^AI^B	blood type AB
i^Oi^O	blood type O

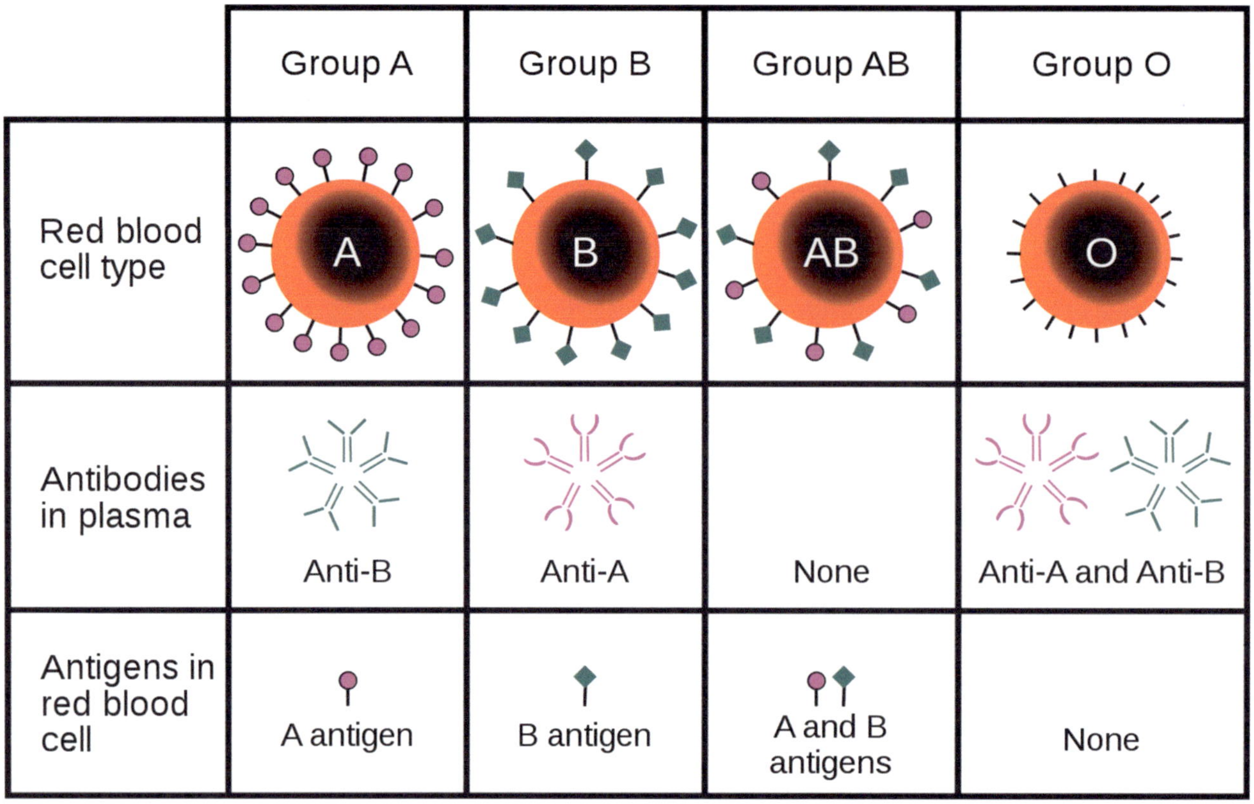

Figure IV.A.15.2: Diagram of the ABO blood groups, the antigens and the antibodies (IgM; BIO 8.2) present in each.

Blood typing is critical before doing a blood transfusion. This is because people with blood type A have anti-B antibodies, those with type B have anti-A, those with type AB have neither antibody, while type O has both anti-A and anti-B antibodies. If a person with type O blood is given types A, B, or AB, the clumping of the red blood cells will occur (= *agglutination*). Though type O can only <u>receive</u> from type O, it can <u>give</u> to the other blood types since its red blood cells have no antigens {type <u>O</u> = universal d<u>o</u>n<u>o</u>r}. Type AB has neither antibody to react against A or B antigens so it can receive blood from all blood types {type AB = universal recipient}.

The only other antigens which have some importance are the <u>Rh factors</u> which are coded by different genes at different loci from the A and B antigens. Rh factors are either there (Rh^+) or they are not there (Rh^-). 85% of the population are Rh^+. The problem occurs when a woman is Rh^- and has been exposed to Rh^+ blood and then forms anti-Rh^+ antibodies (note: unlike the previous case, exposure is necessary to produce these antibodies). If this woman is pregnant with an Rh^+ fetus her antibodies may cross the placenta and cause the fetus' red blood cells to agglutinate (*erythroblastosis fetalis*). This condition is fatal if left untreated.

15.3 Mendelian Genetics

Recall that in gametogenesis homologous chromosomes separate during the first meiotic division. Thus alleles that code for the same trait are segregated: this is **Mendel's First Law of Segregation. Mendel's Second Law of Independent Assortment** states that different chromosomes (*or factors which carry different traits*) separate independently of each other. For example, consider a primary spermatocyte (2*n*) undergoing its first meiotic division. It is not the case that all 23 chromosomes of paternal origin will end up in one secondary spermatocyte while the other 23 chromosomes of maternal origin ends up in the other. Rather, each chromosome in a homologous pair separates *independently* of any other chromosome in other homologous pairs.

However, it has been noted experimentally that sometimes traits on the same chromosome assort independently! This non-Mendelian concept is a result of *crossing over* (recall that this is when homologous chromosomes exchange parts, BIO 14.2). In fact, it has been shown that two traits located far apart on a chromosome are more likely to cross over and thus assort independently, as compared to two traits that are close. The propensity for some traits to refrain from assorting independently is called linkage. Double crossovers occur when two crossovers happen in a chromosomal region being studied.

Another exception to Mendel's laws involves **sex linkage**. Mendel's laws would predict that the results of a genetic cross should be the same regardless of which parent introduces the allele. However, it can be shown that some traits follow the inheritance of the sex chromosomes. Humans have one pair of sex chromosomes (XX = female, XY = male), and the remaining 22 pairs of homologous chromosomes are called **autosomes**.

Since females have two X chromosomes and males have only one, a single recessive allele carried on an X chromosome could be expressed in a male since there is no second allele present to mask it. When males inherit one copy of the recessive allele from an X chromosome, they will express the trait. In contrast, females must inherit two copies to express the trait. Therefore, an X-linked recessive phenotype is much more frequently found in males than females. In fact, a typical pattern of sex linkage is when a mother passes her phenotype to all her sons but **none** of her daughters. Her daughters become *carriers* for the recessive allele. Certain forms of hemophilia, colourblindness, and one kind of muscular dystrophy are well-known recessive sex-linked traits. {In what was once known as Lyon's Hypothesis, it has been shown that every female has a condensed, inactivated X chromosome in her body or somatic cells called a Barr body.}

Let us examine the predictions of Mendel's First Law. Consider two parents, one homozygous dominant (AA) and the other homozygous recessive (aa). Each parent can only form one type of gamete with respect to that trait (*either* A *or* a, *respectively*). The next generation (*called first filial or* $\mathbf{F_1}$) must then be uniformly heterozygotes or *hybrids* (Aa). Now the F_1 hybrids can produce gametes that can be either A *half the time* or a *half the time*. When the F_1 generation is self-crossed, i.e. Aa X Aa, the F_2 generation will be more genotypically and phenotypically diverse and we can predict the outcome in the next generation (F_2) using a Punnett square:

	1/2 A	1/2 a
1/2 A	1/4 AA	1/4 Aa
1/2 a	1/4 Aa	1/4 aa

Here is an example as to how you derive the information within the square: when you cross A with A you get AA (i.e. 1/2 A × 1/2 A = 1/4 AA). Thus by doing a simple *mono*hybrid cross (Aa × Aa) with random mating, the Punnett square indicates that in the F_2 generation, 1/4 of the population would be AA, 1/2 would be Aa (1/4 + 1/4), and 1/4 would be aa. In other words the *genotypic* ratio of homozygous dominant to heterozygous to homozygous recessive is 1:2:1. However, since AA and Aa demonstrate the same *phenotype* (i.e. dominant) the ratio of dominant phenotype to recessive phenotype is 3:1.

Now we will consider the predictions of Mendel's Second Law. To examine independent assortment, we will have to consider a case with two traits (usu. on different chromosomes) or a *di*hybrid cross. Imagine a parent which is homozygous dominant for two traits (AABB) while the other is homozygous recessive (aabb). Each parent can only form one type of gamete with respect to those traits (*either* AB *or* ab, *respectively*). The F_1 generation will be uniform for the dominant trait (i.e. *the genotypes would all be* AaBb). In the gametes of the F_1 generation, the alleles will assort independently. Consequently, an equal amount of all the possible gametes will form: 1/4 AB, 1/4 Ab, 1/4 aB, and 1/4 ab. When the F_1 generation is self-crossed, i.e. AaBb X AaBb, we can predict the outcome in the F_2 generation using the Punnett square:

	1/4 AB	1/4 Ab	1/4 aB	1/4 ab
1/4 AB	1/16 AABB	1/16 AABb	1/16 AaBB	1/16 AaBb
1/4 Ab	1/16 AABb	1/16 AAbb	1/16 AaBb	1/16 Aabb
1/4 aB	1/16 AaBB	1/16 AaBb	1/16 aaBB	1/16 aaBb
1/4 ab	1/16 AaBb	1/16 Aabb	1/16 aaBb	1/16 aabb

Thus by doing a dihybrid cross with random mating, the Punnett square indicates that there are nine possible genotypes (*the frequency is given in brackets*): AABB (1), AABb (2), AaBb (4), AaBB (2), Aabb (2), aaBb (2), AAbb (1), aaBB (1), and aabb (1). Since A and B are dominant, there are only four phenotypic classes in the ratio 9:3:3:1 which are: the expression of both traits (AABB + AABb + AaBb + AaBB = 9), the expression of only the first trait (AAbb + Aabb = 3), the expression of only the second trait (aaBB + aaBb = 3), and the expression of neither trait (aabb = 1). Now we know, for example, that 9/16 represents that fraction of the population which will have the phenotype of both dominant traits.

15.3.1 A Word about Probability

If you were to flip a quarter, the probability of getting "heads" is 50% ($p = 0.5$). If you flipped the quarter ten times and each time it came up heads, the probability of getting heads on the next trial is still 50%. After all, previous trials have no effect on the next trial.

Since chance events, such as fertilisation of a particular kind of egg by a particular kind of sperm, occur independently, the genotype of one child has no effect on the genotypes of other children produced by a set of parents. Thus in the previous example of the dihybrid cross, the chance of producing the genotype AaBb is 4/16 (25%) irrespective of the genotypes which have already been produced. For more about probability, *see* GM 6.1.

15.4 The Hardy-Weinberg Law

The Hardy-Weinberg Law deals with population genetics. A **population** includes all the members of a species which occupy a more or less well defined geographical area and have demonstrated the ability to reproduce from generation to generation. A **gene pool** is the sum of all the unique alleles for a given population. A central component to evolution is the changing of alleles in a gene pool from one generation to the next.

Evolution can be viewed as a changing of gene frequencies within a population over successive generations. The Hardy-Weinberg Law or *equilibrium* predicts the outcome of a randomly mating population of sexually reproducing diploid organisms who are not undergoing evolution.

For the Hardy-Weinberg Law to be applied, the idealised population must meet the following conditions: i) **random mating**: the members of the population must have no mating preferences; ii) **no mutations**: there must be no errors in replication nor similar event resulting in a change in the genome; iii) **isolation**: there must be no exchange of genes between the population being considered and any other population; iv) **large population**: since the law is based on statistical probabilities, to avoid sampling errors, the population cannot be small; v) **no selection pressures**: there must be no reproductive advantage of one allele over the other.

To illustrate a use of the law, consider an idealised population that abides by the preceding conditions and has a gene locus occupied by either A or a. Let p = the frequency of allele A in the population and let q = the frequency of allele a. Since they are the only alleles, p + q = 1. Squaring both sides we get:

$$(p + q)^2 = (1)^2$$

OR

$$p^2 + 2pq + q^2 = 1$$

The preceding equation (= *the Hardy-Weinberg equation*) can be used to calculate genotype frequencies once the allelic frequencies are given. This can be summarised by the following:

	pA	qa
pA	p^2AA	pqAa
qa	pqAa	q^2aa

The Punnett square illustrates the expected frequencies of the three genotypes in the next generation: AA = p^2, Aa = 2pq, and aa = q^2.

For example, let us calculate the percentage of heterozygous individuals in a population where the recessive allele q has a frequency of 0.2. Since p + q = 1, then p = 0.8. Using the Hardy-Weinberg equation and squaring p and q we get:

$$0.64 + 2pq + 0.04 = 1$$

$$2pq = 1 - 0.68 = 0.32$$

Thus the percentage of heterozygous (2pq) individuals is 32%.

A practical application of the Hardy-Weinberg equation is the prediction of how many people in a generation are carriers for a particular recessive allele. The values would have to be recalculated for every generation since humans do not abide by all the conditions of the Hardy-Weinberg Law (i.e. *humans continually evolve*).

15.4.1 Back Cross, Test Cross

A back cross is the cross of an individual (F_1) with one of its parents (P) or an organism with the same genotype as a parent. Back crosses can be used to help identify the genotypes of the individual in a specific type of back cross called a test cross. A test cross is a cross between an organism whose genotype for a certain trait is unknown and an organism that is homozygous recessive for that trait so the unknown genotype can be determined from that of the offspring. For example, for P: AA x aa and F_1: Aa, we get:

Backcross #1: Aa x AA
Progeny #1: 1/2 Aa and 1/2 AA

Backcross #2: Aa x aa
Progeny #2: 1/2 Aa and 1/2 aa

15.5 Genetic Variability

Meiosis and mutations are sources of genetic variability. During meiosis I, crossing over occurs between the paternal and maternal genes which leads to a recombination of parental genes yielding unique haploid gametes. Thus recombination can result in alleles of linked traits separating into different gametes. However, the closer two traits are on a chromosome, the more likely they will be linked and thus remain together, and vice versa.

Further recombination occurs during the random fusion of gametes during fertilisation. Consequently, taking Mendel's two laws and recombination together, we can predict that parents can give their offspring combinations of alleles which the parents never had. This leads to **genetic variability**.

Mutations are rare, inheritable, random changes in the genetic material (DNA) of a cell. Mutations are much more likely to be either neutral (esp. *silent mutations*) or negative (i.e. cancer) than positive for an organism's survival. Nonetheless, such a change in the genome increases genetic variability. Only mutations of gametes, and not somatic cells, are passed on to offspring.

The following are some forms of mutations:

- **Point mutation** is a change affecting a single base pair in a gene
- **Deletion** is the removal of a sequence of DNA, the regions on either side being joined together
- **Inversion** is the reversal of a segment of DNA
- **Translocation** is when one chromosome breaks and attaches to another
- **Duplication** is when a sequence of DNA is repeated.
- **Frame shift mutations** occur when bases are added or deleted in numbers other

than multiples of three. Such deletions or additions cause the rest of the sequence to be shifted such that each triplet reading frame is altered.

A mutagen is any substance or agent that can cause a mutation. A mutagen is not the same as a carcinogen. Carcinogens are agents that cause cancer. While many mutagens are carcinogens as well, many others are not. The Ames test is a widely used test to screen chemicals used in foods or medications for mutagenic potential.

Mutations can produce many types of genetic diseases including inborn errors of metabolism. These disorders in normal metabolism are usually due to defects of a single gene that codes for one enzyme.

15.6 Genetics and Heredity: A Closer Look

The rest of this chapter begins to push into more advanced topics in genetics. However, these topics continue to represent legitimate exam material.

Epistasis occurs when one gene masks the phenotype of a second gene. This is often the case in pigmentation where one gene turns on (or off) the production of pigment, while a second gene controls the amount of pigment produced. Such is the case in mice fur where one gene codes for the presence or absence of pigmentation and the other codes for the colour. If C and c represent the alleles for the presence or absence of colour and B and b represent black and brown then a phenotype of CCbb and Ccbb would both correspond to a brown phenotype. Whenever cc is inherited the fur will be white.

Pleiotropy occurs when a single gene has more than one phenotypic expression. This is often seen in pea plants where the gene that expresses round or wrinkled texture of seeds also influences the expression of starch metabolism. For example, in wrinkled seeds there is more unconverted glucose which leads to an increase of the osmotic gradient. These seeds will subsequently contain more water than round seeds. When they mature they will dehydrate and produce the wrinkled appearance.

Polygenic inheritance refers to traits that cannot be expressed in just a few types but rather as a range of varieties. The most popular example would be human height which ranges from very short to very tall. This phenomenon (many genes shaping one phenotype) is the opposite of pleiotropy.

Penetrance refers to the proportion of individuals carrying a particular variant of a gene (allele or genotype) that also express the associated phenotype. Alleles which are highly penetrant are more likely to be noticed. Penetrance only considers whether individuals express the trait or not. *Expressivity* refers to the variation in the degree of expression of a given trait.

Nondisjunction occurs when the chromosomes do not separate properly and do not migrate to opposite poles as in normal anaphase of meiosis (BIO 14.2). This could arise from a failure of homologous chromosomes to separate in meiosis I, or the failure of sister chromatids to separate during meiosis II or mitosis. Most of the time, gametes produced after nondisjunction are sterile; however, certain imbalances can be fertile and lead to genetic defects. Down Syndrome (Trisomy 21 = 3 copies of chromosome 21 due to its nondisjunction, thus the person has an extra chromosome making a total of 47 chromosomes; *see* Fig. IV.A.15.3 below); Turner and Klinefelter Syndrome (nondisjunction of sex chromosomes); and Cri du Chat (deletion in chromosome 5) are well known genetic disorders. Hemophilia and red-green colour blindness are common sex-linked disorders and are recessive.

Phenylketonuria, sickle-cell anemia and Tay-Sachs disease are common autosomal recessive disorders.

Gene linkage refers to genes that reside on the same chromosome and are unable to display independent assortment because they are physically connected (BIO 15.3). The further away the two genes are on the chromosome the higher probability there is that they will crossover during synapsis. In these cases recombination frequencies are used to provide a linkage map where the arrangement of the genes can be ascertained. For example, say you have a fly with genotype BBTTYY and the crossover frequency between B and T is

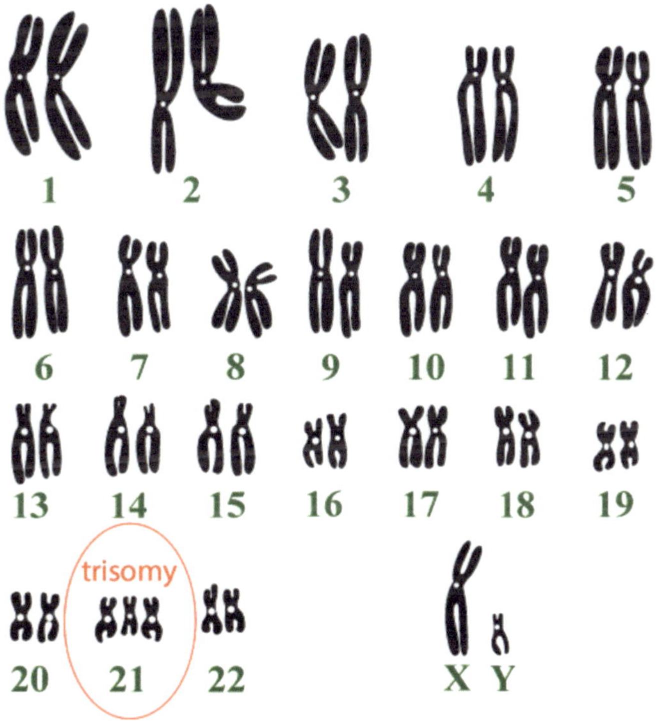

Figure IV.A.15.3: Illustration of a karyotype from a person with Down's syndrome. A karyotype is a picture of one set of chromosomes. First, chromosomes are isolated, then stained, and finally examined under a microscope. A picture of the chromosomes is taken through the microscope. Note the following points regarding the illustration: 47 chromosomes, male, and trisomy 21.

26%, between Y and T is 18% and between B and Y is 8%. Greater recombination frequencies mean greater distances so you know that B and T are the furthest apart. This corresponds to a gene order of B-Y-T and since frequencies are a direct measure of distance you know exactly how far apart each allele is and can easily calculate the map distances.

Twin studies (nature vs. nurture) help to gauge the relative importance of environmental and genetic influences on individuals in a sample. Twins can either be monozygotic ("identical"), meaning that they develop from one zygote (BIO 14.5) that splits and forms two embryos, or dizygotic ("fraternal"), meaning that they develop from two separate eggs, each fertilised by separate sperm cells. Thus fraternal twins are like any 2 siblings from a genetic point of view, but they may share the same environment as they grow up together.

To control for environment, the classical twin study design compares the similarity of monozygotic and dizygotic twins. If identical twins are considerably more similar than fraternal twins (which is found for most traits), this implies that genes play an important role for those specific traits. By comparing hundreds of families of twins, researchers can then understand more about the roles of genetic effects, shared environment, and unique environment in shaping behavior or in the development of disease.

15.6.1 Mitochondrial DNA

Mitochondrial DNA (mtDNA or mDNA) has become increasingly popular as a tool to determine how closely populations are related as well as to clarify the evolutionary relationships among species (= phylogenetics). Mitochondrial DNA is circular (BIO 1.2.2, 16.6.3) and can be regarded as the smallest chromosome. In most species, including humans, mtDNA is inherited solely from the mother. The DNA sequence of mtDNA has been determined from a large number of organisms and individuals (including some organisms that are extinct).

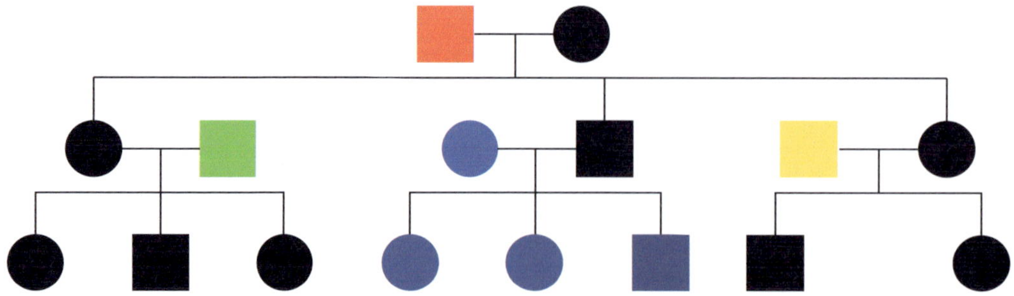

Figure IV.A.15.4: Pedigree ("Family tree"): Maternal inheritance pattern of mtDNA for 3 generations with the grandparents in the top row. As is the standard, circles represent females, squares represent males. Colours show the inheritance of the same mt genome (from mother to offspring, i.e. children). Don't be surprised to see a pedigree of some sort in your practice questions and/or on the real exam.

15.7 DNA Recombination and Genetic Technology

DNA recombination involves DNA that contains segments or genes from different sources. The foreign DNA can come from another DNA molecule, a chromosome or from a complete organism. Most DNA transferred is done artificially using DNA recombination techniques which use restriction enzymes to cut pieces of DNA. These enzymes originate from bacteria and are extremely specific because they only cut DNA at specific recognition sequences along the strand. These recognition sites correspond to different nucleotide sequences and produce sticky and blunt ends when a double stranded DNA segment is cut.

The sticky end is the unpaired part of the DNA that is ready to bind with a complementary codon (sequence of three adjacent nucleotides; BIO 3.0). These cut pieces or **restriction fragments** are often inserted into plasmids (circular piece of DNA that is able to replicate independently of the chromosomal DNA) which are then able to be introduced into the bacteria via transformation (*see* BIO 2.2).

Bacterium and Vector Plasmid

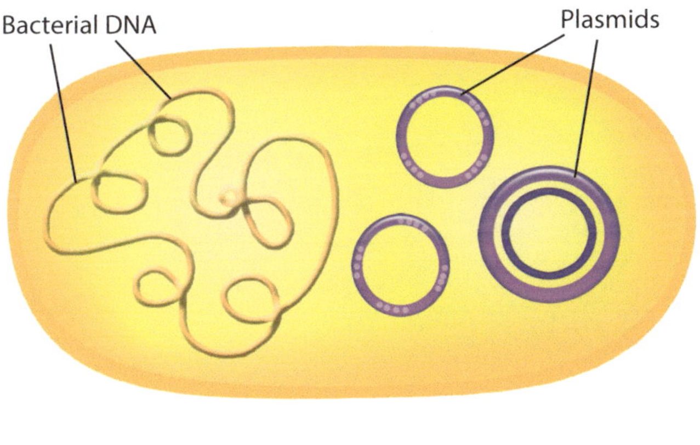

Treating the plasmid, or replicon, with the same restriction enzymes used on the original fragment produces the same sticky ends in both pieces allowing base pairing to occur when they are mixed together. This attachment is stabilised by DNA ligase. After the ends are joined and the recombinant plasmid is incorporated into bacteria, the bacteria become capable of producing copious amounts of a specific protein that was not native to its species (i.e. bacteria with recombinant DNA producing insulin to treat diabetes).

Gel electrophoresis is a method of separating restriction fragments of differing lengths based on their size (as described in the previous section, a restriction fragment is a fragment of DNA cleaved by a restriction enzyme). The DNA fragments are passed through a gel which is under the influence of an electric field. Since DNA is negatively charged it will move towards the cathode (positive electrode). The shorter fragments move faster than the longer ones and can be visualised as a banding pattern using autoradiography techniques.

SDS-PAGE, sodium dodecyl sulfate polyacrylamide gel electrophoresis (ORG 13), also separates proteins according to their electrophoretic mobility. SDS is an anionic detergent (i.e. negatively charged) which has the following effect: **(1)** linearise proteins and **(2)** give an additional negative charge to the linearised proteins. In most proteins, the binding of SDS to the polypeptide chain gives an even distribution of charge per unit mass, thus fractionation will approximate size during electrophoresis (i.e. not dependent on charge).

Restriction fragment length polymorphisms or RFLP is a technique that exploits variations in restriction fragments from one individual to another that differ in length due to polymorphisms, or slight differences in DNA sequences. The process involves digesting DNA sequences with different restriction enzymes, detecting the resulting restriction fragments by gel electrophoresis, and comparing their lengths. In DNA fingerprinting, commonly used to analyse DNA left at crime scenes, RFLP's are produced and compared to RFLP's of known suspects in order to catch the perpetrator.

Sometimes it is necessary to obtain the DNA fragment bearing the required gene directly from the mRNA that codes for the polypeptide in question. This is due to the presence of introns (non-coding regions on a DNA

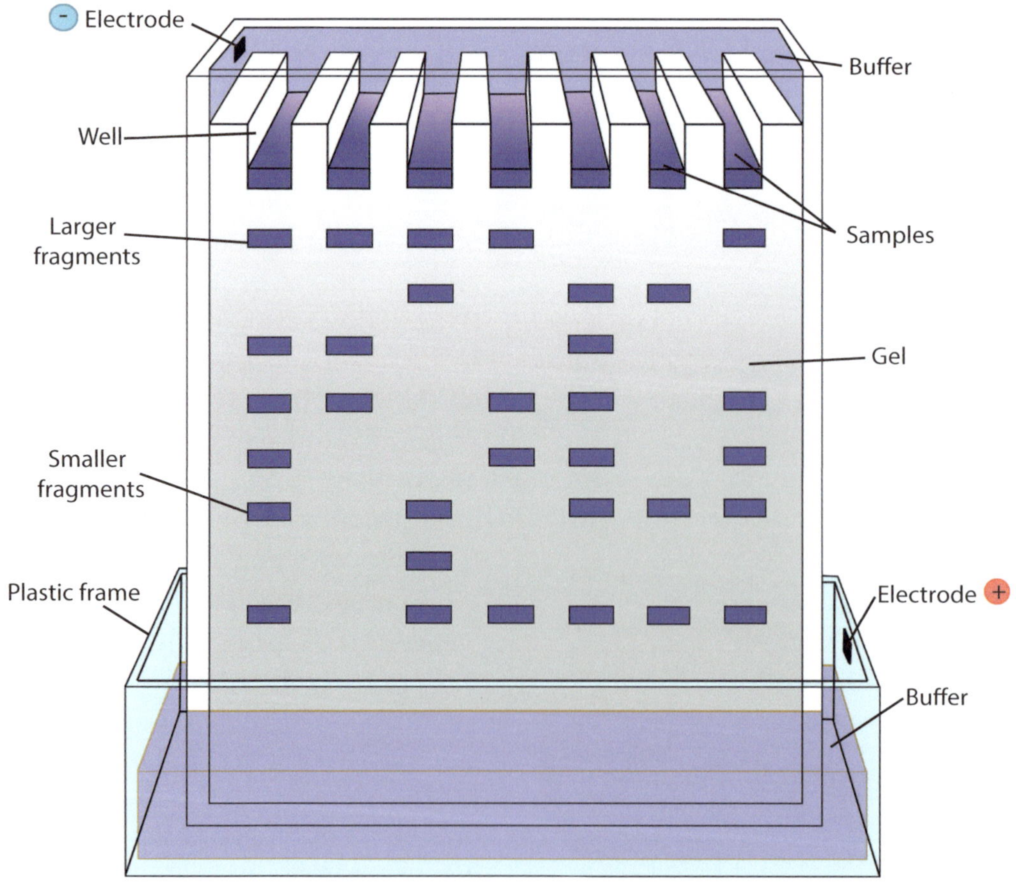

Figure IV.A.15.5: Gel Electrophoresis.

molecule; BIO 3.0) which prevent transcription of foreign genes in the genome of bacteria, a common problem in recombinant technology. To carry this out one can use reverse transcriptase producing complementary DNA (cDNA) which lack the problematic introns.

Rather than using a bacterium to clone DNA fragments, sometimes DNA is copied directly using the polymerase chain reaction (PCR). This method allows us to rapidly amplify the DNA content using synthetic primers that initiate replication at specific nucleotide sequences. This method relies on thermal cycling (repeated heating and cooling) of the DNA primers and can lead to thousands and even millions of copies in relatively short periods of time.

Southern blotting, named after Dr. E. Southern, is the process of transferring DNA fragments from the electrophoresis agarose gel onto filter paper where they are identified with probes. The procedure begins by digesting DNA in a mixture with *restriction endonucleases* to cut out specific pieces of DNA. The DNA fragments are then subjected to gel electrophoresis. The now separated fragments are bathed in an alkaline solution where they immediately begin to denature. These fragments are then placed (or blotted) onto nitrocellulose paper and then incubated with a specific probe whose location can be visualised with autoradiography.

Northern blotting is adapted from the Southern blot to detect specific sequences of RNA by hybridisation with cDNA. Similarly, *Western blotting* is used to identify specific amino-acid sequences in proteins. Since this is not required for you to memorise for the GAMSAT, you may want to set aside this mnemonic for when you are attending medical school: SNOW DROP.

SNOW	DROP
Southern	**D**NA
Northern	**R**NA
O	**O**
Western	**P**rotein

DNA microarray technology (= DNA chip or biochip or "laboratory-on-a-chip") helps to determine which genes are active and which are inactive in different cell types. This technology evolved from Southern blotting and can also be used to genotype multiple regions of a genome. DNA microarrays are created by robotic machines that arrange incredibly small amounts of hundreds or thousands of gene sequences on a single microscope slide. These sequences can be a short section of a gene or other DNA element that is used to hybridise a cDNA or cRNA (also called antisense RNA) sample. The hybridisation is usually observed and quantified by the detection of fluorescent tag.

A *gene knockout* is a genetic technique in which one of an organism's genes is made inoperative ("knocked out" of the organism). The same expression can be used with reference to the organism with a gene knockout (e.g., *a knockout mouse*). Two minus signs on either side of a forward slash (-/-) means that both alleles have been knocked out (*homozygous knockout*). If only one allele is missing, then the non-mutant allele that prevails in natural conditions (= the *wild type* allele) would be represented by a plus sign and, again, the missing or knocked out allele by a minus sign (+/-). This *heterozygous* condition can be achieved by, for example, breeding knockout mice with wild type mice.

NB: The molecular biology techniques of FRAP (BIO 1.5) and ELISA (BIO 8.4) were described earlier in this book. Electrophoresis and chromatography are discussed in Organic Chemistry Chapter 13.

CHAPTER 15: Genetics

GOLD STANDARD FOUNDATIONAL GAMSAT PRACTICE QUESTIONS

1) Although the cloned sheep Dolly contains the exact DNA as her genetic mother, there are a few visible and behavioral differences in Dolly. This is most probably due to:

- **A.** the sheep in which the embryo was implanted.
- **B.** the induction of specific genes not expressed in the mother.
- **C.** mutations caused by incubation in the nutrient-deficient solution.
- **D.** environmental factors.

2) In fruit flies, males have XY sex chromosomes, females have XX, and white eye colour is sex linked. If red-eyed (heterozygous) females are crossed with white-eyed males, what would be the expected eye colours and sexes of the progeny?

- **A.** ¾ white-eyed female and ¼ red-eyed male.
- **B.** ½ red-eyed female and ½ white-eyed male.
- **C.** All red eyed, half male and half female.
- **D.** ¼ red-eyed female, ¼ white-eyed female, ¼ red-eyed male and ¼ white-eyed male.

3) Von Willebrand's disease is an autosomal dominant bleeding disorder. A man who does not have the disease has two children with a woman who is heterozygous for the condition. If the first child expresses the bleeding disorder, what is the probability that the second child will have the disease?

- **A.** 0.25
- **B.** 0.50
- **C.** 0.75
- **D.** 1.00

4) Over 10 million North Americans are treated for thyroid diseases and, overwhelmingly, women are much more likely than men to succumb to these conditions. Is it reasonable to conclude that thyroid disease is sex-linked?

- **A.** No, because thyroid disease appears to be caused by a defect of the immune system and not a defective DNA sequence.
- **B.** No, because if the disease was sex-linked, there would be a high incidence in the male, rather than the female, population.
- **C.** Yes, because the high incidence of the disease in women suggests that a gene found on the X chromosome codes for the disease.
- **D.** Yes, because the same factor increases the risk of women getting the disease, regardless of familial background.

GOLD STANDARD GAMSAT-LEVEL PRACTICE QUESTIONS

Questions 5–7

Sickle cell disease (SCD), also known as sickle cell anemia, describes a group of inherited red blood cell disorders. People with SCD have abnormal hemoglobin, called hemoglobin S or *sickle* hemoglobin, in their red blood cells, while the normal variant is hemoglobin A.

SCD is as an autosomal recessive disorder. Having one copy of HbA produces enough normal hemoglobin to prevent anemia. Thus the heterozygous condition, AS, is a carrier and is described as 'sickle cell trait'.

In humans, blood type is a result of multiple alleles: I^A, I^B, and i^O. A few simple rules of blood-type genetics are that:

- I^A is dominant over i^O,
- I^B is dominant over i^O, and
- I^AI^B are codominant.

5) Consider the case in which two parents are heterozygous for type A blood and have sickle cell trait. What is the genotype of the parents?

A. I^Ai^OAS
B. I^Ai^AAS
C. I^Ai^OSS
D. I^Ai^OAA

6) Which of the following does NOT represent a genotype likely to be present in the gametes of the parents described in the previous question?

A. I^AA
B. i^OA
C. i^OS
D. All of the above are likely.

7) Which of the following ratios best represents the likelihood that the parents previously described would have offspring with blood type O and sickle cell trait?

A. 9/16
B. 3/16
C. 2/16
D. 1/16

8) The genes in the intestinal bacterium *E. Coli*, in alphabetical order: ade, ilv, rad, and trp, all map onto the same chromosome. Pairwise crosses between single mutants give the frequencies of wild type recombinants provided in Table 1. Which of the following represents the most likely correct order in which the four genes lie along the chromosome?

	rad	ade	ilv	trp
rad	0	10.2	7.8	3.4
ade	10.3	0	3.3	4.8
ilv	7.6	4.0	0	2.8
trp	3.1	7.0	2.8	0

Table 1

A. ade-trp-ilv-rad
B. ilv-ade-trp-rad
C. trp-rad-ilv-ade
D. rad-trp-ilv-ade

Questions 9–12

The polymerase chain reaction (PCR) is a powerful biological tool that allows the rapid amplification of any fragment of DNA without purification. In PCR, RNA primers are made to flank the specific DNA sequence to be amplified. These RNA primers are then extended to the end of the DNA molecule with the use of a heat-resistant DNA polymerase. The newly synthesised DNA strand is then used as the template to undergo another round of replication.

The 1st step in PCR is the melting of the target DNA into 2 single strands by heating the reaction mixture to approximately 94 °C, and then rapidly cooling the mixture to allow annealing of the RNA primers to their specific locations (note: annealing is the sticking together of complementary single strands which, of course, involves the formation of hydrogen bonds between the base pairs; BIO 1.2.2). Once the primer has annealed, the temperature is elevated to 72 °C to allow optimal activity of the DNA polymerase. The polymerase will continue to add nucleotides until the entire complimentary strand of the template is completed at which point the cycle is repeated (Figure 1).

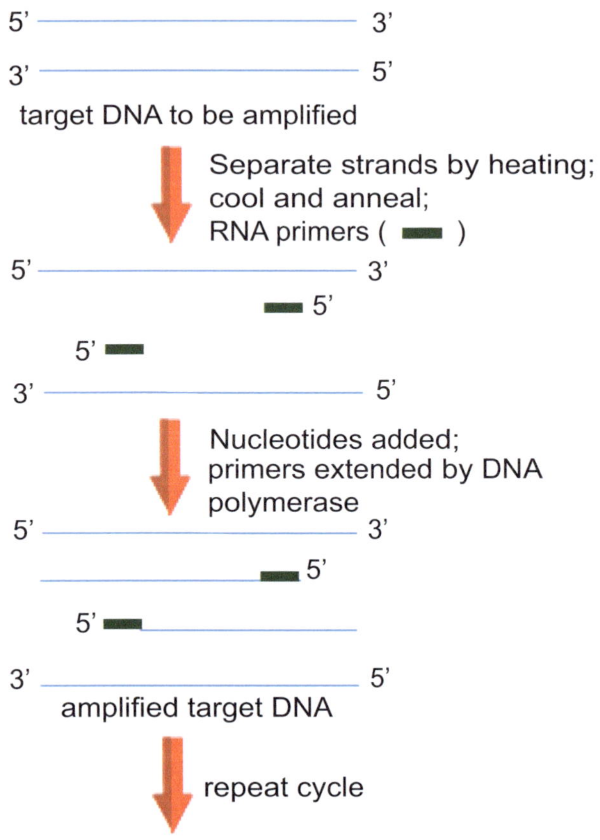

Figure 1

One of the uses of PCR is sex determination, which requires amplification of intron 1 of the amelogenin gene. This gene found on the X-Y homologous chromosomes has a 184 base pair deletion on the Y homologue. Therefore, by amplifying intron 1, females can be distinguished from males by the fact that males will have 2 different sizes of the amplified DNA while females will only have 1 unique fragment size.

9) The polymerase chain reaction resembles which of the following cellular process?

- **A.** Transcription of DNA
- **B.** Protein synthesis
- **C.** DNA replication
- **D.** Translation

10) Why is a heat resistant DNA polymerase required for successive replication in the polymerase chain reaction, rather than simply a human DNA polymerase?

- **A.** The high temperatures required to melt the DNA double strand may denature a normal human cellular DNA polymerase.
- **B.** The high temperatures required to melt the DNA would cause human DNA polymerase to remain bound to the DNA strand.
- **C.** Heat resistant DNA polymerase increases the rate of the polymerase chain reaction at high temperatures whereas human DNA polymerase lowers the rate.
- **D.** Heat resistant DNA polymerase recognises RNA primers whereas human DNA polymerase does not.

11) The use of PCR for sex determination relies on the fact that:

A. the amelogenin gene is responsible for an autosomal recessive trait.

B. the X and Y homologous chromosomes have different sizes of intron 1 of the amelogenin gene.

C. females have an X and Y chromosome and males have two X chromosomes.

D. intron 1 has a different nucleotide length than intron 2.

12) What would PCR amplification of an individual's intron 1 of the amelogenin gene reveal if the individual were male?

A. One type of intron 1 since the individual has one X chromosome and one Y chromosome.

B. Two types of intron 1 since the individual has only one X chromosome.

C. One type of intron 1 since the individual has only one X chromosome.

D. Two types of intron 1 since the individual has one X chromosome and one Y chromosome.

13) The autosomal dominant gene Curly (CY) of the fruit fly *Drosophila melanogaster* results in adult flies with abnormal wings that curl up when the inactive form (*the pupae*) are maintained at 25 °C, but remain uncurled when the pupae are kept at 19 °C. Consider the F_1 generation of a cross between two flies heterozygous for curly wings. What would be the expected percentage of F_1 flies with normal (uncurled) wings when the pupae are maintained at either 19 °C or 25 °C?

A. 100% uncurled at 19 °C; 75% uncurled at 25 °C

B. 100% uncurled at 19 °C; 25% uncurled at 25 °C

C. 75% uncurled at 19 °C; 25% uncurled at 25 °C

D. 25% uncurled at 19 °C; 75% uncurled at 25 °C

Questions 14–15

Sickle cell anemia in humans is an example of a mutation affecting a base in one of the genes involved in the production of hemoglobin. Hemoglobin, in adults, is made up of four polypeptide chains attached to the prosthetic group heme. The polypeptide chains influence the oxygen carrying capacity of the molecule. A change in the base sequence of the triplet coding for one amino acid out of the normal 146 amino acids in the beta chains gives rise to the production of sickle cell hemoglobin. The physiological effect of this is to lower the oxygen-carrying capacity of these red blood cells. In the heterozygous condition individuals show the sickle-cell trait. The red blood cells appear normal and only about 40% of the hemoglobin is abnormal.

A gene represented by two or more alleles within a population is said to be *polymorphic*. Allelic differences are caused by sequence differences, that is, the DNA itself is polymorphic and results in sequence differences between homologous regions of DNA in different individuals. These differences can be detected even when no other differences can be found and knowledge of this polymorphism could be used for the pre- or postnatal diagnosis for the sickle-cell gene.

Rather than directly sequencing a gene, differences called restriction fragment length polymorphisms (RFLPs) can be used to highlight the regions of sequence differences between individuals. The technique depends on a restriction enzyme making a cut at a site on the gene for normal hemoglobin, not present on sickle-cell hemoglobin, causing fragments cut by the given enzyme to be smaller than it is in individuals not possessing the site.

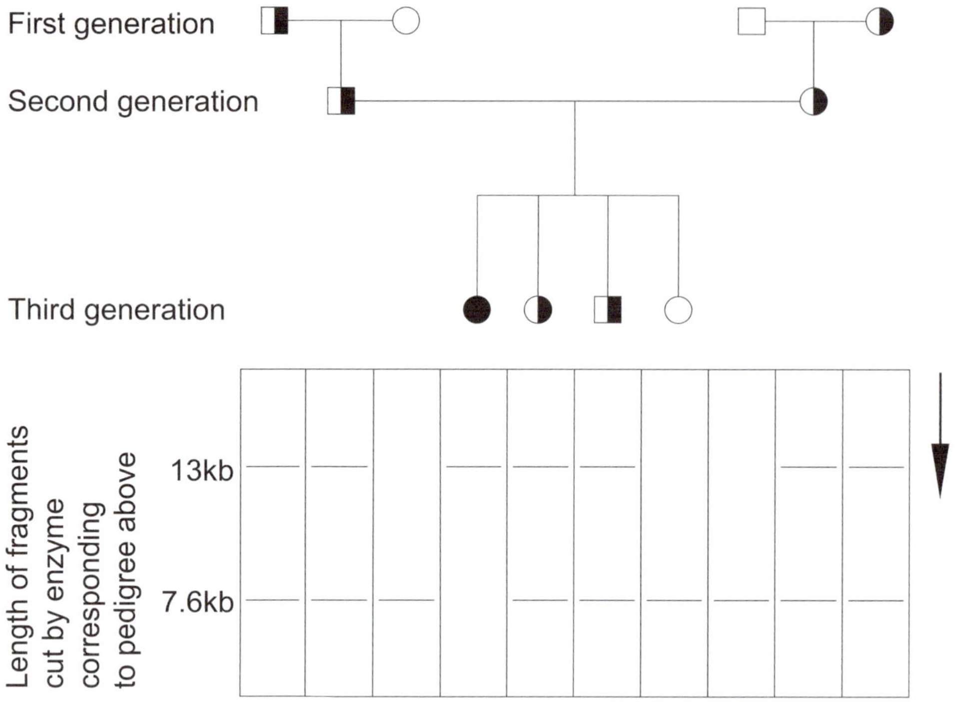

Figure 1: Inheritance pattern of an RFLP associated with sickle-cell disease. Males are represented by squares and females by circles. An open square or circle indicates an individual who is homozygous normal. A half-filled square or circle indicates an individual with sickle-cell trait. A filled square or circle indicates a homozygous individual with sickle-cell disease. The direction of electrophoresis is indicated by an arrow.

14) Figure 1 indicates that the fragment cut by the restriction enzyme in an individual who is homozygous for the sickle-cell condition is:

A. 7.6 kb long.
B. 13 kb long.
C. 20.6 kb long.
D. 5.4 kb long.

15) If the heterozygous male in the first generation in Figure 1 was substituted with a homozygous male for the normal condition, the phenotypes of the third generation would be expected to be in the ratio of:

A. 1 normal : 2 sickle-cell trait : 1 sickle-cell disease.
B. 1 normal : 1 sickle-cell trait.
C. 2 normal : 1 sickle-cell trait : 1 sickle-cell disease.
D. 1 sickle-cell trait : 1 sickle-cell disease.

Bonus Question!

16) The Hardy–Weinberg principle, or law, states that allele and genotype frequencies in a population will remain constant from generation to generation in the absence of other evolutionary influences. For example, consider an idealised population that abides by certain conditions and has a gene locus occupied by either the dominant gene 'A' or the recessive gene 'a'. Let p = the frequency of allele 'A' in the population, and let q = the frequency of allele 'a'. Since they are the only alleles, then p + q = 1. Squaring both sides we get:

$(p + q)^2 = (1)^2$ and thus

$p^2 + 2pq + q^2 = 1$.

Consider Figure 1.

According to Figure 1, what is the frequency of the heterozygous state?

A. 0.36
B. 0.4
C. 0.48
D. 0.6

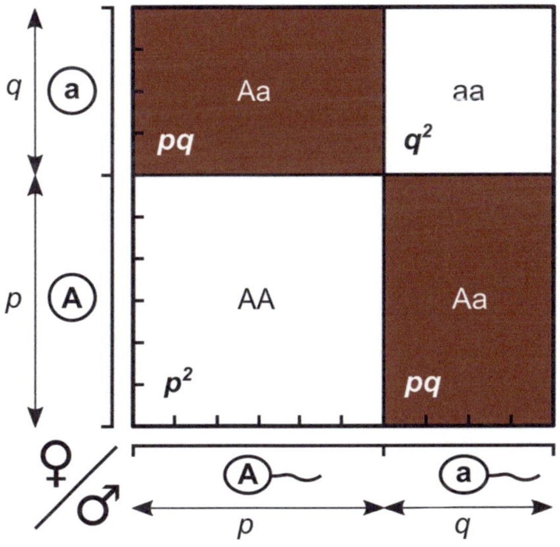

Figure 1: Allele frequencies in a model population

SPOILER ALERT

Gold Standard has cross-referenced the content in this chapter to examples from ACER's official GAMSAT practice materials. It is for you to decide when you want to explore these questions since you may want to preserve some of ACER's materials for timed mock-exam practice.

Examples – Dihybrid cross: Q16-17 of 1; monohybrid cross: Q23-26 of 2; genotype/phenotype: Q1-4 of 3; pedigree with dihybrid cross: Q24-26 of 4; dihybrid cross Q54-56 of 5. Note that "Q" is followed by the question number, and, for example, "of 1" refers to booklet number 1 which is referenced in the Spoiler Alert table at the end of Chapter 1. The 15 full-length GAMSAT practice tests by Gold Standard, HEAPS-1 through HEAPS-15, contain specific cross-references to this chapter within the worked solutions. Note that the dihybrid-cross, sickle-cell unit is a rare treat from HEAPS-1; the pedigree analysis is from HEAPS-7. Side note: HEAPS-1 also has a heavy meiosis/crossing over unit with recurring concepts.

High-level Importance

Chapter Checklist

- ☐ Access your online account to view answers, worked solutions and discussion boards.
- ☐ Reassess your 'learning objectives' for this chapter: Go back to the first page of this chapter and re-evaluate the top 3 boxes and the Introduction.
- ☐ Complete a maximum of 1 page of notes using symbols/abbreviations to represent the entire chapter based on your learning objectives. These are your Gold Notes.
- ☐ Consider your multimedia options based on your optimal way of learning:
    - ☐ Download the free Gold Standard GAMSAT app for your Android device or iPhone.
    - ☐ Create your own, tangible study cards or try the free app: Anki.
    - ☐ Record your voice reading your Gold Notes onto your smartphone (audio files, e.g., *memo* or MP3s) and listen during exercise, transportation, etc.
    - ☐ Try out the Gold Standard GAMSAT online videos at gamsat-prep.com, or you can try other options on YouTube like Khan Academy or Crash Course Biology.
- ☐ Reassess your schedule for your full-length GAMSAT practice tests: ACER and/or HEAPS exams. Ensure that you have scheduled one full day to complete a practice test and 1-2 days for a thorough assessment of worked solutions while adding to your abbreviated Gold Notes.
- ☐ Reassess your progress in scheduling and/or evaluating stress reduction techniques such as regular exercise (sports), yoga, meditation and/or mindfulness exercises (*see* YouTube for suggestions).

How can you distinguish the sex chromosomes? Pull down their genes! :)

EVOLUTION

Chapter 16

Memorise	Understand	Importance
* Define: species	* Natural selection, speciation * Genetic drift * Basics: origin of life * Basics: comparative anatomy * Analogous structures vs. homologous structures	**Low level: 0% of GAMSAT Biology** questions released by ACER are related to content in this chapter (in our estimation). * Note that approximately 75% of the questions in GAMSAT Biology are related to just 7 chapters: 1, 2, 3, 4, 7, 12, and 15.

GAMSAT-Prep.com

Introduction

Evolution is, quite simply, the change in the inherited traits of a population of organisms from one generation to another. This change over time can be traced to 3 main processes: variation, reproduction and selection. The major mechanisms that drive evolution are natural selection and genetic drift. As you have done before, get familiar with the basics and then the practice questions will have you exercising your reasoning and graph-analysis skills which you can apply to many other GAMSAT-question types and topics.

Multimedia Resources at GAMSAT-Prep.com

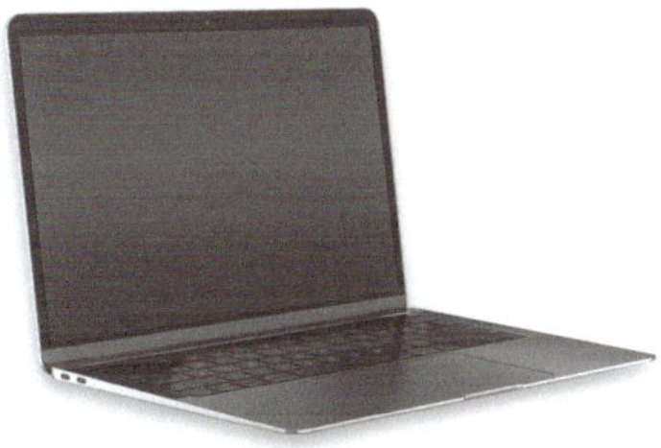

Open Discussion Boards
(*gamsat-prep.com/forum*)

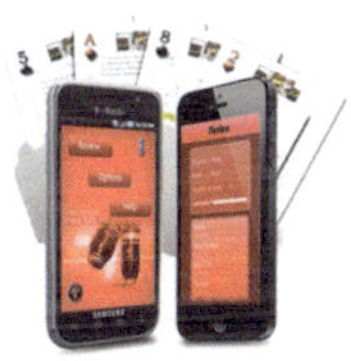

Flashcards

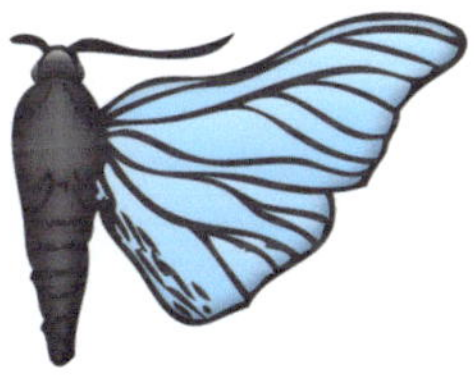

Special Guest

* The real GAMSAT may have advanced-level information presented (i.e. in a passage) but previous knowledge of said information is not required to answer the questions that would follow. Practice questions at the end of this chapter, as well as ACER and GS (HEAPS) practice GAMSATs can help you clarify this point.

16.1 Overview

Evolution is the change in frequency of one or more alleles in a population's gene pool from one generation to the next. The evidence for evolution lies in the fossil record, biogeography, embryology, comparative anatomy, and experiments from artificial selection. The most important mechanism of evolution is the **selection** of certain phenotypes provided by the **genetic variability** of a population.

16.2 Natural Selection

Natural selection is the non-random differential survival and reproduction from one generation to the next. Natural selection contains the following premises: i) genetic and phenotypic variability exist in populations: offspring show variations compared to parents; ii) more individuals are produced than live to grow up and reproduce; iii) the population competes to survive; iv) individuals with some genes are more likely to survive (greater fitness) than those with other genes; v) individuals that are more likely to survive transmit these favorable variations (genes) to their offspring so that these genes become more dominant in the gene pool.

It is not necessarily true that natural selection leads to the the Darwin-era expression "survival of the fittest"; rather it is the genes, and not necessarily the individual, which are likely to survive.

Evolution goes against the foundations of the Hardy-Weinberg Law. For example, natural selection leads to non-random mating due to phenotypic differences. Evolution occurs when those phenotypic changes depend on an underlying genotype; thus non-random mating can lead to changes in allelic frequencies. Consider an example: if female peacocks decide to only mate with a male with long feathers, then there will be a selection pressure against any male with a genotype which is expressed as short feathers. Because of this differential reproduction, the alleles which are expressed as short feathers will be eliminated from the population. Thus this population evolves.

The three forms of natural selection are: i) **stabilising selection** in which genetic diversity decreases as the population stabilises on an average phenotype (*phenotypes have a "bell curve" distribution*). This is the most common form of natural selection. It is basically the opposite of disruptive selection, instead of favoring individuals with extreme phenotypes, it favors the intermediate phenotype; ii) **directional selection** when an extreme phenotype has a selective advantage over the average phenotype causing the allele frequency continually shifting in one direction (*thus the curve can become skewed to the left or right*). It occurs most often when populations migrate to new areas with environmental pressures; iii) **disruptive**

Low-level Importance

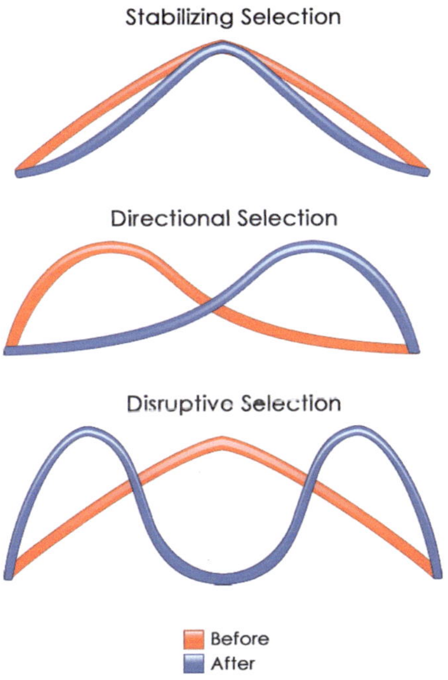

selection where both extremes are selected over the average phenotype; this would produce a split down the middle of the "bell curve" such that two new and separate "bell curves" would result.

For example, if a bird only ate medium sized seeds and left the large and small ones alone, two new populations or groups of seeds would have a reproductive advantage. Thus by selecting against the group of medium sized seeds, two new groups of large and small seeds will result. This is an example of group selection causing *disruptive selection*.

16.3 Species and Speciation

Species can be defined as the members of populations that interbreed or can interbreed under natural conditions. There are great variations within species. A **cline** is a gradient of variation in a species across a geographical area. **Speciation** is the evolution of new species by the isolation of gene pools of related populations. The isolation of gene pools is typically geographic. An ocean, a glacier, a river or any other physical barrier can isolate a population and prevent it from mating with other populations of the same species. The two populations may begin to differ because their mutations may be different, or, there may be different selection pressures from the two different environments, or, *genetic drift* may play a role.

Genetic drift is the random change in frequencies of alleles or genotypes in a population (recall that this is antagonistic to the Hardy-Weinberg Law). Genetic drift normally occurs when a small population is isolated from a large population. Since the allelic frequencies in the small population may be different from the large population (*sampling error*), the two populations may evolve in different directions.

Populations or species can be sympatric, in which speciation occurs after ecological, genetic or behavioral barriers arise within the same geographical boundary of a single population, or allopatric, in which speciation occurs through geographical isolation of

Low-level Importance

groups from the parent population {Sympatric = live together, Allopatric = live apart}. Mechanisms involved in allopatric speciation are represented in the two preceding paragraphs.

The following represents some isolating mechanisms that prevent sympatric populations of different species from breeding together: **i)** habitat differences; **ii)** different breeding times or seasons; **iii)** mechanical differences (i.e. different anatomy of the genitalia); **iv)** behavioral specificity (i.e. different courtship behavior); **v)** gametic isolation (= fertilisation cannot occur); **vi)** hybrid inviability (i.e. the hybrid zygote dies before reaching the age of sexual maturity); **vii)** hybrid sterility; **viii)** hybrid breakdown: the hybrid offspring is fertile but produces a next generation (F_2) which is infertile or inviable.

16.4 Origin of Life

Evidence suggests that the primitive earth had a reducing atmosphere with gases such as H_2 and the reduced compounds H_2O (vapor), $NH_{3(g)}$ (ammonia) and $CH_{4(g)}$ (methane). Such an atmosphere has been shown (i.e. Miller, Fox) to be conducive to the formation and stabilisation of organic compounds. Such compounds can sometimes polymerise (*possibly due to autocatalysis*) and evolve into living systems with metabolism, reproduction, digestion, excretion, etc.

Critical in the early history of the earth was the evolution of: **(1)** the reducing atmosphere powered with energy (e.g. lightening, UV radiation, outgassing volcanoes) converting reduced compounds (water, ammonia, methane) into simple organic molecules (the 'primordial soup'); **(2)** self-replicating molecules surrounded by membranes forming protocells (very primitive microspheres, coacervates assembling into the precursor of prokaryotic cells: protobionts); **(3)** chemosynthetic bacteria which are anaerobes that used chemicals in the environment to produce energy; **(4)** photosynthesis which releases O_2 and thus converted the atmosphere into an oxidising one; **(5)** respiration, which could use the O_2 to efficiently produce ATP; and **(6)** the development of membrane bound organelles (*a subset of prokaryotes which evolved into eukaryotes,* BIO 16.6.3) which allowed eukaryotes to develop meiosis, sexual reproduction, and fertilisation.

It is important to recognise that throughout the evolution of the earth, organisms and the environment have and will continue to shape each other.

16.5 Comparative Anatomy

Anatomical features of organisms can be compared in order to derive information about their evolutionary histories. Structures which originate from the same part of the embryo are called homologous. **Homologous** structures may have similar anatomical features shared by two different species as a result of a common ancestor but with a late divergent evolutionary pattern in response to different evolutionary forces. Such structures may or may not serve different functions. **Analogous** structures have similar functions in two different species but arise from different evolutionary origins and entirely different developmental patterns (*see* Figure IV.A.16.1).

Vestigial structures represent further evidence for evolution since they are organs which are useless in their present owners, but are homologous with organs which are important in other species. For example, the appendix in humans is a vestige of an organ that had digestive functions in ancestral species. However, it continues to assist in the digestion of cellulose in herbivores.

Taxonomy is the branch of biology which deals with the classification of organisms. Humans are classified as follows:

Kingdom	Animalia
Phylum (= Division)	Chordata
Subdivision	Vertebrata
Class	Mammalia
Order	Primates
Family	Hominidae
Genus	*Homo*
Species	*Homo sapiens*

{Mnemonic for remembering the taxonomic categories: King Philip came over for great soup}

The subphyla Vertebrata and Invertebrata are subdivisions of the phylum Chordata. Acorn worms, tunicates, sea squirts and amphioxus are invertebrates. Humans, birds, frogs, fish, and crocodiles are vertebrates. We will examine features of both the chordates and the vertebrates.

Chordates have the following characteristics at some stage of their development: i) a notochord; ii) pharyngeal gill slits which lead from the pharynx to the exterior; iii) a hollow dorsal nerve cord. Other features which are less defining but are nonetheless present in chordates are: i) a more or less segmented anatomy; ii) an internal skeleton (= *endoskeleton*); iii) a tail at some point in their development.

Low-level Importance

Vertebrates have all the characteristics of chordates. In addition, vertebrates have: i) a vertebral column; ii) well developed sensory and nervous systems; iii) a ventral heart with a closed vascular system; iv) some sort of a liver, endocrine organs, and kidneys; and v) cephalisation which is the concentration of sense organs and nerves to the front end of the body producing an obvious head.

16.6 Patterns of Evolution

The evolution of a species can be divided into four main patterns:

1. Divergent evolution – Two or more species originate from a common ancestor.
2. Convergent evolution – Two unrelated species become more alike as they evolve due to similar ecological conditions. The traits that resemble one another are called analogous traits. Similarity in species of different ancestry as a result of convergent evolution is homoplasty. For example, flying insects, birds and bats have evolved wings independently.
3. Parallel evolution – This describes two related species that have evolved similarly after their divergence from a common ancestor. For example, the appearance of similarly shaped leaves in many genera of plant species.
4. Coevolution – This is the evolution of one species in response to adaptations gained by another species. This most often occurs in predator/prey relationships where an adaptation in the prey species that makes them less vulnerable leads to new adaptations in the predator species to help them catch their prey.

16.6.1 Macroevolution

Low-level Importance

Macroevolution describes patterns of evolution for groups of species rather than individual species. There are two main theories:

1. **Phyletic gradualism** – This theory argues that evolution occurs through gradual accumulation of small changes. They point to fossil evidence as proof that major changes in speciation occur over long periods of geological time and state that the incompleteness of the fossil record is the reason why some intermediate changes are not evidenced.
2. **Punctuated equilibrium** – This theory states that evolutionary history is marked

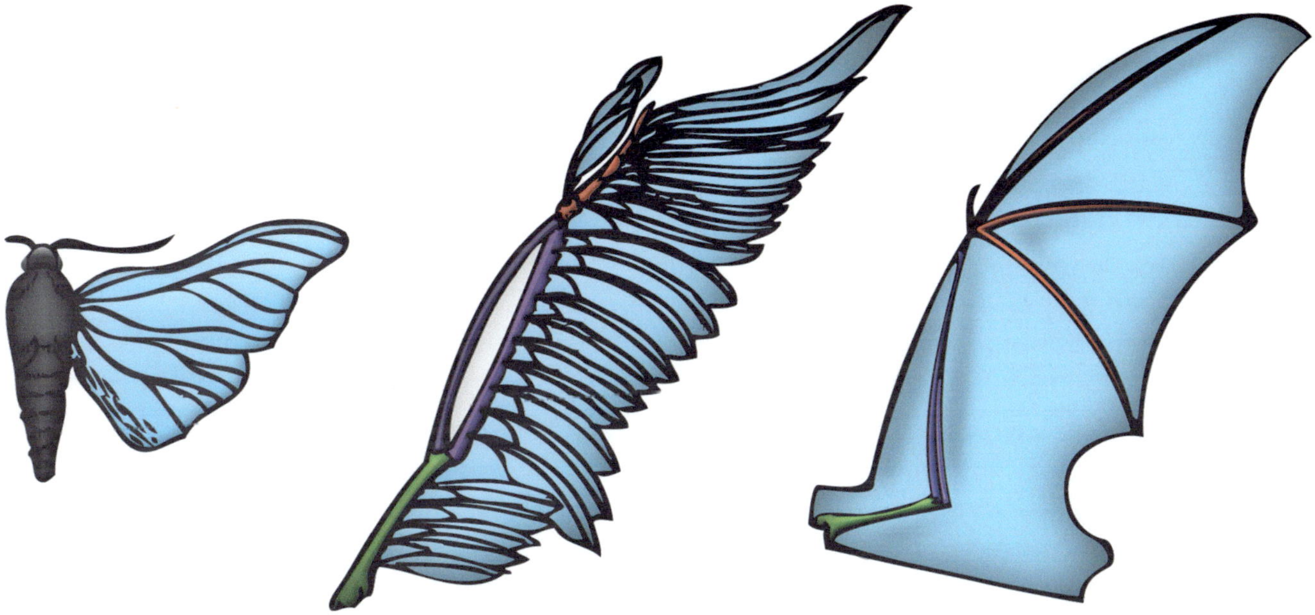

Figure IV.A.16.1: Analogous and homologous structures. The light blue wings represent analogous structures between different species: a flying insect, a bird and a bat, respectively. The bones are homologous structures. For example, green represents the humerus, purple represents the radius and ulna, red represents metacarpals and phalanges. Of course, insects have no bones. *See* the skeleton in BIO 11.3 to remind yourself of the meaning of some of these bony structures homologous in humans.

by sudden bursts of rapid evolution with long periods of inactivity in between. Punctuated equilibrium theorists point to the absence of fossils showing intermediate change as proof that evolution occurred in short time periods.

16.6.2 Basic Patterns for Changes in Macroevolution

1. Phyletic change (anagenesis): gradual change in an entire population that results in an eventual replacement of ancestral species by novel species and ancestral populations can be considered extinct.
2. Cladogenesis: one lineage gives rise to two or more lineages each forming a "clad". It leads to the development of a variety of sister species and often occurs when it is introduced to a new, distant environment.
3. Adaptive radiation: a formation of a number of lineages from a single ancestral species. A single species can diverge into a number of different species, which are able to exploit new environments.
4. Extinction: more than 99.9% of all species are no longer present.

Low-level Importance

16.6.3 Eukaryotic Evolution

Eukaryotes evolved from primitive heterotrophic prokaryotes in the following manner:

1. Heterotrophs first formed in the primordial soup (mixture of organic material) present in the early Earth (BIO 16.4). As the cells reproduced, competition increased and natural selection favored those heterotrophs who were best suited to obtain food.
2. Heterotrophs evolved into autotrophs (capable of making own food) via mutation. The first autotrophs were highly successful because they were able to manufacture their own food supply using light energy or energy from inorganic substrates (i.e. cyanobacteria).
3. As a by-product of the photosynthetic activity of autotrophs, oxygen was released into the atmosphere. This lead to formation of the ozone layer which prevented UV light from reaching the earth's surface. The interference of this major autotrophic resource was caused by the increased blockage of light rays.
4. Mitochondria, chloroplasts, and possibly other organelles of eukaryotic cells, originate through the symbiosis between multiple microorganisms. According to this theory, certain organelles originated as free-living bacteria that were taken inside another cell as endosymbionts. Thus mitochondria developed from proteobacteria and chloroplasts from cyanobacteria. This is the belief of the endosymbiotic theory which counts the following as evidence that it bodes true:
   - A. Mitochondria and chloroplasts possess their own unique DNA which is very similar to the DNA of prokaryotes (circular). Their ribosomes also resemble one another with respect to size and sequence.
   - B. Mitochondria and chloroplasts reproduce independently of their eukaryotic host cell.
   - C. The thylakoid membranes of chloroplasts resemble the photosynthetic membranes of cyanobacteria.

Low-level Importance

16.6.4 The Six-Kingdom, Three-Domain System

Genetic sequencing led to the replacement of the 'old' Five-Kingdom system of taxonomy (BIO 15.5). Under the current system, there are six kingdoms: Archaebacteria (ancient bacteria), Eubacteria (true bacteria; BIO 2.2), Protista (a diverse group of eukaryotic microorganisms), Fungi (BIO 2.3), Plantae ('plants'), and Animalia ('animals'). The Archaea and Bacteria domains contain prokaryotic organisms. The Eukarya domain includes eukaryotes and is subdivided into the kingdoms Protista, Fungi, Plantae, and Animalia.

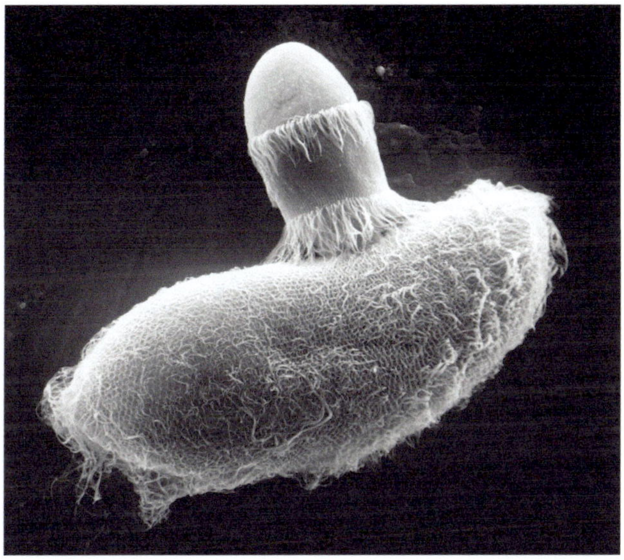
(Antipa, Wessenberg, CIL:39250)

Figure IV.A.16.2: David and Golliath: Two animal-like unicellular, ciliated protists in an epic struggle. The larger of the two carnivores, Paramecium, is attacked from above by the smaller Didinium. In this case, the organisms were preserved for this SEM micrograph (BIO 1.5, 1.5.1) before the outcome could be determined. Like other ciliates (ciliaphora), they can reproduce asexually (binary fission) or sexually (conjugation); osmoregulation is via contractile vacuoles; and, they are also visible using a light microscope.

Six-Kingdom, Three-Domain System

- Archaea Domain
  Kingdom Archaebacteria
- Bacteria Domain
  Kingdom Eubacteria
- Eukarya Domain
  Kingdom Protista
  Kingdom Fungi
  Kingdom Plantae
  Kingdom Animalia

If your study of GAMSAT Section 3 assumed knowledge is complete, it's time to consolidate your Gold Notes, and prepare for full-length (timed) GAMSAT practice exams! Good luck!

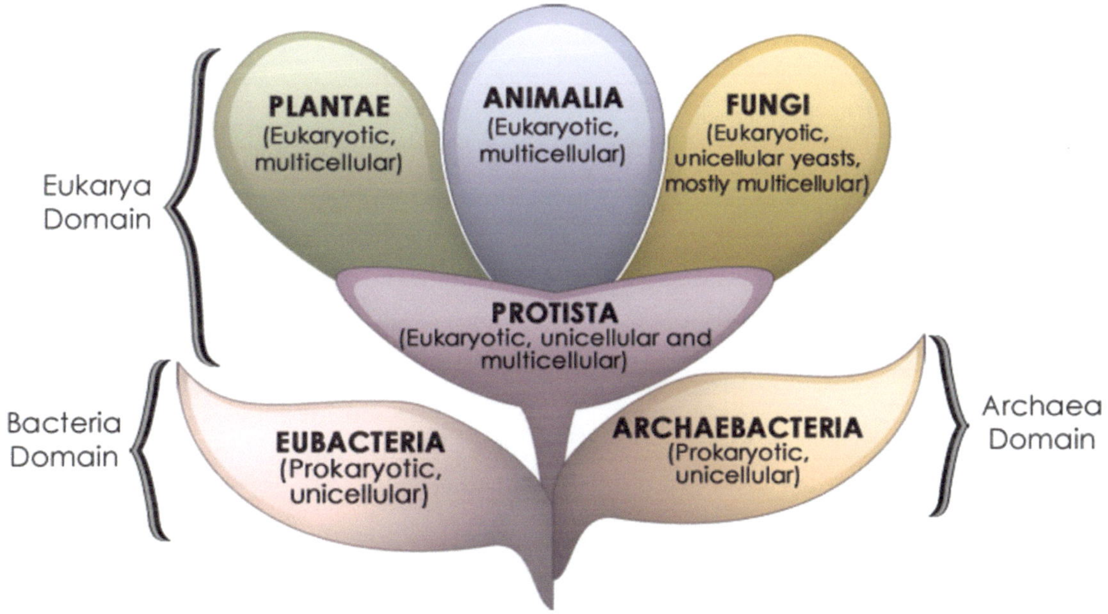

Figure IV.A.16.3: The Six-Kingdom, Three-Domain System.

Low-level Importance

High-level Importance

CHAPTER 16: Evolution

GOLD STANDARD FOUNDATIONAL GAMSAT PRACTICE QUESTIONS

1) During a GAMSAT study session discussing evolution, one of your peer's states: "The giraffe stretched its neck while reaching for higher foliage and then its offspring inherited longer necks as a result." Which of the following would be best to correct your peer's misconception?

   A. Overproduction of offspring leads to a struggle for survival.
   B. Only favorable adaptations have survival value.
   C. Spontaneous mutations can result in the appearance of new traits.
   D. Characteristics acquired during an organism's lifetime are generally not passed on through genes.

2) Which of the following would be the best evidence that two species are related?

   A. Analogous structures
   B. Homologous structures
   C. Similar outward appearance
   D. Similar use of the environment

GOLD STANDARD GAMSAT-LEVEL PRACTICE QUESTIONS

Questions 3–8

Much of the study of evolution of *interspecific* interactions had focused on the results rather than the process of coevolution. In only a few cases has the genetic bases of interspecific interactions been explored. One of the most intriguing results has been the description of "gene-for-gene" systems governing the interaction between certain parasites and their hosts. In several crop plants, dominant alleles at a number of loci have been described that confer resistance to a pathogenic fungus; for each such gene, the fungus appears to have a recessive allele for "virulence" that enables the fungus to attack the otherwise resistant host. Cases of character displacement among competing species are among the best evidence that interspecific interactions can result in genetic change.

Assuming that parasites and their hosts coevolve in an "arms race," we might deduce that the parasite is "ahead" if local populations are more capable of attacking the host population with which they are associated than other populations. Whereas the host may be "ahead" if local populations are more resistant to the local parasite than to other populations of the parasite.

Several studies have been done to evaluate coevolutionary interactions between parasites and hosts, or predators and prey. In one, the fluctuations in populations of houseflies and of a wasp that parasitised them were recorded. The results of the experiment are shown in Figure 1.

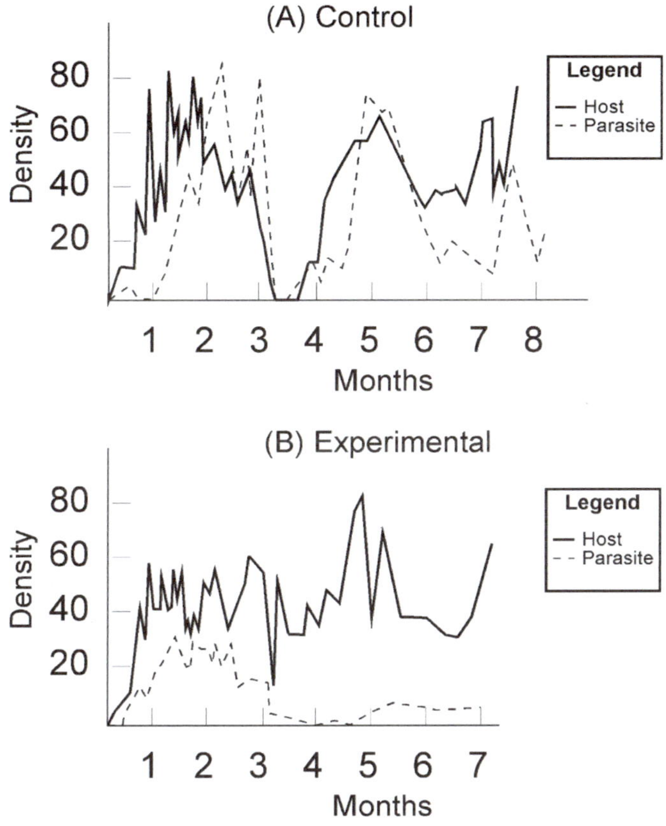

Figure 1

3) A pathogenic fungus is more capable of growth and reproduction on its native population of its sole host, the wild hog peanut, than on plants from other populations of the same species. It is reasonable to conclude that:

A. the fungus, in this instance, was capable of more rapid adaptation to its host than vice versa.

B. the fungus, in this instance, was capable of more rapid adaptation to all populations of the host species than vice versa.

C. the host, in this instance, was capable of more rapid adaptation to the fungus than vice versa.

D. all populations of the host species were capable of more rapid adaptation to the fungus than vice versa.

4) Allopatric refers to areas isolated geographically from one another whereas sympatric populations occupy the same or overlapping geographical areas. The passage suggests that one result of interspecific interactions might be:

A. genetic drift within sympatric populations.

B. genetic drift within allopatric populations.

C. genetic mutations within sympatric populations.

D. genetic mutations within allopatric populations.

5) According to Figure 1, the experiment showed that over time:

A. coevolution caused a decrease in both the host and parasite populations.

B. coevolution caused both a decrease in fluctuation of the host and parasite populations, and a lowered density of the parasite population.

C. coevolution caused a marked increase in the fluctuation of only the host population, and lowered the density of the parasite population.

D. coevolution caused a decrease in the population density of the parasite population but caused a marked increase in the density of the host population.

6) The control in the experiment likely consisted of:

A. members from different populations of the host and parasite species used in the experimental group, that had a short history of exposure to one another.

B. members of the host and parasite species used in the experimental group, that had a long history of exposure to one another.

C. members of the host and parasite species used in the experimental group that had no history of exposure to one another.

D. members from different populations of the host and parasite species used in the experimental group, that had a long history of exposure to one another.

High-level Importance

7) Which of the following is the least likely explanation of the results obtained for the control group in Figure 1?

A. A low parasite population results in a lowered host population by the sheer virulence of the parasite.
B. A low host population can increase a parasite population by forcing the parasite to seek an alternate source for food.
C. A high parasite population destroys the host population resulting in a lowered host population.
D. A high host population creates a breeding ground for parasites thus increasing the parasite population.

8) Penicillin is an antibiotic which destroys bacteria by interfering with cell wall production. Could the development of bacterial resistance to Penicillin be considered similar to coevolution?

A. Yes, a spontaneous mutation is likely to confer resistance to Penicillin.
B. No, an organism can only evolve in response to another organism.
C. Yes, as antibiotics continue to change there will be a selective pressure for bacterial genes which confer resistance.
D. No, bacteria have plasma membranes and can survive without cell walls.

9) Phytoplankton are photosynthesising microscopic organisms that inhabit the upper sunlit layer of almost all oceans and bodies of fresh water. Consider the following graph corresponding to four different species of phytoplankton identified as Q, R, S and T. These four species were collected from different depths of the sea and their rate of photosynthesis was measured. Which of the four species of phytoplankton was collected at the greatest depth?

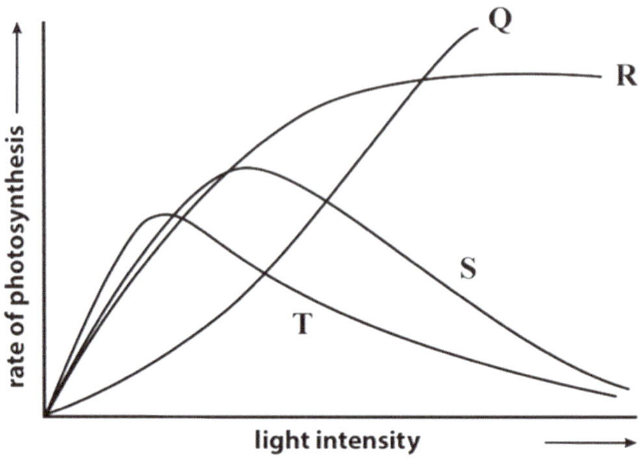

A. Q
B. R
C. S
D. T

10) Hummingbirds have an exceptionally high daytime metabolic rate which results in the need to feed every few minutes. They have evolved a process that occurs at night called 'torpor'. That is to say, their metabolism and body temperature decline markedly, and they become extremely sluggish and inactive. Which of the following life processes is likely to be LEAST affected during nighttime torpor?

A. Insulatory heat exchange
B. Metabolic heat production
C. Responsiveness to external stimuli
D. Need for food

SPOILER ALERT

Gold Standard has cross-referenced the content in this chapter to examples from ACER's official GAMSAT practice materials. It is for you to decide when you want to explore these questions since you may want to preserve some of ACER's materials for timed mock-exam practice.

Examples – None. Although 'Evolution' is an important introductory-level topic, the knowledge from Chapter 16 is not necessary to respond to the over 400 Section 3 practice questions that ACER has released. However, as mentioned in the Introduction for this chapter, the reasoning and graph-analysis skills which you exercise in the GAMSAT-level practice questions will be helpful for many other GAMSAT-question types and topics. The 15 full-length GAMSAT practice tests by Gold Standard, HEAPS-1 through HEAPS-15, contain specific cross-references to this chapter within the worked solutions. Note that the phytoplankton curves are from HEAPS-5, and the interspecific evolution passage is from HEAPS-6.

Chapter Checklist

- ☐ Access your online account to view answers, worked solutions and discussion boards.
- ☐ Reassess your 'learning objectives' for this chapter: Go back to the first page of this chapter and re-evaluate the top 3 boxes and the Introduction.
- ☐ Complete a maximum of 1 page of notes using symbols/abbreviations to represent the entire chapter based on your learning objectives. These are your Gold Notes.
- ☐ Consider your multimedia options based on your optimal way of learning:
  - ☐ Download the free Gold Standard GAMSAT app for your Android device or iPhone.
  - ☐ Create your own, tangible study cards or try the free app: Anki.
  - ☐ Record your voice reading your Gold Notes onto your smartphone (audio files, e.g., *memo* or MP3s) and listen during exercise, transportation, etc.
  - ☐ Try out the Gold Standard GAMSAT online videos at gamsat-prep.com, or you can try other options on YouTube like Khan Academy or Crash Course Biology.
- ☐ Reassess your schedule for your full-length GAMSAT practice tests: ACER and/or HEAPS exams. Ensure that you have scheduled one full day to complete a practice test and 1-2 days for a thorough assessment of worked solutions while adding to your abbreviated Gold Notes.
- ☐ Reassess your progress in scheduling and/or evaluating stress reduction techniques such as regular exercise (sports), yoga, meditation and/or mindfulness exercises (*see* YouTube for suggestions).